Mental Health Nursing

An Introductory Text

Mental Health Nursing

An Introductory Text

BARBARA B. BAUER, RN, MSN

Adjunct Instructor
Northeast Wisconsin Technical College
Green Bay, Wisconsin

SIGNE S. HILL, RN, BSN, MA

Formerly Instructor, Practical Nurse Program
Northeast Wisconsin Technical College
Green Bay, Wisconsin

W.B. SAUNDERS COMPANY

A Division of Harcourt Brace & Company
Philadelphia London Toronto
Montreal Sydney Tokyo

W.B. SAUNDERS COMPANY
A Division of Harcourt Brace & Company

The Curtis Center
Independence Square West
Philadelphia, Pennsylvania 19106

Library of Congress Cataloging-in-Publication Data

Bauer, Barbara B.
Mental health nursing : an introductory text / Barbara B. Bauer,
Signe S. Hill.

p.   cm.

Some material previously appeared in Essentials of mental health
care.

Includes bibliographical references and index.

ISBN 0–7216–7753–3

1. Psychiatric nursing.   I. Hill, Signe S.   II. Essentials of
  mental health care.   III. Title.
  [DNLM: 1. Mental Disorders—nursing.   2. Mental Disorders—therapy
  Nurses' Instruction.   3. Patient Care Planning Nurses' Instruction.
  WY 160 B344m 2000]

RC440.B353 2000   610.73'68—dc21

DNLM/DLC   99–29020

MENTAL HEALTH NURSING: AN INTRODUCTORY TEXT   ISBN 0–7216–7753–3

Printed in the United States of America

Last digit is the print number: 9   8   7   6   5   4   3   2   1

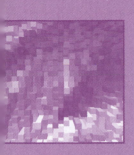

Reviewers

SUZANNE ARMSTRONG-EI MSAIH, MN, BS, BA
Renton Technical College
Renton, Washington

SHARON BEASLEY, MSN, RN
Rend Lake College
Ina, Illinois

MARY M. BLACK, MSN, RN
Moraine Park Technical College
Fond du Lac, Wisconsin

L. LEE BOYLES, RN, MS
Psychiatric Nursing Coordinator
Neosho Community College
Counsel Therapist, Private Practice
Ottawa, Kansas

REITHA CABANISS, MSN, RN
Bevill State Community College
Sumiton, Alabama

CYNTHIA D. CASEY, BSN, RN
Hinds Community College
Jackson, Mississippi

MELANIE ANNE DANIEL, MSN, RN
Psychiatric Clinical Nurse Specialist
Bevill State Community College
Sumiton, Alabama

MONICA G. DeCARLO, MSN, RN
Indiana County Area Vocational-Technical
    School
Indiana, Pennsylvania
Armstrong County Memorial Hospital
Kittanning, Pennsylvania

JEWEL K. DILLER, RN, MSEd
IVY Technical State College, Region 03
Fort Wayne, Indiana

JANET DUNN, BSN, RN
Virginia Beach Career and Technical
    Education Center
Virginia Beach, Virginia

MARILYN LEA FISHER, RN
Northwest Technical Institute
Springdale, Arkansas

NANCY M. GLASSGOW, BSN, RN, BA
Western Dakota Technical Institute
Rapid City, South Dakota

CAROL A. GOFF, MSN, RN
Warren County Area Vocational-Technical
    School
Warren, Pennsylvania

JANE M. HARMON, MSN, RN, CS, PMHNP
Trinity Valley Community College
Kaufman, Texas
Psychiatric Mental Health Nurse Practitioner
Private Practice
Greenville, Texas

DONNA LEACH KANE, RN, BS
Louisiana Technical College
South Louisiana Campus
Houma, Louisiana

JANICE A. KOLVEK, BSN, RN, BS, MPA
IVY Technical State College
Gary, Indiana

We owe our knowledge and skills
to the clients who have allowed us to work with them.
We appreciate the struggle that they are making to function
independently in society while facing the continual stigma, shame,
and guilt that are associated with mental illness.

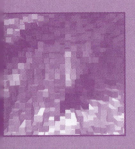

Preface for the Instructor

Together we have 70 years of experience as psychiatric nurses and nursing instructors, during which we developed innovative community support and follow-up programs. Our personal approach to clients continues to be modified as we grow in our profession. *Mental Health Nursing: An Introductory Text* shares some of that knowledge. It also includes the most current information basic to care of persons with mental and emotional problems.

With decreased length of hospital stays, nurses often question whether they can make a difference with a client. We believe that the answer is "yes, one client at a time." This text focuses on the value of each contact with the client, regardless of where it occurs: in the hospital, clinic, community site, nursing home, or home.

A major focus of this text is to provide information that the student can apply while dealing with the emotional issues of a client's illness. Throughout the text, the student is encouraged to think critically and develop an understanding of the concepts through self-exploration. Multiple-choice review questions are provided at the end of each chapter. Answers for these chapter review questions are printed on the inside back cover.

The text is divided into four units. It can be used in any order desired by the instructor. Unit 1, *Perspectives in Mental Health Care,* includes information on milestones in the mental health movement and also addresses funding, legislation, and parity. Biological and other theories are included, as are spiritual and cultural considerations relating to psychiatric care. Stigma, a continuing problem with mental illness, is discussed, and the legal and ethical issues that relate to mental illness are also covered.

Unit 2, *Multidisciplinary Approach,* introduces the psychiatric treatment team members. Communication information is included, with content on managing conflict. The challenge of developing a therapeutic milieu in outpatient, inpatient, and community settings is explored. Critical thinking questions and situations (called *Reality Checks*) appear throughout the chapters. Chapter 8, *Data Collection,* applies critical thinking to nursing process in the care of clients with psychiatric disorders. An initial assessment tool is included, as well as definitions of common psychiatric terms. The multidisciplinary plan as a shared planning tool for all professions involved in the care of the client is reviewed.

Unit 3, *Nursing Responses to Specific Disorders,* consists of 12 chapters that discuss specific disorders and behaviors. The needs of the beginning nurse are the focus of these chapters, with an emphasis on keeping the information practical. Accepted interventions are included. Chapter 19, *Mental Health Problems in Non-*

Psychiatric Settings, reminds students that psychiatric nursing is not limited to the psychiatric unit. This chapter discusses loss and grief, intensive care unit (ICU) psychosis, domestic violence, suicide, and human immunodeficiency virus/acquired immunodeficiency syndrome (HIV/AIDS). Chapter 20, *Older Adults and Mental Health,* introduces content on current issues, such as scams, compulsive gambling, and elder abuse.

Unit 4, *Interventions,* contains reference tables for identifying physical care, nutrition, work, activity and recreation needs, and interventions. Information on psychotherapies and psychopharmacology is introduced.

Inpatient stays are brief, and care often continues in the community. Chapter 29, *Community Reentry,* addresses community treatment and types of advocacy, including self-help and support groups. Chapter 30, *Behaviors That Challenge the Nurse,* is a quick reference for behaviors, goals, approaches, and rationales.

Helpful appendices, such as the *JCAHO Criteria for the Therapeutic Milieu, DSM-IV Classification,* and *Suggestions for Further Reading* (Appendixes A-C, respectively) conclude this text. Appendix D contains student evaluation exercises.

Mental Health Nursing: An Introductory Text emphasizes the importance of sensitivity to client needs and teaches the student how to assist in fulfilling these needs. Thus the nurse becomes an advocate for the client in working as a member of the multidisciplinary team.

An *Instructor's Manual* with a printed test bank of approximately 600 multiple-choice questions is available free to adopters of the text.

BARBARA B. BAUER
SIGNE S. HILL

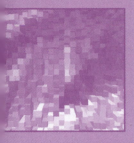

Preface for the Student

We wish to challenge you, the student, to use your skills in assisting clients with mental illness to adjust more effectively to life changes. Your goals in client care need to include the following:

- *A sense of control in life*. In an institutional, outpatient, or community setting, where it seems like everyone else controls his or her own life, there are ways to give some control back to the client. (1) Permit the client to participate in planning and approving goals and interventions. (2) Encourage the client to continue to do whatever he or she can to use his or her own strengths to deal with weaknesses. (3) Share with the client your observation of his or her abilities, using positive reinforcement.
- *Learning and testing skills through meaningful activity*. Eventually there may be a job or volunteer position for the client. Meanwhile, look at the skills the client needs to become more socially acceptable. Ask the client, if necessary. For example, a young mother, hospitalized for depression, experienced feelings of inadequacy because she did not know what to do when her toddler scraped his knee or had some other minor injury, so she took him to the emergency room. A student taught her basic first aid, including how to clean and cover the cut, and when to change the bandage. The client also learned when an injury was serious enough for medical intervention.
- *Close supportive relationships*. Often lacking is a strong support system. Although we do not advocate crossing the line to become personally involved, there are numerous professional alternatives. Many clients lack a support system because of a lack of social skills. They may have worn out their welcome with family and friends. Perhaps no one likes to be around them because of inappropriate behavior. (1) Teach by example. Treat each client with respect and as an equal. Your personal example is powerful. Confront destructive manipulation using "I"-centered statements. Encourage the client to do likewise. Role play possible dialogue. Being listened to and heard may be an entirely new experience. (2) Teach clients how to avoid expressing delusions and hallucinations in social situations. (3) Encourage clients to become involved in community support groups and drop-in centers. Furnish information on how and when to become involved. (4) Encourage contact with their sources of spiritual beliefs, including clergy and parishioners. Because of the continuing stigma involved with mental and emotional problems, clients often feel isolated.
- *Learning to lighten-up and find humor*. For many clients, this is a new experi-

ence. Life for them is basically a struggle. First of all, clients need to learn the difference between a hostile interchange (spiteful teasing) and humor. They also need to know that if the other person involved ends up with hurt feelings, it was not funny after all. It is important to laugh *with* the person and not at them. Collecting silly jokes and cartoons is a safe place to start.

- *Opportunity to help others by direct interaction*. The great Viennese psychiatrist Viktor Frankl said he always asked his clients who were depressed to volunteer their time regularly at a nurs-

ing home. Doing something directly with and for others made a dramatic difference in their mood and recovery. Frankl said it made people think and feel outside of themselves.

We all have the same basic drives in life, but we may communicate these needs in different ways. It is how we go about fulfilling these needs that determines how we function in life.

Good luck in your relationships with others.

BARBARA B. BAUER
SIGNE S. HILL

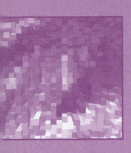

Acknowledgments

We wish to thank the contributors to our previous work, *Essentials of Mental Health Care: Planning and Interventions*. They include Amy Bauer, Paula Lamberg, Michael Hill, Paul Schanen, Terri Timmers, and our husbands, Frank Hill and the late George Bauer. Their input and ideas helped our dream become a reality.

As we complete this edition, we are grateful to the following individuals:

- Ilze Rader, our editor for *Essentials of Mental Health Care,* who put in motion the ground work for this new text.
- Terri Wood, our present editor, who has inspired and challenged us with new ideas.
- Marie Thomas, Editorial Assistant, who was always available to answer questions and guide us through the maze.
- The nursing instructors and directors of nurses who responded to our survey with helpful hints.
- Dennis Henkel, a social worker, who encouraged including more on the care of people with mental illness living in the community.

- Mona Kempfert, our devoted transcriber, who met all of our deadlines.
- Amy Bauer, who followed in her father's footsteps with editing and transcribing.
- Anne Ryan, Nancy Henry, and Helen Smits, used their creative talents in the development of the *Instructor's Manual for Mental Health Nursing*.
- Virginia, who so willingly shared her struggles and successes with mental illness.

We are particularly appreciative of the nurse educators who reviewed the text and offered many meaningful suggestions. Their contributions added to the clarity and comprehensiveness of the content. We thank you all.

Finally, we acknowledge a friendship and professional relationship—ours—that has withstood the test of working closely together and continually evaluating each other's work.

BARBARA B. BAUER
SIGNE S. HILL

NOTICE

Nursing is an ever-changing field. Standard safety precautions must be followed, but as new research and clinical experience broaden our knowledge, changes in treatment and drug therapy become necessary or appropriate. Readers are advised to check the product information currently provided by the manufacturer of each drug to be administered to verify the recommended dose, the method and duration of administration, and the contraindications. It is the responsibility of the treating licensed prescriber, relying on experience and knowledge of the patient, to determine dosages and the best treatment for the patient. Neither the publisher nor the editor assumes any responsibility for any injury and/or damage to persons or property.

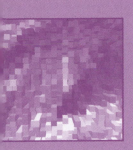

Contents

Mental Health Nursing

An Introductory Text

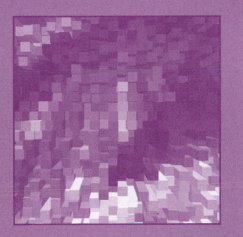

Perspectives in Mental Health Care

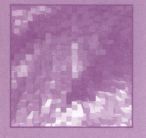

Chapter ONE

A Brief Historical Perspective of the Mental Health Movement

Outline

- **Ancient Civilization**
- **Middle Ages**
- **Renaissance and Reformation**
- **Modern Era**
  European Pioneers in Treating Mental
    Illness
  American Pioneers in Treating Mental
    Illness
  Mental Health Care in the Early 1900s
- **Legislation Resulting From World
  War II**
- **Recent Developments in Mental Health
  Care**
  Deinstitutionalization
  Mental Health Systems Act of 1980
  The Omnibus Budget Acts
  Mental Health Care in the 1990s

Key Terms

- **Action for Mental Health**
- **ADA**
- **bedlam**
- **deinstitutionalization**
- **managed care**
- **Mental Health Parity Act**
- **Mental Health Systems Act**
- **National Mental Health Act**
- **OBRA**

Objectives

Upon completing this chapter, the student will be able to:

1. Identify three treatment approaches for people with mental illness and explain how these treatments reflect the values of the time during which they were used.
2. Name five people who contributed to the mental health movement.
3. Identify federal legislation that attempted to improve the care of people with mental illness.
4. Name two reports that contributed to increased public awareness of mental health problems.

his history of the mental health movement focuses on areas that continue to be significant in the treatment of mental illness today. Like other things in life, each type of treatment reflects the predominant values of the time during which it was applied (Angrist, 1963, p. 20). The values and beliefs in early years alienated, isolated, and confined people with mental illness. Despite this harsh treatment, some people brought hope and promise through their writings and research on mental illness.

ANCIENT CIVILIZATION

During the age of primitive humans, all things good and evil were believed to have been caused by spirits. Incantations, spells, and charms were used to prevent or cure disease. Sorcerers were employed to cast out demons that were believed to cause all illness.

Four centuries before Christ, Hippocrates (460–370 BC) discarded the old theories and denied that mental illness was sacred. He believed that mental disorders, like other diseases, had natural causes and required treatment. There was some public care for people with mental disorders, which dated back to the temples of healing in Greece in the sixth century BC. Ancient Rome had public provisions for the mentally ill by the fourth century BC. During the third century BC, Egyptian temples were the sites of purification treatment, as well as various other activities for people with mental disorders. However, such facilities were rare. In general, people still believed that demons caused mental illness (Angrist, 1963, p. 20).

MIDDLE AGES

Little improvement occurred in caring for the mentally ill between 400 AD and the Renaissance (1450–1650). Troubled minds were thought to be influenced by the moon, hence the word *lunacy*. However, with the advent of Christianity, the Church began to provide more humane treatment in its monasteries.

Also during this time, a system of colony (family) care for people with mental illness was instituted at Gheel in Belgium. According to legend, an Irish princess named Dymphna was slain in the area of Gheel in AD 600. The king—her insane, widowed father—killed her after she refused his request to marry him. Many people flocked to Dymphna's tomb in the hope that she might intercede on behalf of the ill. Miraculous cures were reported, and as the Dymphna legend spread, Gheel became increasingly renowned as a center for the treatment of persons with mental illness (Aring, 1974). As more and more people came to the village, they began taking housing with the townsfolk. Many were given jobs to do, which gave them structure and meaningful work. Thus the people of Gheel became used to caring for persons with mental illness, and since 1246 AD the colony of Gheel has been a haven for people with mental illness. The colony also served as a model for community care in the United States.

Also earning its place in the history of mental health care, although under a somewhat dubious distinction, was the Hospital of St. Mary of Bethlehem in London. At this hospital, little was done for persons with mental illness except to house them, so a very chaotic environment developed. The hospital's name was later shortened to "Bedlam," and the term **bedlam** entered the language in its present sense: a scene of uproar and confusion.

RENAISSANCE AND REFORMATION

The Renaissance and the Reformation (1517) brought changes in the care of people with mental illness. For example, during the reign of King Edward II, a law was enacted that directed the property of "lunatics" to be vested in the crown.

One of the most important contributors to mental health policies during this time was Johann Weyer (1515–1588), a physician some consider to have been the first psychiatrist. He spoke out against the belief that witchcraft and possession by demons caused mental disorders. He described abnormal behaviors of these people as symptoms of mental illness. Weyer advised that qualified physicians be called in to treat people accused of witchcraft. He suggested that the origin of this behavior could be found by obtaining detailed information about the sufferer. Weyer was successful in treating some of these people by sitting alone and talking with them for long periods (Kolb and Brodie, 1982, p. 4).

MODERN ERA

The period from the early eighteenth century to the present comprises the "modern era." The following paragraphs highlight people, institutions, and legislation that have affected the treatment of people with mental illnesses. For a synopsis of these and other events, refer to Table 1–1.

European Pioneers in Treating Mental Illness

In 1792, Philippe Pinel (1745–1826), a psychiatrist in Paris, liberated more than 50 residents of a mental hospital in less than a week. Some of these people had been in chains for up to 30 years. Dr. Pinel believed that they were unmanageable only because they had been robbed of their freedom. He provided workshops with light and air instead of the darkness and smell of the dungeons. The results of his actions proved that he was correct.

In England, two people made contributions to the care of people with mental illness. William Tuke (1732–1822) founded the York Retreat, an asylum for Quakers with mental illnesses. John Conolly (1794–1866) became an enthusiastic advocate of nonrestraint. In 1856, Dr. Conolly published a book called *The Treatment of the Insane Without Mechanical Restraint,* which established a new principle in hospital management. He wrote, "Restraints and neglect may be considered as synonymous; for restraints are merely a general substitute for the thousand attentions required by troublesome patients" (Conolly, 1856; reprint 1973, p. 261). After 5 years as superintendent of an asylum in England, during which time no mechanical restraint was used, he wrote, "there is no asylum in the world in which all mechanical restraints may not be abolished, not only with perfect safety, but with incalculable advantage" (Conolly, 1856; reprint 1973, p. 261).

American Pioneers in Treating Mental Illness

Before the middle of the eighteenth century, many people with mental illness in America were confined to poorhouses and jails. There they were treated as paupers and common criminals. The first American hospital to care for clients with mental illnesses along with other patients was the Pennsylvania Hospital in Philadelphia, established in 1752. In 1773, the Eastern Lunatic Asylum in Williamsburg, Virginia, became the first public institution in the United States designed solely for the care of clients with mental illness.

Dr. Benjamin Rush (1745–1813) was the first American physician to make a serious study of mental disorders. He is considered the father of American psychiatry. Along with Philippe Pinel and William Tuke, he was influential in spreading the doctrine of moral treatment. These physicians advocated treating mental illness with kindness.

In spite of reform movements for separate institutions and moral treatment, facilities for the care of people with mental illness remained overcrowded and inadequate throughout the first part of the nineteenth century. In the mid-1800s, Dorothea Lynne Dix (1802–1887), a retired schoolteacher, agreed to teach Sunday School classes to women inmates in prison. She was shocked at the filth, the apparent neglect and brutality, and the number of women locked in cells. She aroused public awareness of the treatment of people with mental illness and campaigned for more and larger institutions for their care.

Toward the end of the nineteenth century, Linda Richards graduated as the first psychiatric nurse in the United States. She organized nursing services and educational programs in several state mental hospitals in Illinois (Murray and Huelskoetter, 1991, p. 94).

Mental Health Care in the Early 1900s

At the beginning of the twentieth century, people with mental illness were usually cared for and

Table 1–1 **Milestones in the Mental Health Movement**

Period in History	Event
Ancient civilization	Sorcerers used to cast out demons that were believed to cause all illnesses
4th century BC (460–370 BC)	Hippocrates denied that mental health was sacred; like other diseases, mental illness had natural causes and required treatment
3rd century BC	Egyptian temples were sites of purification treatment
Middle Ages (1000–1450)	Church provided care for people with mental illness in monasteries
1246	Gheel, Belgium: Dymphna legend led to community care for people with mental illness; future model for community care in United States
1247	Hospital of St. Mary of Bethlehem (London) began providing care for people with mental illness
Renaissance (1450–1650) and Reformation (1517) eras	Lunacy legislation in England directed that the property of lunatics be vested in the crown
	Johann Weyer denounced witchcraft; advocated getting detailed information about sufferers and spending time talking to them
Modern Era (1700s)	More active advocacy for people with mental illness
1752	Pennsylvania Hospital in Philadelphia was the first American hospital to care for persons with mental illness
1773	Eastern Lunatic Asylum at Williamsburg, Virginia, became the first public institution solely for the care of persons with mental illness in the United States
1792	Philippe Pinel of Paris liberated persons with mental illness from chains
1796	William Tuke of England founded the York Retreat for sick Quakers
1745–1813	Dr. Benjamin Rush was the first American physician to make a serious study of mental disorders; he is considered the father of American psychiatry
Modern Era (1800s)	
1802–1887	Dorothea Lynne Dix advocated better conditions and treatment of persons with mental illness in prisons
1856	Dr. John Conolly published *The Treatment of the Insane Without Mechanical Restraint*
1880	Linda Richards became the first graduate psychiatric nurse in the United States
1856–1926	Emil Kraepelin described mental illnesses and gave them names
1856–1939	Sigmund Freud founded psychoanalysis
Modern Era (1900s)	Clifford W. Beers founded the Connecticut Society for Mental Hygiene, later known as the *National Mental Health Association*
1920	First psychiatric nursing textbook was written by Harriet Bailey
1933	Manfred Sakel of Vienna introduced insulin coma therapy
1936	Egas Moniz and Almidia Lima of Portugal performed prefrontal lobotomies
1938	Ugo Cerletti and Luciano Bini of Italy initiated electroshock therapy
1946	Passage of National Mental Health Act provided federal aid for research, training, and community service
1948	National Institute of Mental Health was created
1950s	Psychotherapeutic drugs were introduced
1950s–1960s	Major psychiatric nursing contributions were made by Hildegard Peplau, Gwen Tudor, June Mellow, and Ida Orlando
1961	Action for Mental Health Report was published by the Joint Commission on Mental Illness and Health

Table continued on following page

Table 1–1	Milestones in the Mental Health Movement *Continued*

Period in History	Event
1963	The Mental Retardation Facilities and Community Mental Health Centers Construction Act provided funds for establishing a network of community mental health centers
	Deinstitutionalization began
1977	President's Commission on Mental Health was established to review mental health needs and determine how best to meet them
1980	Mental Health Systems Act was implemented
1981	Omnibus Budget Reconciliation Act repealed the Mental Health Systems Act of 1980 and gave each state block grants to care for people in need
1987	Omnibus Budget Reform Act (OBRA) prevented inappropriate placement of people with mental illness in nursing homes
1990	"Decade of the brain" focused on the relationship of brain anatomy and physiology to behavior and mental illness
	ADA prohibits discrimination against people with disabilities
1996	Mental Health Parity Act passed

treated in large state-run institutions. These institutions were often located outside the city, with the explanation that the clients needed the fresh country air. Frequently, however, it was the fear and stigma associated with mental illness that determined the location of the institutions.

A number of people made significant contributions to psychiatry during the first part of the twentieth century. For example, Emil Kraepelin (1856–1926) described mental illnesses and gave them names. He is sometimes referred to as "the great descriptive psychiatrist." Sigmund Freud (1856–1939), the founder of psychoanalysis, introduced the idea that unconscious motivation is important in causing mental illness.

Another significant figure in the mental health movement was Clifford W. Beers (1876–1943), a graduate of Yale University who spent 3 years in mental hospitals. After his recovery, he was determined to do something about the conditions that existed in these hospitals. He accomplished this in 1908 by writing an account of his experiences, entitled *A Mind That Found Itself*. His exposure of mental institutions contributed directly to the organization of the mental hygiene move-

ment. On May 6, 1909, Beers founded the Connecticut Society for Mental Hygiene. The chief purpose of the society was the following (Beers, 1948, p. 304):

. . . to work for the conservation of mental health; to help prevent nervous and mental disorders and mental defects; to help raise the standards of care for those suffering from any of these disorders or defects; to secure and disseminate reliable information on these subjects; to cooperate with federal, state, and local agencies or officials and with public and private agencies whose work is in any way related to that of a society for mental hygiene.

The following year, the National Committee for Mental Hygiene was organized. In 1950, it merged with the National Mental Health Foundation and the Psychiatric Foundation to form the National Mental Health Association. The symbol of the National Mental Health Association is the Mental Health Bell, which was cast from shackles and chains that once restrained people in mental hospitals (Fig. 1–1). The 300-lb bell, housed in Arlington, Virginia, bears the inscription: *Cast from the shackles which bound them, this bell shall ring out hope for the mentally ill and victory over mental illness.*

The first psychiatric nursing textbook, *Nursing Mental Disease,* was published by Harriet Bailey in 1920. It focused on the disease rather than the client (Murray and Huelskoetter, 1991, p. 94). Descriptive psychiatry provided the knowledge base for treatment. People with mental disorders were slotted into the various diagnostic categories according to their symptoms. The treatments given were classified as physical or medical therapies. These included insulin coma therapy, introduced by Manfred Sakel of Vienna in 1933; electroshock therapy for artificial production of convulsive seizures, initiated by Ugo Cerletti and Luciano Bini of Italy in 1938; and prefrontal lobotomy, begun by Egas Moniz and Almidia Lima of Portugal in 1936. Hydrotherapy continued to be used as it was in ancient times to relax the body.

Legislation Resulting From World War II

World War II brought about public and professional awareness of the effects of psychological stress and the widespread need for rehabilitation of war veterans. The public also recognized that mental illness was costing the taxpayers millions of dollars each year and that facilities were nonetheless inadequate. These factors led to the passage

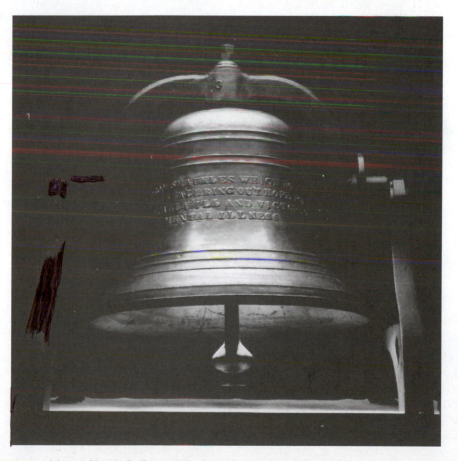

FIG. 1–1   Mental Health Bell, symbol of the National Mental Health Association. (Courtesy National Mental Health Association.)

of **The National Mental Health Act** in 1946. Its purpose was to provide federal aid for research, training, and community service. In 1948, the National Institute of Mental Health, located at the Clinical Center of the National Institutes of Health in Bethesda, Maryland, was created.

RECENT DEVELOPMENTS IN MENTAL HEALTH CARE

During the 1950s, psychotherapeutic drugs were introduced as a treatment for people with mental illness. They were not a "cure" for mental illness; instead, they made the person more receptive to other forms of psychotherapy. As a result of medication, these clients began to move out of the large institutions. In 1961, the Joint Commission on Mental Illness and Health published a report entitled **Action for Mental Health.** The report placed strong emphasis on community-based services by calling for a reduction in the size of large state hospitals and the development of mental health services in local communities (Joint Commission, 1961, p. 268).

The Mental Retardation Facilities and Community Mental Health Centers Construction Act of 1963 provided funds for establishing a network of publicly supported community mental health centers throughout the country. Major nursing contributions were made during this time by Hildegard Peplau, Gwen Tudor, June Mellow, and Ida Orlando. They stressed the importance of the interpersonal/therapeutic relationship (Murray and Huelskoetter, 1991, pp. 94, 95).

Deinstitutionalization

A movement called **deinstitutionalization** began in the early 1960s. Deinstitutionalization is an on-going social policy in which large numbers of persons with mental illness have been moved out of state hospitals into the community. Many of these people have found themselves in worse condition than when they were institutionalized because the communities were not prepared to receive them.

Near the beginning of this movement, clients were not taught living skills such as shopping, handling money, and finding housing—skills that most people take for granted. People with mental illnesses who did not have these skills had difficulty surviving. Those with chronic mental illness became homeless or, if they needed rehospitalization, were placed in nursing homes. In fact, nursing homes were called "the new mental hospitals of America" (Pfeiffer, 1983, p. 17). Concepts of deinstitutionalization, rehabilitation, and long-term care of people with severe mental illness are key components of the mental health system today.

Mental Health Systems Act of 1980

In 1977, the President's Commission on Mental Health was established to review the mental health needs of the nation and to make recommendations about how those needs might best be met. Its report in 1978 focused on the following areas:

- Development of networks of high-quality mental health services at the local level, coordinating mental health services with other human services
- Adequate financing of mental health services with public and private funds
- Appropriately trained personnel
- Services for populations with special needs
- Setting a national priority to meet the needs of people with chronic mental illness
- An increased base of knowledge about the nature and treatment of mental disabilities
- Protection of human rights and guaranteed freedom of choice
- Prevention of mental diseases

These recommendations were part of the **Mental Health Systems Act** passed by Congress in 1980.

The Omnibus Budget Acts

Before the Mental Health Systems Act could be implemented, a new president took office, and mental health care reform changed again. As a result of these changes, federal funding for all mental health services was reduced. The Omnibus Budget Reconciliation Act of 1981 (Community Services Block Grant Act) in essence repealed the Mental Health Systems Act of 1980. This bill resulted in each state receiving a designated amount of money to cover treatment for alcohol and drug abuse and mental health services. It was up to the state to determine where and how the money would be spent. This led to severe financial restrictions, and many long-term clients were transferred to nursing homes.

To prevent inappropriate placement of people with mental illness in nursing homes, the Omnibus Budget Reform Act of 1987 (**OBRA**) was passed. This legislation required that all persons, regardless of age, be screened before admission to a nursing home. If the results indicated that the person was mentally ill and not in need of medical care, he or she could not be admitted. OBRA required that states find alternative solutions for the care of persons with mental illness. Many communities have since developed crisis shelters, group homes, and supportive apartment living. The institution, with increasing costs of care, provides short-term hospitalization for persons with acute mental illness, usually for medication evaluation or suicide precautions.

Mental Health Care in the 1990s

Four dominant trends characterize the mental health movement in the 1990s. They include research on the physiology of the brain, antidiscrimination legislation, insurance parity, and managed care for mental illness. Each of these trends is discussed here.

Research

Advances in technology allow more research on understanding the chemistry of the brain. Studies focus on the relationship of brain anatomy and physiology to behavior and mental illness. Because of this emphasis on brain structure and function, the 1990s have become known as the "decade of the brain" (Varcarolis, 1998, p. 16).

Reality Check

Discuss what is meant by the "decade of the brain."

Legislation

On July 26, 1990, President George Bush signed the Americans with Disabilities Act (**ADA**). This was the first comprehensive federal civil rights law for people with mental and physical disabilities. The ADA prohibits discrimination against people with disabilities in employment, public transportation, public accommodations, and telecommunications.

Insurance Parity

Another landmark piece of legislation was the **Mental Health Parity Act** of 1996. This act requires insurance companies to have the same annual and lifetime limits for mental health services as they do for general medical illnesses. When President William Clinton signed the law, he said, "No more double standards; it's time that the law and insurance practices caught up with science . . ." (Boroughs, 1996, p. 3). Although the law is another historic victory, it only provides partial parity. It does *not* require group insurance to include mental health services. Also, insurers may charge higher premium levels for mental health services.

Managed Care

One way of controlling health care costs has been through **managed care.** Under this system, an enrollee has one doctor who is in charge of a client's care. This method of care began in the private sector; major cuts in health and social service programs have moved managed care into the public sector. Providing this kind of care for people with serious mental illness is a huge task, requiring informed advocacy that allows people with mental disabilities access to appropriate mental health care.

SUMMARY

The history of the mental health movement depicts a continuous struggle to treat people with mental illness as human beings. In ancient times, people believed that all maladies were caused by spirits. Hippocrates, however, denied that mental illness was sacred. He maintained that mental illness, like other diseases, required treatment.

During the Dark Ages, little improvement was made in caring for people with mental illness. The city of Gheel in Belgium became a haven for these people, as well as a model for later community care in the United States. Belief in witchcraft and possession by demons persisted during the Renaissance and Reformation eras. The physician Johann Weyer spoke out against such practices and demonstrated ways to treat people with mental illness more humanely.

The Modern Era brought more active advocacy for people with mental illness. Those who were influential in spreading the doctrine of moral treatment, including kindness and humanitarianism, are listed in Table 1–1.

During the 1950s, psychotherapeutic drugs were introduced. Many clients who were mentally ill were able to leave the hospitals. However, communities usually lacked the resources to care for all of the discharged clients. As a result, many people with mental illness became homeless. Legislation passed in 1980 provided money for research, training, and community service. However, changes in federal administration led to severe fiscal restraints; the care of the mentally ill thus continues to be a challenge. Nurses need to join other disciplines to advocate for access to quality care for people who are mentally ill.

Critical Thinking Activities

1. Discuss areas in the mental health movement that continue to be significant in the care of persons with mental illness today.
2. How has specific legislation influenced the care of people with mental illness?
3. Investigate ways you can advocate for legislation to improve the care of persons with mental illness (see Chapter 29).

Review Questions

Multiple Choice—Choose the best answer to each question.

1. Legislation that prohibits discrimination against people with disabilities in employment is the
   a. Mental Health Systems Act.
   b. Americans with Disabilities Act.
   c. Mental Health Parity Act.
   d. Omnibus Budget Reform Act.
2. An advocate for nonrestraint who wrote that "restraints and neglect may be considered synonymous" was
   a. Sigmund Freud.
   b. Benjamin Rush.
   c. Emil Kraepelin.
   d. John Conolly.
3. The person who began the mental health movement with the founding of the Connecticut Society for Mental Hygiene was
   a. Dorothea Lynne Dix.
   b. Emil Kraepelin.
   c. Clifford W. Beers.
   d. Benjamin Rush.
4. Psychotherapeutic drugs were introduced during the
   a. 1940s.
   b. 1950s.
   c. 1960s.
   d. 1970s.
5. The first graduate psychiatric nurse in the United States was
   a. Linda Richards.
   b. Harriet Bailey.
   c. Gwen Tudor.
   d. Hildegard Peplau.

References

Angrist S: The mental hospital: its history and destiny. Perspect Psychiatr Care 1(6):20–26, 1963.
Aring C: Gheel revisited. JAMA 239(7):849, 1974.
Beers C: A Mind That Found Itself, 7th ed. New York, Doubleday and Co, 1948.

Boroughs L: Victory for mental health parity. The BELL, the newsletter of the NMHA 2(4):3, 1996.

Conolly J: Treatment of the Insane Without Mechanical Restraints. London, Smith, Elder and Co, 1856. Reprinted by photolithography in 1973 by Dawson of Pall Mall, London.

Joint Commission on Mental Illness and Health: Action for Mental Health. New York, John Wiley and Sons, 1961, p. 268.

Kolb C, Brodie H: Modern Clinical Psychiatry, 10th ed. Philadelphia, WB Saunders Co, 1982.

Murray RB, Huelskoetter MMW: Psychiatric Mental Health Nursing: Giving Emotional Care, 2nd ed. Norwalk, Conn, Appleton & Lange, 1991.

Pfeiffer E: Assessments: The long-term issue of the '80s. Coordinator July:17, 1983.

Varcarolis EM: Psychiatric nursing: past, present, future. In: Varcarolis EM (ed): Foundations of Psychiatric Mental Health Nursing, 3rd ed. Philadelphia, WB Saunders Co, 1998.

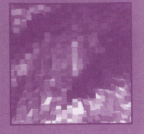

Influences on Mental Health Services

Outline

- **Biological Factors**
  - Chemical Imbalance
  - Physical Brain Changes
  - Endocrine Triggers
  - Immune System
  - Genetics/Heredity
- **Psychoanalytical/Psychosexual Theories**
  - Levels of Awareness

- Personality Structure
- Anxiety and Defense Mechanisms
- Psychosexual Stages
- **Psychosocial Theory**
- **Human Needs and Behavior**
  - Humanistic Theory
  - Maslow's Hierarchy of Needs
- **Other Theorists**

Key Terms

- biological model
- ego
- humanistic theory
- id
- neurons
- neuroses
- neurotransmitters

- pleasure principle
- psychosocial theory
- reality principle
- self-actualization
- superego
- synapses

Objectives

Upon completing this chapter, the student will be able to:

1. Discuss two factors most theorists believe contribute to the potential for developing mental illness.
2. Explain how stress may affect the immune system.
3. Name two mental illnesses that may have a family (genetic) basis.
4. Name the person credited as the founder of psychoanalysis.
5. Define *id, ego,* and *superego*.
6. Provide a real-life example for five defense mechanisms.
7. Give a brief explanation of Freud's five developmental stages.
8. Discuss Erikson's eight stages of man.

Objectives—cont'd

9. Give an example of each level of needs according to Maslow's hierarchy:
   - physical/survival (physiological)
   - safety and security
   - love and belongingness
   - self-esteem
   - self-actualization

Intervention for mental illness continues to be an inexact science. The causes of mental illness are complex and difficult to pinpoint. Many theorists believe that mental illness is related to genetic or inherited factors and family environment during the formative years. Selected theories are reviewed briefly in this chapter.

BIOLOGICAL FACTORS

The **biological model** views psychiatric illness like any other disease. Mental illness is thought to be related to changes in the brain. Reasons include genetic or inherited potential, nutritional factors, infections, and other biochemical changes in the brain.

Interest in biological factors started with the studies of Sigmund Freud. Despite his psychoanalytic orientation, he supported the possibility of biological factors in mental illness. With the discovery of psychotherapeutic drugs in the 1950s, interest in biological factors reawakened. Serious interest in biological research emerged in the 1970s, 1980s, and 1990s.

Emphasis has been primarily on genetic studies and the central nervous system (CNS). Biological research has caused a major move toward using only a psychopharmacological approach to treat clients with mental illness. However, although medications help relieve psychiatric symptoms, the underlying problems still need to be dealt with by integrating a psychological approach as part of the total treatment.

Chemical Imbalance

Brain studies have indicated that mental illness may be associated with the amount of neurotrans-mitters produced or available in the brain. **Neurotransmitters** are chemicals that are needed to transmit messages at the **synapses** (fluid-filled spaces between **neurons,** or nerve cells). When an impulse (message) arrives at a synapse, it triggers the release of a neurotransmitter. The neurotransmitter allows the impulse to travel from one neuron to the next without physical contact between the cells (Fig. 2–1). The following are examples of neurotransmitters (Sanford, 1995, p 31):

- *Dopamine:* Decrease may cause severe depression; increase may be related to mania or schizophrenia
- *Norepinephrine:* Thought to be involved primarily in anxiety and addiction
- *Serotonin:* Appears to be involved primarily in anxiety, schizoaffective disorders, mood disorders, and violence
- *Gamma-aminobutyric acid (GABA):* Lower levels of GABA may lead to development of anxiety disorders

The purpose of the prescribed psychotropic medications is to correct the neurotransmitter imbalance. Some medications block the neurotransmitter, some increase its level in the body, and others limit the amount of neurotransmitter that is released in the brain (see Chapter 22).

Physical Brain Changes

Animal studies and postmortem evaluations provide most of the physical information for biological research. Many questions remain regarding physical brain changes and mental illness because animal responses may be different than human responses. Also, the condition of the brain before

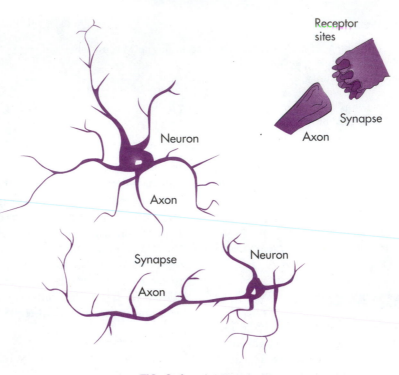

FIG. 2–1 A synapse.

the onset of the illness in a person is often unknown.

Endocrine Triggers

Anxiety or depression accompany some endocrine disorders. Examples include depression and anxiety in people with hypothyroidism and depression in people with diabetes, Cushing's syndrome, and Addison's disease. The fact that light therapy is effective for some people with seasonal affective disorder suggests a neuroendocrine imbalance related to light and temperature. The exact relationship is still a mystery. Does the endocrine disorder trigger the depression or anxiety, or do the depression and anxiety trigger changes in the endocrine system?

Immune System

Biological research has shown that the immune system communicates with the brain. There is evidence that stress affects the immune system and

may make some people vulnerable—or invulnerable—to illness. These illnesses are thought to include arthritis, ankylosing spondylitis, diabetes, narcolepsy, rheumatoid arthritis, multiple sclerosis, and systemic lupus erythematosus.

Reality Check

As you continue to learn about illnesses, be alert to depression, anxiety, confusion, emotional lability, and/or other mental symptoms listed. Is the illness considered an autoimmune disorder (one in which the body attacks its own immune system)?

Genetics/Heredity

Some mental illnesses have a family (genetic) basis. Depression, bipolar disorders, schizophrenia, and some anxiety disorders are included. This does not mean that the person will become mentally ill just because there is a family history of mental illness. As with genetic physical disorders, environmental conditions play an important role. For example, a person who inherits a tendency for schizophrenia is most at risk if physical stress is present. This might include, but is not limited to, complications at birth, a viral illness, or a head injury.

PSYCHOANALYTICAL/ PSYCHOSEXUAL THEORIES

Understanding human development provides information useful in distinguishing the client's chronological age and his or her level of functioning. Interest in observing and defining stages of development dates back to Hebrew, Chinese, and Greek writings of 2000 years ago.

Sigmund Freud, an Austrian psychiatrist, is considered the founder of psychoanalysis. His work set into motion the study of human development, motivation, and thought. Since that time his theories have been modified and have stimulated the development of new theories.

Originally, Freud's work (most of which was with adults) was intended to describe how people develop **neuroses** (anxiety disorders). Later, his work became a general theory about human personality development. The major parts of his theory included levels of awareness, personality structure, anxiety and related defense mechanisms, and psychosexual stages of development.

Levels of Awareness

According to Freud, the levels of awareness include the following (Trubowitz, 1994, p 11–12):

- *Conscious:* The thinking, feeling, and actions a person is aware of and is able to control. Freud considered the conscious mind to be logical and based on the **reality principle.** This means that a person is able to postpone satisfaction to meet greater needs.
- *Preconscious* (subconscious): Thoughts, feelings, and desires below the surface that a person

is to recall to consciousness. The purpose of this level is to censor and/or repress certain thoughts and feelings that cause discomfort.
- *Unconscious:* Thoughts, feelings, desires, and memories that are repressed. Freud considered the unconscious to be illogical and governed by the **pleasure principle** ("I want what I want when I want it.") The unconscious contains impulses that would create great anxiety, contradictions in feelings, intense emotions, and strong sexual urges. Unconscious material can be brought to consciousness with special drugs or hypnosis. It sometimes shows up in dreams or slips of the tongue, causing the person to think or say "Where did that come from?!"

Personality Structure

Freud described personality structure in terms of the id, the ego, and the superego.

- *Id:* The **id** includes primitive urges and instincts such as sexual desires and aggression. Although the id is unconscious, it may have observable effects on a person's thinking, feelings, and actions. Freud stressed the unconscious nature of motivation and the powerful effect of this hidden source of human behavior. Dreams can offer clues to unconscious motivation. The id, being unconscious, intrudes into our dreams and becomes an important source of revealing a person's fundamental motives.
- *Ego:* A person's **ego** is conscious and operates on the reality principle. It provides some control over the id, which wants to satisfy its every whim (pleasure principle) and would destroy the person in its continued demand to satisfy its urges. Consequently, the ego's function is to control impulses and to guide behavior toward long-term goals. The ego mediates between the id and the superego.
- *Superego:* The **superego** is sometimes referred to as the *conscience.* It is actually more than that. It is the place where the ego finds the rules it uses to control the id. The superego is primarily unconscious, incorporating the va

of human society, and acts as a sensor for the id. Example:

Id: "I want what I want when I want it."

Superego: "You can't have it."

Ego: "Why not wait and see what tomorrow brings?"

The id, ego, and superego are not fixed. They depend on personal human experience and the balance a person achieves between instinctual urges and the demands of society.

Anxiety and Defense Mechanisms

Anxiety is a part of living. Moderate anxiety is an excellent motivator. Without anxiety, people would not be motivated to get up, get dressed, go to class or work, and so on. Excessive anxiety threatens to overwhelm a person. Freud believed that the ego develops defense mechanisms to help protect people from excessive anxiety. These defense mechanisms offer protection to the ego. It is only when defense mechanisms become too extreme in distorting reality (thinking, feeling, and acting) that they interfere with healthy living. Table 2–1 provides descriptions and examples of common defense mechanisms.

Psychosexual Stages

Freud believed that stages of human development from infancy to adulthood are related to the primary source of gratification for each age. Each stage has a primary conflict and task that must be mastered. He saw the mother–father–child triangle as the greatest influence during development. He identified the following stages of human development, sources of satisfaction, and ages at which the stage is experienced:

1. *Oral* (mouth-sucking, biting, chewing) 0 to 1 year
2. *Anal* (expulsion and retention of feces) 1–3 years
3. *Phallic* (masturbation) 3–6 years
4. *Latency* (tapering off of conscious biological and sexual urges) 6–12 years
5. *Genital* (sexual intercourse) 13–end of puberty

PSYCHOSOCIAL THEORY

Erik Erikson, an American psychoanalyst, developed his **psychosocial theory** of personality development from studying children. His theory of growth and development included the influences of Freud (biological, instinctual drives, and libido) and the influences of Harry Stack Sullivan (a student of Freud's who focused on social experience with significant people who mold identity). The theories of Freud and Erikson have concepts in common, as well as outstanding differences. Erikson placed more emphasis on the need to solve problems at each stage of personality development (Erikson, 1963). He believed that social and environmental (cultural) factors influence personality development. Table 2–2 offers a comparative look at Freud's and Erikson's theories of personality development.

HUMAN NEEDS AND BEHAVIOR

Basically, all the theorists agree that development occurs in an orderly progression through specific stages from conception through death. This progression is a dynamic process for each person, based on his or her uniqueness. This uniqueness is a combination of the person's inherent potential, past experiences, and environment. All the factors create specific needs within the person's life. The effectiveness with which a person moves through the life cycle depends on how he or she deals with these needs. Therefore a basic understanding of needs is essential to plan care for clients who are experiencing psychiatric problems. This is the basis of **humanistic theory.**

Humanistic Theory

Needs are like holes in a person's life that, when filled, result in an increased feeling of well being. A goal is a point toward which a person directs his or her efforts to fulfill a need. The action that a person takes toward a goal to fulfill a need is one description of behavior. Figure 2–2 diagrams what happens when a person encounters an obstacle along the pathway to a goal. He or she experiences

Table 2–1   Common Defense Mechanisms

Defense Mechanism	Description	Example
Compensation	Covering for real or imagined inadequacy by developing or exaggerating a desirable trait	An undersized boy develops his intellectual ability instead of participating in sports
Conversion	Channeling of anxiety into physical symptoms	A woman develops a headache on the evening she is scheduled to present a paper at a convention and is unable to make her presentation
Denial	Rejection of things, events, or feelings as they actually are, thus eliminating the need for anxiety	The alcoholic denies his/her alcoholism: "I am a social drinker and can stop anytime"
Displacement	Feelings toward an object are distorted and transferred to a less threatening object	A boy, angry at the weather, which he cannot control, kicks his cat
Dissociation	Painful ideas, situations, or feelings are separated from awareness	A man has forgotten details of the accident in which a loved one was killed
Fantasy	Using the imagination to solve problems; on a conscious level, fantasy is used to reduce stress through relaxation; on the unconscious level, fantasy is used as a retreat from a threatening environment	Children work through situations they will encounter in adult life by assuming parental roles and using pets as children
Identification	An individual takes on the characteristics and values of someone he admires	A teenager dresses like his favorite singing star
Introjection	Incorporating or internalizing of conflicting values, standards, people, objects, or attitudes so that they are no longer an external threat	A political candidate professes to represent every interest group so that no one can attack his platform
Projection	Attributing to other people or objects motives and emotions that are unacceptable to oneself	An overweight woman blames her 2-year-old child for her condition, saying he makes her nervous
Rationalization	Logical-sounding excuses that conceal the real reason for actions, thoughts, or feelings	A young boy explains why he left for school without feeding the dog. "I did it because Johnny came over and told me we had to leave right away"
Reaction formation	Sometimes viewed as an overcompensation; a means of disguising from the self an unacceptable desire or drive by developing its exact opposite to an exaggerated degree	The wife is angry at her husband for the attention he gives the dog, but acts overly sweet
Regression	A retreat to an earlier, less stressful time of development	An adult has a temper tantrum
Repression	Unconscious withholding of unpleasant thoughts, feelings, or experiences	A woman is unable to remember the name of a demanding neighbor when she meets her at the market
Sublimation	Substituting acceptable behavior for an unacceptable or unattainable desire	A person channels feelings of fear into creating vivid paintings
Suppression	Conscious forgetfulness of painful thoughts and experiences	A woman with a growth on her groin ignores it until she can no longer sit down
Undoing	An attempt to conceal negative action by other positive action	A father offers his son an allowance after punishing him

Table 2–2 A Comparative Look at Freud's and Erikson's Theories of Personality Development

Age 0–1 Year

	Freud	Erikson
Stage or task	Stage 1: Expresses needs and satisfaction through mouth: sucking, biting, chewing, noises, crying, breathing Oral stage; beginning of ego development	Stage 1: Expresses needs through crying; dependent on others to meet needs quickly and gently Trust versus mistrust
Commendable quality	Weaning	Hope
Undesirable behavior	Oral habits later in life such as overeating, drinking, cigarette smoking, nail-biting, gum chewing	Frustration, fear, despair
Significant others	Mother or mothering person	Mother or mothering person

Age 1–3 Years

	Freud	Erikson
Stage or task	Stage 2: Toilet training, first experience with mastery, considered first experience with creativity Anal stage	Stage 2: Learns to "do it himself" (i.e., eating, walking, toileting) Autonomy versus self-doubt and shame
Commendable quality	Toilet training, self-control, responsibility	Willpower
Undesirable behavior	Parsimony, compulsiveness, obstinacy, possessiveness	Feels dirty or bad; reckless bravado, shamelessness
Significant others	Mother and father	Mother and father

Age 3–6 Years

	Freud	Erikson
Stage or task	Stage 3: Interest in genital area (masturbation); begins to understand sexual differences Phallic stage; beginning of superego development Ages 5–6: Time of conflict; needs to resolve attraction to opposite parent and identify with same parent	Stage 3: Still self-centered; shows off, looks for approval Initiative versus guilt
Commendable quality	Satisfaction with self as a sexual being, positive control over self-identity with same parent	Purpose, develops conscience, accepts consequences of acts
Undesirable behavior	Guilt and dissatisfaction with self as a sexual being	Feels morally bad; difficulty with decisions
Significant others	Mother and father, playmates	Mother and father, playmates

Table 2–2	A Comparative Look at Freud's and Erikson's Theories of Personality Development *Continued*

	Ages 6–12 Years	
	Freud	**Erikson**
Stage or task	Stage 4: Moral teaching from parents; confused in unfamiliar settings; needs direction, approval, praise; sexual interest dormant Latency; growth of ego functions	Stage 4: Seeks achievement; interacts with others, sometimes competes Industry versus inferiority
Commendable quality	Sense of moral responsibility (superego)	Competence; completes activities that are begun
Undesirable behavior	Confusion regarding expectations	Feels mediocre; withdraws, acts out
Significant others	Peers, other adults	Peers, other adults

	Ages 13 Years and Over	Ages 12–18 or 21 Years
	Freud	**Erikson**
Stage or task	Stage 5: Puberty; biological changes and drugs, sexual intercourse, time of confusion and turmoil; education and economic goals are important, drives take second place Genital; developing satisfying relationships with opposite sex, emancipation from parents	Stage 5: Great physical and emotional changes; anxiety and mood swings typical Identity versus role confusion
Commendable quality	Control of biological drives	Fidelity; learns who he is and what he can and cannot do; knows what others think of him
Undesirable behavior	Unresolved confusion and turmoil regarding biological changes and drives	Problems with sexual role; delinquent behaviors, delinquent in choosing a career or vocation; problems with interpersonal relationships
Significant others	Peers, adult role models	Peers, adult role models

		Erikson
		Ages 21–35 or 40 Years
Stage or task		Stage 6: Establishes intimate personal relationships with friends; establishes intimate love relationship with one person Intimacy versus isolation *Table continued on following page*

Table 2–2 A Comparative Look at Freud's and Erikson's Theories of Personality Development *Continued*

	Erikson
	Ages 21–35 or 40 Years
Commendable quality	Love; mature relationship with member of opposite sex; suitable marital partner; performs work and socializes in acceptable ways
Undesirable behavior	Isolation from others; unable to share feelings, thoughts, and needs on emotionally mature level
Significant others	Spouse, children
	Erikson
	Ages 35 or 40–65 Years
Stage or task	Stage 7: Marriage, family, or fulfillment through career, religious vocation, etc.; children leave home; begins to be concerned about what will happen to future generations Generativity versus stagnation
Commendable quality	Care; involvement in helping activities; creative, caring, productive
Undesirable behavior	Overly concerned with bodily changes and self; selfish; exploits others; parasitic existence
Significant others	Community, other generations
	Erikson
	Ages 65 Years to Death
Stage or task	Stage 8: Satisfaction with one's achievements Integrity versus despair
Commendable quality	Wisdom; reviews life realistically; accepts past failures and future limitations; helps younger generation view life realistically; accepts death with dignity
Undesirable behavior	Sees past as total failure; fears death
Significant others	Self

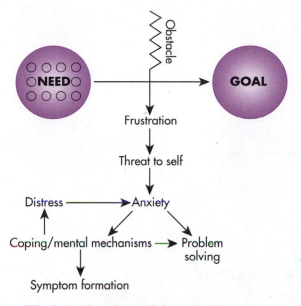

FIG. 2–2   Bauer's model for goal achievement.

frustration and anxiety. These feelings are normal reactions to obstacles throughout the life cycle. As vague and uncomfortable as these feelings may be, they can be growth-producing if dealt with in a constructive, problem-solving way. If the person does not use constructive methods, he or she may experience distress and find destructive ways of coping with the discomfort. At this point, the nurse must intervene and help the person develop problem-solving skills.

Reality Check

The nurse is reassigned to another unit in which she does not feel competent. She is afraid to share this information with the nurse manager for fear of receiving a poor evaluation. Later, the nurse goes home with a headache (symptom formation). Unless the nurse risks confronting the nurse manager and working through this problem, she will continue to have physical symptoms. What defense mechanism is the nurse using?

All behavior is purposeful and meaningful. Observation of behavior, including one's own, is a source for assessing individual needs. Needs can be categorized in many ways. One way is to consider them in relation to the physical, emotional, social, intellectual, and spiritual aspects of a person's life.

- *Physical needs,* sometimes referred to as *biological needs,* are closely related to body function and are necessary for survival. They include food, water, air, clothing, shelter, sex, exercise, and sensory and motor stimulation. At each stage of development, the person finds new ways to satisfy these needs. In the infant, the mother or mother substitute provides food, warmth, and stimulation. As the child grows, he or she finds other ways to meet basic physical needs based on previous experiences.
- *Emotional needs* are "the need to love and be loved and the need to feel we are worthwhile to ourselves and to others" (Glasser, 1965, p. 9). It is through love that the person receives approval and esteem; it is through feeling worthwhile that a person develops self-respect and feels that he or she is a contributing member of society.
- *Social needs* evolve from the person's cultural group. The most common social need is identification or belonging. During adolescence, belonging to a peer group is very important.
- *Intellectual/learning needs* begin at birth. Survival and security are related to learning specific tasks during the various stages of development.
- *Spiritual needs* are also related to the person's cultural influences and can have a significant effect on behavior.

Maslow's Hierarchy of Needs

Another approach to understanding human needs was developed by Abraham Maslow, a psychologist. He developed a hierarchy of needs that evolved into a humanistic theory. He focused on the whole person, including the qualities that make people distinctive and how these qualities develop. Maslow developed a pyramid to show the relation-

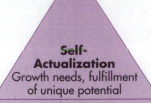

FIG. 2–3   Abraham Maslow's hierarchy of needs.

ship among the five levels of the hierarchy (Fig. 2–3). The base of the pyramid consists of the powerful basic needs—those of physical survival, such as food, water, shelter, sex, sleep, and air. After the needs of this level are reasonably satisfied, the person moves to the next higher level of safety and security. As these needs are satisfied, the person moves up to the next level, and so on up the pyramid until the person reaches **self-actualization**—the fulfillment of unique potential and the highest level in the hierarchy. According to Maslow, the first four levels cover basic needs. Self-actualization relates to a person's growth or fulfillment needs.

In reality, a person may be functioning on more than one level of needs at one time. For example, when a crisis occurs, a person may function on a lower level until the needs precipitated by the crisis are met. Maslow's theory is a "fluid process," in which people move from one level to another throughout each day and throughout their lifetime, depending on their situations and personal needs.

Reality Check

To put this in perspective for yourself, identify the level(s) at which you are currently functioning. If you have had a crisis in your life (e.g., health, accident, financial, marital, illness, loss), what was your primary level of functioning at that time according to Maslow?

OTHER THEORISTS

It is worth noting that other theorists have contributed a great deal of knowledge about personality development as well.

- *Harry Stack Sullivan,* in his interpersonal theory, emphasized the importance of self-esteem. He believed that many mental disorders result from anxiety caused by inadequate communication.
- *Jean Piaget's* contribution was a cognitive theory. Most of his research concerned how children learn and how they use what they learn in the adult world.
- *B. F. Skinner* is the person associated with behaviorism in the United States. His theory of operant conditioning implied that behavior is predictable but is also influenced by experience, interest, and ability.
- *Thomas Wolpe's* behavior therapy used the knowledge gained from the behavior theorists to change behavior through positive reinforcement (see Chapter 25).
- *Rollo May* emphasized the person's individuality and identified the significance of recognizing a higher order of being.

, Kohlberg - moral development

SUMMARY

Many theorists believe that mental illness is related to genetic, inherited factors and family environment during the formative years. Beginning with Freud, many theorists have supported the possibility of biological factors in mental illness. The development of psychotherapeutic medications in the 1950s rekindled interest in biological factors. The role of neurotransmitters has been of special interest. Some endocrine diseases frequently include emotional symptoms, especially depression and anxiety. Researchers still do not understand whether the illness triggers the emotional symptoms or vice versa. Similar questions remain about the relationship between immune disorders and emotional symptoms. Some mental disorders involve a genetic connection. At this time, it seems that environmental triggers play a role in developing family-related illnesses.

Freud, the founder of psychoanalysis, set into motion the study of human development, motivation, and thought. His psychosexual theory became a general theory of personality development. Many theorists began as students of Freud and modified his theories. Among these was Erik Erikson's upbeat psychosocial theory of growth and development. His eight stages of man provide a birth-to-death guideline for both positive and negative stages of growth and development.

Abraham Maslow took another approach to understanding human needs. He developed a hierarchy of needs, which evolved into a humanistic theory. His hierarchy continues to be a practical way of looking at individual needs based on a person's level of functioning.

Critical Thinking Activities

1. Turn to Table 2–1 on defense mechanisms (p. 17). Read the definition and example of each defense mechanism. Write a *new* example for each. (Clue: It is often helpful to think of your own behavior or that of someone you know.)
2. Turn to the comparison of Freud's and Erikson's theories in Table 2–2 (p. 18). Review each of Freud's stages of personality development.
   a. Circle all the positive and negative characteristics with which you *identify*.
   b. Which of these characteristics work for you? Which get in the way?
3. Using Table 2–2, review each of Erikson's eight stages of man.
   a. Circle the characteristics that are most like you at your current stage of development.
   b. Why is Erikson's way of looking at personal growth and development considered more positive than Freud's?
4. Review Maslow's hierarchy of needs in Figure 2–3 (p. 22).
   a. At which of Maslow's five levels are you currently functioning? Give a specific example to support your conclusion.
   b. Give an example of a time when you functioned at a higher or lower level of needs.

Review Questions

Multiple Choice—Choose the best answer to each question.

1. Which theory of mental illness relates to changes in the brain?
   a. Cognitive theory
   b. Existential theory
   c. Biological theory
   d. Psychosocial theory
2. How does stress affect the immune system?
   a. There is a relationship between behavioral changes and amount of dopamine
   b. An immune system imbalance related to light and temperature creates stress
   c. A family history of mental illness affects the immune system reaction
   d. Stress affects the immune system, making some people vulnerable to illness
3. Which is an example of the id?
   a. "You cannot have it"
   b. "Why not wait and see what tomorrow brings?"
   c. "I want what I want when I want it"
   d. "I'm not OK, you're not OK, and that's OK"
4. How did Freud view personality development?
   a. Placed emphasis on the need to solve problems at each stage of development
   b. Viewed development of mental disorders as a result of anxiety due to inadequate communication
   c. Saw each stage of development relating to the primary source of gratification for that age
   d. Believed that development was needs-based, beginning with physical survival
5. Which of the following is an example of rationalization?
   a. Smoking to fit in with a peer group
   b. Becoming angry out of proportion to the incident
   c. Ignoring symptoms of illness as a way of coping
   d. Not doing homework because someone came to visit

References

Erikson E: Childhood and Society, 2nd ed. New York, W Norton Co, 1963.

Sanford M: Concepts of psychiatric care. In: Antai-Otong D (ed): Psychiatric Nursing: Biological and Behavioral Concepts. Philadelphia, WB Saunders Co, 1995.

Trubowitz J: Historical overview, personality theories and classification of mental illness. In: Varcarolis EM (ed): Foundations of Psychiatric Mental Health Nursing, 2nd ed. Philadelphia, WB Saunders Co, 1994.

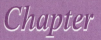

THREE

Spiritual and Cultural Considerations

Outline

- **Spirituality and Religion**
- **Collecting Data on Spiritual Needs**
    - Nonverbal Data
    - Verbal Data
    - Interpersonal Relationships
    - Environment
- **Needs Related to Health Care**
- **Cultural Considerations**
    - Space
    - Touch
        - Time
        - Voice
- **Addressing the Client**
- **Culturally Related Mental Health Issues**
    - African American
    - Native American
    - Asian American
    - Latino American
    - Euro-American

Key Terms

- culture
- deity
- religion
- spirit
- spirituality

Objectives

Upon completing this chapter, the student will be able to:

1. Differentiate between spiritual needs and religion.
2. List four possible areas to include when collecting data about spiritual needs.
3. Identify a spiritual belief or practice related to mental illness for each of the major belief systems important to clients in the area where the student will practice nursing.
4. Discuss how the nurse benefits from including spiritual beliefs as part of data collection.
5. Explain why it is helpful to learn about broad cultural differences.
6. Discuss why additional data collection during admission is needed to verify or dispute broad cultural assumptions.
7. List a cultural consideration regarding mental illness for people representing major cultures in the area where the student will practice nursing.

Reality Check

Before continuing, take some time to think about your personal definitions of spirituality and religion. Of what importance is knowledge of spirituality, religion, and culture in providing client care?

Florence Nightingale recognized that addressing the needs of the spirit are a part of nursing. The North American Nursing Diagnosis Association (NANDA) includes spiritual care as a nursing diagnosis. A nurse who does not understand customs can easily misinterpret a situation. Yet nurses are often reluctant to ask the questions leading to information about a client's spiritual needs during data collection. Some psychiatric nurses consider questions about spiritual needs a taboo in psychiatric care centers. Some have ongoing concerns and confusion regarding spiritual care and support of religious delusions. Sometimes the nurse's own spiritual discomfort may get in the way of integrating spiritual care as a part of total care.

Spiritual caregiving assumes the presence of spiritual needs in both nurse and client. "A nurse need not have a perfect understanding of spirituality; one need only be a receptive listener" (Price, Stevens, LaBarre, 1995, p. 6).

SPIRITUALITY AND RELIGION

Organized religion is not the only way of expressing spirituality, but it is a significant way for many clients. What does spirituality mean? How does it differ from religion?

Religion comes from the Latin root "to tie fast" and implies linking the person to a **deity** (God or higher being). The lifestyle of the person is to be lived in a manner pleasing to the deity. **Spirit,** on the other hand, derives from the Latin root "breath," which suggests the broader concept of that which gives life. Additional definitions include "the core of my being," "all that I am and will become," "my reason for being," etc. Some definitions specifically refer to a relationship with the deity. **Spirituality,** or one's concept of spirit, is one dimension of culture.

LeGere (in Gerardi, 1991, p. 76) differentiates between religion and spirituality as follows: Spirituality is not a religion. Spirituality has to do with experience; religion has to do with giving form to that experience. Spirituality focuses on what happens in the heart. Religion tries to make rules and capture that experience in a system.

COLLECTING DATA ON SPIRITUAL NEEDS

Many spiritual needs are exactly the same for clients with psychiatric disorders as they are for those with other illnesses. The focus in this chapter will be primarily on the client with a psychiatric disorder.

When a client who is experiencing psychosis (major mental illness) is first admitted, completing a written spiritual needs data collection is not a priority. The nurse can, however, make some observations while the client's thinking, feeling, and behavior are being stabilized. Later, the nurse can use these perceptions to guide a more in-depth data collection.

Nonverbal Data

The nurse should observe the client's behavior. For example, does the client pray during the day, watch religious TV programs, look at religious materials?

Verbal Data

The nurse should listen to what the client is saying. Is the client making references to God, such as asking for help, being unworthy of God's love, being punished, or being abandoned by God? Does the client indicate that he or she wants to go to church? Does the client ask for a pastor, a Bible, or other religious material? As part of the verbal assessment, the nurse should separate verbalizations that may be delusional (e.g., "I am God,", "I am Jesus," "I am the creator of the universe"). Behind these pronouncements are both spiritual and psychological needs. The best response is usually to be an effective listener.

Interpersonal Relationships

Another avenue for assessment is to determine who accompanied the client to the facility. Was it a family member, a friend, or a religious representative? Was the client supported and comforted by this person or upset by his or her presence?

Environment

Direct observation is another key to spiritual assessment. The nurse who admits the client should notice if he or she has a Bible, prayer book, Koran, or other special spiritual reading materials. Did the client bring religious medals, pins, or other symbols to be worn on the person? Did he or she insist on keeping on an undergarment or keeping the head covered? Did the client bring any pictures, tapes, letters, or other materials to help keep his or her spirits up?

Most of the data mentioned in this section can be collected merely by looking and listening during the initial admission period. Later, it will be appropriate to continue collecting data through conversations with the client. For example, the nurse may collect further information on religious practices and whether a need exists to continue these practices. With some thought, the nurse can often make it possible for a client to continue prayers and other practices with supervision, even when acutely ill.

The nurse's approach to spiritual data collection needs to be accepting, and the timing needs to be right. "It is important for nurses to be aware that just as spirituality may not be the easiest topic for them to explore with the client, it is often a difficult area for the client to discuss. The best approach avoids asking one question after another; instead, questions are used to respond to verbal and nonverbal clues that indicate the presence of a spiritual need" (Carson, 1989, p. 157).

Reality Check

List additional observations you can make about spiritual needs by *looking* and *listening.*

NEEDS RELATED TO HEALTH CARE

Because limited information about the relationship of religion and psychiatric illness is available, knowledge of basic beliefs and practices of various religious groups is essential for nurses. On occasion, nurses are quick to blame clergy for not showing up to minister to their members. Nurses should remember that sometimes clergy may not even be aware that a member has been hospitalized. In the psychiatric area, clergy can be called only with permission of the client. In addition to the client's own clergy, a pastoral care representative, or chaplain, may be a member of the team in the hospital setting. It is appropriate to ask if the client wishes to see a member of the clergy, whether it be the hospital chaplain or the client's own clergy. Rules of confidentiality continue to apply, regardless of whether clients see their own clergy or a hospital chaplain.

Whenever possible, dietary rules, care of religious objects, observance of special days, and other practices must be respected. On psychiatric units, staff members are accustomed to removing a client's valuables for safekeeping. There is a reason to rethink these rules in the realm of spiritual needs. For example, if the client is not posing a danger to self or others, is it necessary to remove the gold medallion? In this generation, most Muslims wear gold medallions such as a gold form with the Arabic word *Allah* or a prayer or quote from the Koran. According to their beliefs, it should not be removed. It takes tact, gentleness, courtesy, and listening skills to discover a client's spiritual needs. The nurse should also review his or her own belief system and be comfortable with it. Otherwise, a client's belief system, when different from the nurse's, may feel threatening to the nurse. There is even some evidence that spiritual caregiving can revitalize a nurse's professional life, preventing burnout and flight from the profession (Price, Stevens, LaBarre, 1995, p. 8).

Reality Check

Take a moment to identify religious articles you may want to keep while hospitalized. Ask someone else of a different religion what he or she would keep.

CULTURAL CONSIDERATIONS

Culture involves the total of all the ideas, beliefs, values, attitudes, and objects that a group of people possesses. It includes *ways of doing things*. Reviewing cultural differences provides general guidelines only. The significant differences are personal. The nurse identifies these differences by observing, listening, and using other data-collection skills.

The nurse must respond to subcultures created by the behaviors related to mental illness. At the same time, the nurse must continue to be aware of traditional cultural beliefs, even though these may sometimes conflict with behaviors caused by mental illness. Traditional beliefs often affect a client's preferences and customs involving "personal space," concepts of touch and time, and speaking customs.

Space

Nurses invade clients' personal space on a regular basis to provide care. Clients experiencing a mental illness may be less tolerant of automatic nursing practices. For example, suppose a client with a paranoid disorder is exhibiting a suspicious pattern of behavior. Moving into the client's personal space too quickly may be perceived as a threat. On the other hand, a client with a major depression whose primary behavior pattern is withdrawal/ isolation may welcome the closeness and yet feel unworthy of this attention.

The nurse must deal with other spatial issues at the same time. For example, the size of a client's personal space may depend on the client's cultural background. For many African American clients, this space may be approximately an arm's length. An African American client may not believe that he or she knows you well enough to invite you into this area. A client with Asian roots may want you even further away until inviting you in. Understanding cultural beliefs about personal space helps the nurse respond with sensitivity.

Touch

Nurses are taught that touching is a way of expressing caring, but touching may not be appropriate with a client experiencing mental illness. Even if touch is considered appropriate, if a client is of the Thai culture, the nurse must recall that the head is considered sacred and not to be touched. If a treatment or examination of the head of a Thai client is necessary, the nurse should carefully explain the process and ask the adult for permission.

The location of touch may have implications for people of other cultures as well. Patting someone on the knee or thigh is an intimate gesture and may have sexual connotation. A nurse should proceed with caution, especially with a client who is acutely ill. Touching the hand or arm is usually acceptable. However, a Euro-American male in an authority position may interpret the touching as demeaning. This supports the saying, "the diagnosis is not the person."

Clients experiencing a schizophrenic disorder usually exhibit withdrawal as their major behavior pattern. Rushing to touch such a client may create fear and further withdrawal. When mixed behavior patterns exist, the nurse must make a judgment call based on the major behavior pattern. Cues should be taken from the client, as well as from what the nurse knows about specific behaviors and cultures.

Time

Are clients resistive to treatment when they show up late for their appointments? Perhaps. There may also be cultural reasons. Time is interpreted and valued differently by people of various cultures. For example, Euro-Americans tend to be sticklers for time and can become easily irritated when having to wait. Clients with Asian, Arab, and Latin American roots tend not to live by schedules in the same rigid manner.

All cultures value time for celebrations and rituals with family, religious, or cultural significance. For example, in remembrance of a deceased loved one, Filipinos are expected for family prayers for nine consecutive evenings after the person's death. This is especially important for those with strong traditions of ancestor worship. The inability to comply with expected cultural norms honoring the deceased may lead to mental health problems (Carson and Arnold, 1996, p. 310).

Planned use of time can be of value in working therapeutically with some clients. For example, a client with a suspicious pattern of behavior has difficulty trusting anyone, including the nurse. It is often helpful to set up a time schedule for approaching the client. The nurse might use the following procedures to help gain a client's trust:

- Approach the client and maintain a respectful distance.
- Stay for a short period of time dictated by the clues observed about the client's comfort level.
- When leaving, state a specific time when the nurse will return.
- Return at *exactly* the given time.
- Continue this procedure. If the nurse is a minute early or late, the client will say so!

Voice

Nurses may interpret voice tones common to other cultures as being suspicious, threatening, or insulting. For example, an African American client has family members visiting. In an attempt to encourage and cheer the client, the visitors carry on a loud conversation. A nurse who does not understand this cultural tactic may make an incorrect assumption that the situation is threatening. "The use of loud verbalization has long been misunderstood in Latinos and African Americans: It is often misla-

beled as threatening" (Lovett-Scott and Ullman, 1994, p. 73).

The nurse's tone of voice makes a difference in penetrating the world of the client experiencing psychosis. For example, Danny, age 18, was experiencing an acute psychosis with auditory hallucinations (hearing voices). The voices told him to protect himself. Playing catch with beanbags was a way to help focus the young, strong client. Sometimes when the nurse would be picking up a beanbag, she would look up to see a beanbag aimed at her head. A firm, somewhat louder, "Stop that, Danny. You do not want to hurt me," would stop Danny from throwing the beanbag. To be effective, commands must not sound like a question.

A nurse sitting next to a client experiencing a depressive behavioral pattern may choose to sit quietly initially. As the relationship progresses, the nurse may thumb through a magazine, pointing out pictures while making brief, quiet comments to the client.

ADDRESSING THE CLIENT

The easiest way to avoid blunders in addressing a client is never to assume how a client wishes to be addressed, and to ask when in doubt. Sometimes clients who become mentally ill see their title as being "all that is left." The nurse may wish to address these clients formally (e.g., Mr., Ms., Mrs.), by title (e.g., Doctor, Professor, Congressman, Judge, Ambassador), or by rank (e.g., General, Captain, Admiral). This can be a boost for the client's self-respect, which is something nurses want to support. If the client wishes to be addressed in a different manner, he or she will let you know. For example, a client who developed a severely incapacitating obsessive-compulsive disorder became ill while he was a full professor at a university. He did not respond to the available treatments and ultimately was admitted to a long-term psychiatric facility. He addressed himself as Professor, and staff reciprocated by addressing him as Professor. He dressed daily in a white shirt, slacks, and tie, reflecting his former profession. A bonus: The introduction as Professor always alerted newcomers to a positive topic of conversation: his previous work. He could speak on the topic with a sense of accomplishment.

Reality Check

Take some time to think about cultural relationships to specific mental illnesses. Write down one or more statements about culture and mental illness that you believe to be true. How will your beliefs affect client care?

CULTURALLY RELATED MENTAL HEALTH ISSUES

This section addresses broad guidelines based on studies of various cultural groups. The nurse should use this information only as a guideline, because multiple individual differences exist. For example, it makes a difference how many generations a family has lived away from the country of origin, how strictly the practice of family customs has continued from generation to generation, whether members of the family have intermarried with people of other cultural groups, and so on. These factors, as well as personality differences unique to each person, have a large effect on each person's cultural values and beliefs.

African American

Limited studies show African Americans distrust "the system" and believe that one should not share personal information with outsiders. Studies also seem to indicate that among African Americans the following statements are true:

- Alcohol abuse is the number one problem
- Schizophrenia is misdiagnosed and overdiagnosed
- Depression is underdiagnosed
- More sleep paralysis, post-traumatic stress disorders, and simple phobias exist

Native American

Although the incidence of alcoholism has decreased, it is still a problem in the Native American population. Alcoholism is directly related to suicide, sexual assault, family violence, homicide, and child abuse. In addition, a high rate of developmental disorders and learning disabilities in Native Americans is thought to be related to fetal alcohol syndrome and otitis media. The best treatment plan for many Native American clients may be to use a holistic approach involving Native American healers. The role of nature, earth, and stewardship of natural resources is an integral part of successful treatment. Additional helpful information is available by reading *Black Elk Speaks* and *Lakota Myth,* both published by the University of Nevada Press.

Asian American

Limited information exists for this diverse cultural group. Some Asian Americans believe that physical illness causes emotional stress. Therefore they tend to seek treatment for somatic (physical) symptoms. Depending on the belief system, depression may be viewed as atonement for some misdeeds in life. Asian Americans seem to have fewer depression-related suicides.

Schizophrenia is seen among people of all social classes in Asian Americans. Variations seem to be related to fluency (able to express self verbally with ease): delusion is more prevalent in the fluent, and more catatonic symptoms are seen in the less fluent.

Some culture-bound syndromes are more frequent in Asian Americans. Examples include the following (Lovett-Scott and Ullman, 1994, p. 82):

- *Latah* in southeast Asian women: minimal stimuli elicit an exaggerated startle response, often with swearing
- *Anthropophobia* among the Japanese, especially men: easy blushing, anxiety with face-to-face contact, and fear of rejection
- *Koro,* especially in Asian men: fear that the penis will withdraw into the abdomen, causing death
- *Amok* among southeast Asian men: sudden mass assault, usually including homicide and sometimes the death of the perpetrator

Latino American

Mental problems are highly stigmatizing in the Latino American culture. This may partially account for the lower rate of referrals, which seem to be primarily for depression and suicide evaluation. This does not mean that Latino Americans experience more mood disorders. Actually, they experience more adjustment disorders than Caucasian or African Americans (Lovett-Scott and Ullman, 1994, p. 84). Overall, more women experience depression and more men experience alcoholism in this culture.

Euro-American

More studies exist for some backgrounds than for others. *Irish Americans* have experienced problems related to alcoholism and depression. Problems in *Italian Americans* appear to vary according to the region of origin. Strong family and religious ties either support good mental health or propel people toward depression. Those with Sicilian roots are more concerned with placating the power of Satan, "the evil eye," or overcoming magic (Carson and Arnold, 1996, pp. 312–313). *Finnish Americans* seem more prone to problems related to seasonal affective disorder and alcoholism.

SUMMARY

Observing and listening are keys to data collection about the client's spiritual and cultural needs. Knowledge of a client's spiritual and cultural beliefs is valuable, especially when coupled with knowledge of the client's individual differences and preferences. Spirituality is a broad, vague concept related to one's essence of being. Religion is an organized form of expressing spiritual feelings and beliefs. Not all spirituality is expressed through religion.

Although spiritual needs are recognized as a part of nursing care, they are sometimes omitted. This may be because of the nurse's lack of comfort with his or her own spiritual needs. Including spiritual care has been found to affect nurses positively.

When thinking about cultural needs, it is important to think about needs created by the subculture of mental illness. Issues of space, touch, time, and voice, as well as how the client is addressed, are connected both to cultural roots and to patterns of behavior related to mental illness.

Mental illness affects people of all cultures. Studies assist nurses in learning about trends and related issues, but nurses should view these studies only as broad, general guidelines to help them begin to assess a client's cultural and spiritual needs.

Critical Thinking Activities

1. What are your family's spiritual or cultural beliefs regarding mental illness? Which practices could be continued during hospitalization?
2. Consider your own preferences about space, touch, time, voice, and how you wish to be addressed. Focus on the cultural aspects of your preferences. How does this provide insight for dealing with clients in relation to their cultural needs?

Review Questions

Multiple Choice—Choose the best answer to each question.

1. What is spirituality?
   a. A set of beliefs that are followed by a particular church
   b. A way of living that is pleasing to the deity within a belief system
   c. A broad concept such as "core of my being" or "my reason for being"
   d. A dimension of culture unrelated to client care
2. Which statement about religious articles applies to psychiatric clients?
   a. All items should be removed at time of admission
   b. The client is permitted to keep all items while hospitalized
   c. The hospital chaplain is called in to make a decision regarding religious items

d. The decision of whether to remove religious items should be based on safety issues

3. Which is an example of response to touch in a client who is experiencing schizophrenia?
   a. Rushing to touch the client may lead to further withdrawal
   b. Touching is considered a comforting sign of acceptance
   c. The head is sacred and is touched only when necessary
   d. Touching within the client's personal space is acceptable

4. How does conversation reflect cultural variation?
   a. Loud conversation signals hostility and a threat to the client's safety
   b. Muted conversation implies that plans are being made to leave the hospital without permission
   c. Use of a moderate, clear voice is a universal way to penetrate the world of someone who is psychotic
   d. Loud conversation may reflect cheerful encouragement within an African American or Latino American group

5. Which is the most correct conclusion about a culturally related mental health issue?
   a. *Amok* is found among Latino Americans
   b. African Americans are taught to share information with outsiders
   c. The best treatment response for many Native Americans includes cultural healers
   d. Euro-Americans are unaffected by cultural differences

References

Carson VB: Spiritual Dimensions of Nursing Practice. Philadelphia, WB Saunders Co, 1989.

Carson VB, Arnold EN: Mental Health Nursing: The Nurse-Client Journey. Philadelphia, WB Saunders Co, 1996.

Gerardi R: Western spirituality. In: Carson VB: Spiritual Dimensions of Nursing Practice. Philadelphia, WB Saunders Co, 1991.

Lovett-Scott M, Ullman MA: Cultural diversity in mental health nursing. In: Varcarolis EM (ed): Foundations of Psychiatric Mental Health Nursing, 2nd ed. Philadelphia, WB Saunders Co, 1994.

Price JL, Stevens HO, LaBarre MC: Spiritual caregiving in nursing practice. J Psychosoc Nurs 33(12):5–9, 1995.

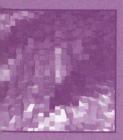

Stigma and Related Legal and Ethical Issues

Outline

- Nature and Sources of Stigma
- Impact of Stigma on Consumers of Mental Health Services
- Overcoming Stigma
    - Contribution of Mental Health Professionals
    - Homelessness and Mental Illness
- Legal Rights of People With Mental Illness
- Voluntary and Involuntary Admissions
- Ethical Issues

Key Terms

- client's rights
- involuntary commitment
- myths
- stereotyping
- stigma
- stigmatization
- voluntary admission

Objectives

Upon completing this chapter, the student will be able to:
1. Describe the nature and sources of stigma.
2. Relate personal experience with stigma to more general concerns.
3. Identify some impacts of stigma on consumers of mental health services.
4. Describe strategies that may be used to reduce the frequency and impact of stigmatization.
5. List six rights of people who are mentally ill.
6. Describe an ethical dilemma that may occur in working with a person who is mentally ill.

Throughout history, people with mental illnesses have been stigmatized. Fear, misunderstanding, and superstition about mental disorders result when people do not understand what is happening. Despite considerable research, these ideas are slow to die.

NATURE AND SOURCES OF STIGMA

In ancient Greece, when a sign was burned into the flesh of a thief, the scar was called a *stigma*. It announced to everyone that the person was discredited in the eyes of the community. Today, a **stigma** is a characteristic that marks a person as different from others. It is selected by a social group to imply that an individual is flawed in some way. Any personal characteristic can be a basis for **stigmatization,** or the development of a stigma. Most stigmas belong to one of three broad classes (Baker, 1993):

- Physical differences (e.g., size, shape, clothes, hair)
- Blemishes of character (e.g., homelessness, unemployment)
- Tribal stigmas (e.g., race, nationality, religion)

The stigma is *not* the characteristic itself, but the choosing of that characteristic by a dominant social group or person to gain power over another group or person. Stigmas become labels. Once a stigma is applied, it guides the way people process information. Stereotyping, or labeling someone because of characteristics such as race, creed, gender, or illness is central in stigmatization. Stigmas shape emotions such as fear and anger. They also direct behavior. A person can respond by attack, withdrawal, or performing the minimum required within his or her role.

Everyone feels stigmatized at some time. People have been too fat, too young, too ugly, too old. They have been marked as different, and hence deficient. Some are stigmatized more frequently or for greater periods because of their appearance or behavior. Those who are prey to frequent or prolonged stigmatization often view themselves differently from other people.

Reality Check

Describe your personal experience with stigma, and discuss any effect that it might have had on you.

IMPACT OF STIGMA ON CONSUMERS OF MENTAL HEALTH SERVICES

In a mental health context, stigmatization involves shunning people and treating them as though they have less value because of their mental illness. This attitude often extends to families with loved ones who are mentally ill, and to those who trust people who have mental illnesses. People with mental illness often experience shame, embarrassment, and/or social isolation as a result of stigma. People with mental illness may be viewed as weak, dangerous, or responsible for their own plight. Although there has been some improvement, those people who are stigmatized as mentally ill still have difficulty with employment, education, housing opportunities, and health-care coverage. Stigmatization may even cause a person to delay seeking mental health treatment.

The prejudice and negative reactions encountered by people with mental illness result from ignorance about the nature and causes of mental illness. Common misconceptions, or **myths,** about mental illness include the following:

Myth: "Mental illnesses are not real diseases like heart disease and cancer" (NMHA, 1996).

Fact: There are many causes for psychiatric disorders. Some can be linked to a biological origin, and some may be situational and temporary, caused by stress or life changes.

Myth: "A person who has had a mental illness can never lead a normal life" (NMHA, 1996).

Fact: Many people with mental illnesses can go on to lead more enriched and accomplished lives. Examples include the following:

- Abraham Lincoln, 16th President of the United States, was plagued throughout his life with mood disorders and insomnia.
- Mark Twain, America's greatest humorist, "episodically retreated into depression, and then came back raging into the world" (California Alliance for the Mentally Ill, p. 6).
- Sir Winston Churchill, Prime Minister of Great Britain, was plagued by what he called his "black dog," his term for depression.
- George Frederic Handel, composer, suffered from manic-depressive illness. During one of his bursts of creativity, he wrote his masterpiece *The Messiah*.

Myth: "Mentally ill people are dangerous" (NMHA, 1996).

Fact: "While less than 3% of mentally ill patients could be categorized as dangerous, 77% of mentally ill people depicted on prime-time television are presented as dangerous" (Dubin and Fink, 1992, p. 3). Unfortunately, the media are responsible for many of the misconceptions people have about mental illness. Newspapers often stress a history of mental illness when reporting crimes of violence. Comedians use mental illness as a source of humor, and movies sensationalize people with mental illness, leaving a negative image. At the same time, the media can be a positive force for eliminating stigma. The media has the power to educate and influence public opinion (NMHA, 1996). Some movies that have attempted to do this are *Rainman* and *As Good As It Gets*.

Myth: "Recovered mental patients can work low-level jobs, but aren't suited for really important or responsible positions" (NMHA, 1996).

Fact: The willingness of people with mental illness to share their experiences has in-

creased public awareness. Mike Wallace, CBS News correspondent, has freely talked about his bouts with depression. He has testified before Congress, calling for more federal research funds and drawing national attention to the illness. The actress Patty Duke discussed her bipolar depression in her autobiographical made-for-TV movie *Call Me Anna*. Former New York Chief Justice Sol Wachtler detailed episodes of his behavior during periods of bipolar depression in *After the Madness: A Judge's Own Prison Memoir*.

OVERCOMING STIGMA

A major problem in combating stigma is the lack of public awareness regarding progress that has been made in the treatment of mental illness. We now possess a greater knowledge of brain chemistry, and we understand better how certain medications help the person who is mentally ill. But the lingering myth that holds families at fault continues. As a result, "many families focus exclusively on mental illness being a brain disease, leaving out the mind. . . . treatment involves not only biological intervention but also social rehabilitation and environmental stimulation" (Dubin and Fink, 1992, p. 5). The development of advocacy groups, such as the National Alliance for the Mentally Ill, has helped support and educate families of those who are mentally ill.

Families who participate in support groups have an opportunity to vent their feelings. By sharing their experiences, group members learn new ways of dealing with difficult situations. They share resource material and support one another's strengths. Many regulatory agencies require family participation in treatment and discharge planning. This involvement serves to decrease the previous sense of helplessness and despair.

Education is another way to overcome stigma. Through public involvement and advocacy for needs and rights of people who are mentally ill, stigma can be reduced. Many resources are available to anyone who wishes to know more (see

Chapter 30). Box 4–1 highlights some positive ways in which people can help reduce the stigma of mental illness.

Contribution of Mental Health Professionals

If the stigma of mental illness is going to be changed, then it must start with the changing of the attitudes and perceptions of mental health professionals.

Anonymous (1993, p. 20).

Dr. Kay Redfield Jamison, in her book *An Unquiet Mind,* relates the reaction of a colleague when she told him of her illness. "He thought I was so wonderful, so strong: How could I have attempted suicide? What had I been thinking? It was such an act of cowardice, so selfish" (Jamison, 1995, p. 200). Some psychiatric nurses reinforce that stigma. Table 4–1 lists interactions with clients that convey dehumanization (the deprivation of a person's individuality) and perpetuate stigma.

BOX 4–1	**Positive Ways to Reduce Stigma**

1. Educate yourself about mental illness.
2. Talk to each other about mental illness "in the terms of illness."
3. Correct false statements about mental illness and people with mental illness.
4. Write letters to the media, offering to send accurate information.
5. Relate to people who are mentally ill as individuals. Avoid stigmatizing people; look at the contents behind the label.
6. Advocate for equal rights in housing, employment, and health care coverage. Mental illnesses are considered a disability under the Americans with Disabilities Act (ADA).
7. Support the efforts of people with mental illnesses to empower themselves by becoming involved in self-help and support groups for these people.
8. Support the consumer mental health movement.

Homelessness and Mental Illness

A very vulnerable group are homeless people who are mentally ill. The negative perceptions of homelessness, added to the stigma of mental illness, only make it more difficult to escape a tough situation. The National Resource Center on Homelessness and Mental Illness is involved in research and programs for homeless people. Programs are aimed at building trust, meeting basic needs, and fostering peer support and empowerment.

Reality Check

Name a way in which you can contribute to the destigmatization of mental illness.

LEGAL RIGHTS OF PEOPLE WITH MENTAL ILLNESS

A definition of rights for people with mental illness is one tool to decrease stigmatization and end discrimination. **Client's rights** are legal provisions that ensure more effective client care. In 1973, the American Hospital Association (AHA) first adopted A Patient's Bill of Rights. The bill included 12 provisions designed to ensure more effective client care. These rights are presented in Table 4–2.

Psychiatric facilities are required to have a client's Bill of Rights posted in a visible area. There is concern that people with mental illnesses and substance-use disorders are being overlooked in the changing health care system. Nine health care organizations issued A Bill of Rights in February 1997 to ensure that all people with mental illness receive quality health care. This document emphasizes that individuals have a right to know pertinent information. Box 4–2 details the 1997 Mental Health Bill of Rights.

VOLUNTARY AND INVOLUNTARY ADMISSIONS

Voluntary admission is initiated by a person seeking help for his or her problems. This person is

Table 4–1	Interactions With Clients That Convey Dehumanization and Perpetuate the Stigma of Mental Illness
Interaction	**Example**
1. Talking about the client in his or her presence.	Saying to the family member who is returning the client from a weekend pass, "Did Joey behave himself while he was home?"
2. Reminding a client that he or she will not do something negative (e.g., hit another person).	"You'd better not hit anyone today!"
3. Threatening a client (showing the client "who is boss").	"If you give me any trouble today, I'll restrict you to the unit."
4. Referring to a client by room number or diagnosis.	"I have that new 'schizophrenic' today."
5. Disregarding the client's plan of care and arbitrarily changing rules or routine.	"I don't know who came up with that dumb rule. Of course you can go home this weekend."
6. Not listening to clients.	"Oh, don't worry about that; we'll take care of you."
7. Demeaning, discounting, or belittling clients.	"What's the use of talking to him. He's in his own little world."
8. Teasing clients.	"Maybe I won't give you your cigarettes this time."
9. Provoking guilt in clients.	"How can you be like that? Your daughter does so much for you."
10. Displacing angry feelings onto clients.	Yelling at clients, shouting directions, being impatient with clients' requests.

aware that support is needed to deal with troubling situations. Because of the person's willingness to go to the hospital, he or she usually becomes an active participant in the treatment plan. Legally, the voluntary client is able to leave the hospital at any time.

Involuntary admission is initiated by someone other than the person needing help, such as police or the person's family. This type of admission is called **involuntary commitment** or *civil commitment*. Each state has specific guidelines for hospitalizing a person against his or her will. These guidelines usually include the following behaviors:

- The person displays a substantial probability of physical harm to self as demonstrated by recent threats or attempts at suicide or serious bodily harm.
- The person displays substantial probability of physical harm to others as demonstrated by recent homicidal or other violent behavior or threats to do serious harm.
- The person fails to care for self because of a mental condition so that a danger of physical harm to self is created.

The patient's rights law applies to a person under involuntary commitment. Especially impor-

Table 4–2	1973 AHA Patient's Bill of Rights
Respectful care	Complete information about his or her condition
Informed consent	Right to refusal of treatment
Privacy	Confidentiality
Requested hospital services	Right to refuse experimental treatment
Continuity of care	Information about his or her bill, and information about the hospital's affiliation with other institutions
Knowledge of the hospital's rules and regulations that apply to his or her conduct	

Data from American Hospital Association: A Patient's Bill of Rights, revised. Chicago, AHA, 1992.

TDO – 72 hrs

BOX 4–2   1997 Mental Health Bill of Rights

Benefits

The right to be provided with information from the purchasing entity and the insurance/third-party payer describing the nature and extent of their mental health and substance abuse treatment benefits. This information should include details on procedures to obtain access to services, on utilization management procedures, and on appeal rights.

Professional Expertise

The right to receive full information from the potential treating professional about that professional's knowledge, skills, preparation, experience, and credentials. The right to be informed about the options available for treatment intervention and the effectiveness of the recommended treatment.

Contractual Limitations

The right to be informed by the treating professional of any arrangements, restrictions, and/or covenants established between a third-party payer and the treating professional that could interfere with or influence treatment recommendations. The right to be informed of the nature of information that may be disclosed for the purpose of paying benefits.

Appeals and Grievances

The right to receive information about the methods used to submit complaints or grievances regarding the provision of care by the treating professional to that profession's regulatory board and to the professional association. The right to be provided information about the procedures they can use to appeal benefit utilization decisions to the third-party payer system, to the employer or purchasing entity, and to external regulatory entities.

Confidentiality

The right to be guaranteed the protection of confidentiality in a client's relationship with his or her mental health and substance abuse professionals, except when laws or ethics dictate otherwise. Any disclosure to another party will be time-limited and made with full written, informed consent of the individuals. Individuals shall not be required to disclose confidential, privileged, or additional information other than that necessary for diagnosis, prognosis, type of treatment, time and length of treatment, and cost. Entities receiving information for the purpose of benefits determination will maintain information in confidence, subject to the same penalties for violation as the direct provider of care.

Choice

The right to choose any duly licensed/certified professional for mental health and substance abuse services. The right to receive information about treatment options (including risks and benefits) and cost implications to make an informed choice regarding the selection of care deemed appropriate by the individual and the professional.

Determination of Treatment

Recommendations regarding mental health and substance abuse treatment shall be made only by a duly licensed/certified professional in conjunction with the individual and his or her family, as appropriate. Treatment decisions should not be made by third-party payers.

Parity

The right to receive benefits for mental health and substance abuse treatment on the same basis as other illnesses, with the same provisions, co-payments, lifetime benefits, and catastrophic coverage in both insurance and self-funded/self-insured health plans.

Discrimination

Individuals who use mental health and substance abuse benefits shall not be penalized when seeking other health insurance or disability, life, or any benefit.

Benefit Usage

The right to receive the entire scope of the benefits within the benefit plan that will address his or her clinical needs.

Benefit Design

Whenever both federal and state law and/or regulations are applicable, the professional and all payers shall use whichever affords the individual the greatest level of protection and access.

Treatment Review

The right to be guaranteed that any review of a client's mental health and substance abuse treatment shall involve a professional having the training, credentials, and licensure required to provide treatment in the jurisdiction in which it will be provided.

Accountability

Treating professionals may be held accountable and liable to individuals for any injury caused by gross incompetence or negligence on the part of the professional. Payers and other third parties may be held accountable and liable to individuals for any injury caused by gross incompetence or negligence or by clinically unjustified decisions.

Data from Mental Health Bill of Rights Project. Washington, DC, February 20, 1997.

tant is that the individual has the right to receive prompt and adequate treatment, rehabilitation, and educational services.

ETHICAL ISSUES

Many ethical dilemmas arise in protecting the rights of people who are mentally ill. Autonomy is one ethical principle that often causes conflict. For instance, what happens to an individual who is hearing voices or is severely depressed, who is not dangerous, but who refuses all forms of treatment? Is this person truly autonomous, or is the decision to refuse treatment a reflection of his illness? One governor has included in his budget the recommendation to create non-treatment facilities for competent adults who refuse certain treatment while committed to psychiatric facilities (WCILC, Spring 1997, No. 6, p. 3). Is this a violation of client autonomy, and is justice being served?

Reality Check

How would you respond to a professional who told you that you were just wasting your time trying to talk to a client who was hearing voices, and urged instead that you should wait until the medication took effect?

Nurses must be aware of the legal and ethical issues involved in treating people who are mentally ill. They need to justify their decisions based on ethical reasoning. When the nurse respects another's rights and cultural beliefs (see Chapter 3), he or she treats that person with dignity and respect. The legal and ethical concepts learned in basic nursing apply to psychiatric nursing, such as standards of care, confidentiality, accountability, charting guidelines, and so on.

SUMMARY

Stigma is a mark that labels a person as different and less attractive than others. Many in society view people with mental illness as being responsible for their own condition. People find the loss of intellectual control difficult to understand; they fear loss of the control of their own mental ability. These fears lead to many misconceptions or myths about mental disorders. People with mental illness are stereotyped. In general, society still believes that a person who has had a mental illness cannot lead an independent life. Opinions are formed without adequate information.

One way to overcome stigma is through public education and advocacy. Nurses, along with their peers from other disciplines, need to speak out when they witness discrimination against people with mental illness. This practice may help improve the quality of life for people with mental illness and their families.

By implementing and enforcing the legal rights of people with mental illnesses, stigma and discrimination against them can be decreased. The 1997 Mental Health Bill of Rights Project encourages states to review and revise their laws to ensure services and protection of people with mental illness.

Respect for a client's dignity, autonomy, cultural beliefs, and privacy is of particular concern when working in the mental health field. Many ethical dilemmas arise in the treatment of people with mental illness. Nurses need to advocate for clients and protect them from unethical behavior.

Critical Thinking Activities

1. What attitudes have you encountered about people with mental illness?
2. What television programs portray people with mental illness or noticeable behavior abnormalities in a negative way?
3. Collect newspaper articles that emphasize the mental illness of a person.
4. What are your observations of the application of clients' rights in the clinical area? Were any rights violated?

Review Questions

Multiple Choice—Choose the best answer to each question.

1. An impact of stigma on consumers of mental health services is
   a. encouragement to seek treatment.
   b. motivation to seek education.
   c. shame, embarrassment, and/or social isolation.
   d. willingness to extend themselves to others.
2. Which of the following is a myth about mental illness?
   a. Mental illness is a real disease like heart disease
   b. People with mental illness are dangerous
   c. People with mental illness can lead productive lives
   d. People with mental illness can be responsible citizens
3. A positive way to reduce the stigma associated with mental illness is to
   a. remind the client that he or she will not do something negative.
   b. talk about the client in his or her presence.
   c. support the efforts of the client to empower him or herself.
   d. discount, belittle, and not listen to the client.
4. Client's rights are
   a. obstacles to effective client care.
   b. an invasion of the rights of health providers.
   c. difficult to implement within the institutional setting.
   d. ways of decreasing stigmatization and discrimination.
5. An ethical principle that often causes conflict in working with a person who is mentally ill is
   a. preventing harm and removing harm to the client.
   b. allowing the client to maintain control over health care decisions.
   c. treating the client's family despite their behavior.
   d. remembering that what you hear, see, and read remains confidential.

References

Anonymous: Coming out: my experience as a mental patient. J Psychosoc Nurs 31(5):20, 1993.

Baker B: Identity and Stigmatization. Workshop, March 1993.

California Alliance for the Mentally Ill: Mark Twain. The Journal 1(4):1–12, 1990.

Dubin W, Fink P: Effects of stigma on psychiatric treatment. In: Fink P, Tasman A (eds): Stigma and Mental Illness. Washington, DC, American Psychiatric Press Inc, 1992.

Jamison K: An Unquiet Mind. New York, Alfred A. Knopf Inc, 1995.

National Mental Health Association: Stigma: Awareness and Understanding of Mental Illness, pamphlet #231, Alexandria, Vir, NMHA, 1996.

The Wisconsin Coalition of Independent Living Centers (WCILC). Eye on the Capitol, No. 6, Spring 1997.

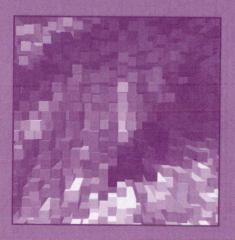

Multidisciplinary Approach

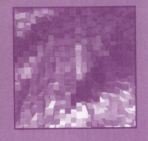

Team Members

Outline

Key Terms

- continuum
- gentle self-defense
- NCLEX-PN
- NCLEX-RN
- psychiatric treatment team

Objectives

Upon completing this chapter, the student will be able to:

1. Explain what is meant by the mental health–mental illness continuum.
2. Discuss psychiatric nursing as a part of all nursing care.
3. Summarize the role of each of the following team members:
    - psychiatric nurse—generalist and clinical specialist
    - psychiatrist
    - psychiatric social worker
    - clinical psychologist
    - psychiatric nursing assistant
4. Describe how the role of psychiatric professionals has been influenced by shortened inpatient treatment stays.

Nurses sometimes think of their work only in terms of their individual specialty areas. Psychiatric nursing is rarely limited to the psychiatric unit. It is a part of *all* nursing care. Mental health–mental illness forms a **continuum** (various degrees of a single concept) for all clients wherever they are hospitalized, or even if they are not in a hospital setting.

```
MENTAL                    MENTAL
HEALTH |_____| ILLNESS
```

Where a person functions on this imaginary line depends on stressors and the person's ability to cope with them. Stressors of all kinds—emotional, physical, and spiritual—produce positive and negative stress. The person's position on the mental health–mental illness continuum may vary on a day-to-day basis. Movement along the continuum may be sharply distinct or a subtle evolution of reactions to stress.

TEAM APPROACH

The **psychiatric treatment team** is made up of many persons, each with his or her own contributions to make (Fig. 5–1). Individually, team members all gain bits and pieces of a puzzle. Only when they can talk and work together can they come up with a satisfying plan of care for each client. To be an effective member of a team, whether in a facility or a community, some characteristics stand out:

- Team members must know what other professionals are capable of doing by virtue of their education.
- They must be willing to share responsibility for the common good of the client.

Psychiatric nurses are an important part of this team. Psychiatric/mental health nursing involves the ability of all nurses, wherever they practice, to see themselves as part of a psychiatric treatment team. The team effort begins at the time of initial

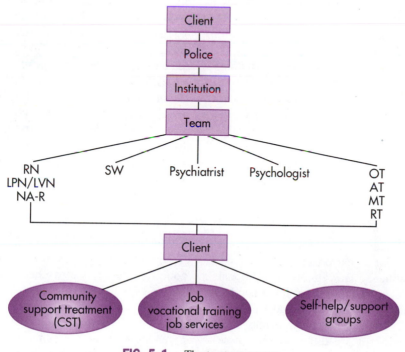

FIG. 5–1   The treatment team.

client contact, *wherever the contact takes place.* The team approach is completed when the client is functioning at potential—emotionally, physically, spiritually, and socially.

CASE STUDY

Mr. D's Story

The rest of this chapter is a case study of a client that demonstrates how the psychiatric treatment team works together for the client's benefit. The case study includes a brief description of traditional psychiatric hospital staff education and responsibility. Note that the roles and assignments my vary according to state, local, and hospital policies.

Background

Mr. D's boss has become increasingly concerned because of behavioral changes he has observed in Mr. D during the last few days. When Mr. D fails to return from lunch today, his boss goes looking for him. He finds Mr. D heading for the highway, yelling "The voices have told me it's time to die." Some other employees nearby come to help. "Call 911" shouts Mr. D's boss.

Alerted by the nature of the call, 911 operators dispatch two police officers trained in dealing with people who are mentally ill. Communities have worked for greater cooperation between law enforcement officers, mental health professionals, and psychiatric hospitals. In some communities, crisis workers or mental health delegates perform this service.

Members of the Treatment Team
Police

The male and female police officers who respond have each attended a 2-year police science course at a technical college. They received additional on-site training on how to recognize and respond to people who exhibit symptoms of mental illness. In this community, they also learned gentle self-defense techniques that are different from those taught in traditional police training. **Gentle self-defense** involves specific defensive (not offensive) techniques to prevent the client from harming self or others. The training also includes legal issues and instruction on decision-making skills needed to decide whether to take the person home, to jail, or to the emergency room or psychiatric hospital (Foster, 1979).

This additional training was provided by a master's-prepared psychiatric nurse. In many communities, involuntary admission of clients involves the police. Although psychiatric clients are not usually suspected of criminal activity, the client's behavior may warrant the special training of law enforcement officers.

Clinical Nurse Specialist

In this case, the police decide that Mr. D presents a danger to himself and that hospitalization should be considered. After they seat Mr. D inside the patrol car, the police notify the clinical nurse specialist at the hospital of the pending admission. The clinical nurse specialist notifies the unit and the psychiatrist. The clinical nurse specialist would also be available during admission as needed. The police also contact Mr. D's wife.

The nurse received a bachelor's degree in nursing (BSN or BAN) from a 4-year college or university. He successfully completed the **NCLEX-RN** (National Council Licensure Examination for Registered Nurses) to become a registered nurse (RN). He then completed a 2-year master's degree in a psychiatric nursing program. To become an instructor, he took additional training in gentle self-defense. Based on his education, this master's-prepared psychiatric nurse may go on to become a clinical nurse specialist/psychiatric mental health nurse practitioner.

Psychiatric Nursing Supervisor

On arrival at the psychiatric hospital, Mr. D and the police are met by the psychiatric nursing supervisor, an LPN/LVN, and a psychiatric assistant. The psychiatrist on call will be arriving shortly. The nursing supervisor extends her hand to Mr. D. Extending her hand is more than a greeting. It is the beginning of a psychiatric nursing assessment.

Mr. D's response to her greeting begins to provide some information about his current mental status. When Mr. D does not extend his hand, the nurse drops her hand without comment. This gives information about Mr. D's discomfort with touch and will be respected. The supervisor goes on to introduce the LPN/LVN and the psychiatric assistant. Taking their cue from the supervisor's experience, they do not extend their hands.

The supervisor, an RN, attended a 3- or 4-year nursing program and successfully completed the NCLEX-RN. She worked as a psychiatric staff nurse and charge nurse before assuming the supervisory role. The psychiatric team in this hospital decided that the supervisor will assume responsibility for the admission (intake) assessment. Assessment is performed by several team members. Communication between the team members is essential to discuss the plan of care for the client. This communication might involve conferences, rounds, reports, and so on.

The supervisor's other duties include supervision of all nursing care of psychiatric clients on the adult treatment units. She is immediately responsible for all five steps of the nursing process (see Chapter 8).

LPN/LVN

To become licensed, the LPN/LVN completed a 9- to 12-month nursing education program in a vocational school or a bi-level program at a community college. She also had to complete the **NCLEX-PN** (National Council Licensure Examination for Practical Nurses) successfully. Because these programs incorporate mental health concepts as a part of the total nursing program, she has limited experience in dealing with people who are mentally ill. Her orientation to the psychiatric hospital included a course on mental health concepts, specific behaviors of people who are mentally ill and ways to respond, effects and side effects of psychotherapeutic medications, and gentle self-defense.

The LPN/LVN's education, skill in data collection, and assisting in all parts of the nursing process set her apart from unlicensed personnel. She was initially assigned to buddy with an experienced LPN/LVN. Both were under the supervision of an RN. As part of the psychiatric care team, her assignments involve assisting the RN with the nursing process, completing one-to-one client assignments, giving medications, performing admitting and discharge duties, and other assignments within the LPN/LVN scope of practice.

Psychiatric Nursing Assistant

The nursing assistant received a minimum of 85 hours of training through a vocational program. After successfully completing a test to be listed in a registry, the assistant was employed by the hospital as a registered nursing assistant (NA-R). Because of limited focus during training on mental illness, the assistant was required to attend a series of classes as part of his orientation. Classes included basic mental health concepts, specific behaviors and approaches, safety issues, and gentle self-defense. The nursing assistant was then assigned to buddy with an experienced LPN/LVN. Both were supervised by an RN. Responsibilities assigned to the NA-R usually depend on the facility. In this hospital, the assistant's responsibilities include the following (Dept. of Labor, 1991):

- Accompanying clients to shower rooms and assisting with bathing, dressing, and grooming
- Accompanying clients to examinations and treatments
- Measuring vital signs
- Recording information on client charts
- Assisting clients in becoming accustomed to unit routine
- Encouraging clients to participate in social and recreational activities to promote rehabilitation
- Observing clients to ensure that they do not wander from the unit or designated area
- Assisting at mealtime, following guidelines on nutritional needs based on diagnosis and behavioral pattern (see Chapter 26), recording reasons for rejecting food or overeating, modifying approach as directed by the RN
- Observing client to detect unusual behavior, aiding in preventing client injury to self or others

- Escorting clients off-grounds to appointments or events
- Cleaning rooms, changing linens, etc.

Today, some of the tasks described here take place in community mental health facilities (see Chapter 29). A brief hospitalization for behavior stabilization is followed by treatment in a community setting. In some settings, the NA-R receives additional training and gives prescribed medications to clients.

Psychiatrist

The psychiatrist makes the final decision regarding emergency admission for Mr. D. This decision is based on a mental status examination of Mr. D, the intake information obtained by the nursing supervisor, and the police account of behavior observed at the work site. The psychiatrist is a medical doctor who completed a 2- to 4-year residency in psychiatry.

The psychiatrist is the professional who heads the psychiatric treatment team. The psychiatrist's major responsibility is diagnosis and treatment of clients with mental, emotional, and behavioral problems. Included in this responsibility is the following (Dept. of Labor, 1991):

- Organizing data concerning the client's family, medical history, and onset of symptoms; this information is obtained from the client, relatives, and other sources, including the nurse, psychiatric social worker, psychologist, and other team members
- Examining the client to determine the general physical condition (remember that some physical illnesses include mental symptoms); in some facilities, the physical examination is performed by a general practitioner
- Ordering laboratory and diagnostic tests and evaluating these data
- Determining the nature and extent of the mental disorder and heading the formation of a treatment program
- Making a formal diagnosis

- Treating or directing client treatment using a variety of psychotherapeutic methods and medications

Psychiatric Social Worker

The social worker (SW) meets with Mrs. D when she arrives at the hospital. In some psychiatric facilities, the psychiatric social worker is the person who does the admission (intake) interview. The SW received his knowledge and skill in casework methods through a master's degree program at a school of social work. Responsibilities of the SW include the following (Dept. of Labor, 1991):

- Providing social work assistance to clients with mental or emotional illness in hospital, clinic, and community treatment settings, and working with other team members to develop a treatment plan
- Investigating the client's family and social background as appropriate to diagnosis and treatment, and then sharing the information with the psychiatrist and other team members
- Interpreting psychiatric treatment to the client's family to help reduce fear and other attitudes that may get in the way of accepting treatment and continuing care
- Serving as a link between the client, the psychiatric agency, and the community
- Providing direct treatment to clients individually or in groups
- Referring the client or the client's family to other community resources
- Assisting in adjustment leading to and after discharge

Clinical Psychologist

The clinical psychologist is asked to administer specific tests to help establish Mr. D's diagnosis. The clinical psychologist attended a master's or doctoral program in clinical psychology and successfully completed an examination to become licensed. Once licensed, the clinical psychologist practices independently or as part of a psychiatric team. The psychologist does not prescribe medication. Her work includes the following (Dept. of Labor, 1991):

- Testing and test interpretation, including intelligence, achievement, interest, personality, and other psychological tests, which aid in diagnosis and development of treatment plans
- Treating mental and emotional disorders using various psychological techniques, including individual and group psychotherapy, play therapy, hypnosis, psychodrama, and milieu therapy

Other Members of the Treatment Team

Numerous other professionals may become part of the treatment team, depending on the nature of Mr. D's illness, the hospital and community treatment available, financial factors, and client and family motivation. The roles of some of these therapists follow.

Occupational Therapist

The registered occupational therapist (OTR) educational program includes 4 years of college, a 1-year internship, and a test to become registered. The OTR is qualified to plan, organize, and conduct therapy in a hospital or community setting. Occupational therapy has traditionally been considered a part of a client's total therapy in an acute or long-term setting. Because hospitalizations are brief, many clients no longer experience this valuable aspect of a total therapeutic plan. Some community mental health treatment programs have incorporated occupational therapy as part of continuing treatment for people who have chronic mental illness.

Today, many occupational therapists have also become recreational therapists, playing a dual role on the treatment team. For the purpose of clarity, each role is described separately in this chapter. OTRs involve clients in activities according to their behavior and needs. These activities may include the following (Dept. of Labor, 1991):

- Manual arts and crafts
- Practice in functional, prevocational, vocational,

and homemaking skills and activities of daily living
- Participation in sensorimotor, educational, recreational, and social activities designed to help clients develop or regain mental functioning

The activities an OTR chooses for a client are based on physical capacity, intelligence, and interest level. OTRs work with clients both individually and in groups according to prescribed goals.

Recreation Therapist

The recreation therapist (RT) has a bachelor's degree in recreational therapy. The RT's overall responsibility is to plan, organize, and direct medically approved recreation programs for clients. As a member of the treatment team, the RT's duties include the following (Dept. of Labor, 1991):

- Involving clients in activities such as sports, dramatics, games, and arts and crafts. This helps the client develop interpersonal relationships, socialize effectively, and develop confidence to participate in group activities. Client activities are based on client capabilities, needs, interests, and therapeutic issues.
- Instructing clients in relaxation techniques (e.g., deep breathing, concentration) to reduce stress and tension
- Providing leisure counseling
- Organizing, coordinating, and accompanying clients to special outings to make them aware of recreational resources
- Keeping other treatment-team members informed of client reaction, progress, or regression

Vocational Rehabilitation Counselor

The counselor is a master's-prepared professional who works with clients on job placement. Originally a part of hospital staff, the vocational counselor is now usually part of a public or private rehabilitation company. Vocational counselors are usually invited to participate as part of the treatment team by referral from a psychiatrist, social worker, insurance company, or employer. Duties of the vocational rehabilitation counselors include the following (Dept. of Labor, 1991):

- Interviewing and evaluating clients
- Conferring with medical and professional personnel to determine the type and degree of handicap, eligibility for rehabilitation services, and feasibility of vocational rehabilitation
- Determining a suitable job consistent with client desires and attitudes, as well as physical, mental, and emotional limitations
- Planning and arranging for the client to study or train for a job
- Assisting the client with personal adjustment throughout the program
- Promoting and developing job openings and placing qualified applicants in jobs
- Reporting back to the referring professional and/or team

Because vocational rehabilitation counselors are rarely part of direct hospital staff, they rely heavily on cooperation of in-house staff for pertinent information. This helps them make the best possible decisions for the client's job placement.

Art Therapist

The art therapist (AT) has a bachelor's degree in art therapy. As a member of the treatment team, the AT is involved in determining the psychological needs of the client. Duties of the art therapist include the following (Dept. of Labor, 1991):

- Devising art therapy programs to rehabilitate clients with mental illness
- Instructing individuals and groups in the use of various art materials
- Evaluating the client's art projections and recovery progress and sharing these findings with other team members

Music Therapist

The music therapist (MT) has a bachelor's degree in music therapy. The MT plans, organizes, and directs medically prescribed music therapy activities. As a member of the treatment team, the MT's duties include the following (Dept. of Labor, 1991):

- Using an individual assessment as the basis of planning
- Directing instrumental and vocal music activities designed to meet the client's psychological needs, capabilities, and interests; these might include solo or group singing, rhythmic and other creative music activities, music listening, and attending concerts
- Instructing clients individually or in groups in prescribed instrumental or vocal music
- Teaching projective techniques such as guided imagery, progressive relaxation, and awareness of conscious feelings
- Studying and analyzing client reactions to various experiences
- Reporting progress or regression to the treatment team

Other Professionals

At different points in time, other professionals become a part of the treatment team, either formally or informally. For example, a teacher or school counselor may become involved at a conference in behalf of a child. Crisis workers, public health nurses, and emergency room or intensive care unit nurses may also become involved. The team assists in identifying and coordinating governmental and community resources to address issues of medical care, housing, and legal and financial assistance. All nurses on all units need to apply mental health concepts as a part of total client care. By doing this, nurses are continuing members of the psychiatric team. ▲

Reality Check

Name three additional professionals outside of the hospital who may influence client care.

CASE STUDY REVISITED

So, what happened to Mr. D? A variety of scenarios are possible, depending on the acuteness and nature of his illness, diagnosis, financial considerations, available treatment and staff, and the all-important plan of care. Mr. D, for example, may have been hospitalized briefly until he was stabilized on medication. He may have been referred to an outpatient therapist for individual or group psychotherapy. Mr. D may have been scheduled to see a psychiatrist for regular medication evaluation. He may have seen a psychologist for testing or been referred to a vocational counselor for job evaluation.

Reality Check

List one possible scenario from the perspective of where you live and the treatment available. Clue: Ask clinical staff to help you identify community resources.

Approximately one third of the clients who become mentally ill will need a lifetime of supervision. The other two thirds recover and go on with their lives. To put this in perspective, it is helpful to think of people you know who experience a physical illness. Some recover fully; others need a lifetime of help. The team approach continues to be important in providing comprehensive care to clients with mental health problems.

SUMMARY

Nurses sometimes believe mistakenly that psychiatric nursing is limited to the psychiatric unit. Mental health nursing concepts are an integral part of all nursing, wherever it takes place. A person's status on the mental health–mental illness continuum varies according to stressors and the ability to cope with the stressors. The traditional psychiatric treatment includes the psychiatrist as the head of the team. In addition to the many professionals who are involved in direct care, the client is influenced by all the staff within the facility. The team members may or may not be employed by the hospital. Referral to professionals in the community is a common practice today.

Critical Thinking Activities

1. Write a reasonable story about someone who becomes mentally ill for the first time.
2. Discuss the client you identified in question 1 from the standpoint of the profession you represent. Be sure to consider the viewpoint of the client and the other treatment team members.
3. Develop a treatment plan that is acceptable to the client in your scenario. Write out this plan.
4. What is your greatest frustration in working with members of the team in this scenario?

Review Questions

Multiple Choice—Choose the best answer to each question.

1. What is meant by the mental health–mental illness continuum?
   a. The process that the client goes through to recover from mental illness
   b. A system of care from initiation of intervention to involvement in community care
   c. The psychiatric treatment team involving all professionals who deal with the client
   d. An imaginary line of functioning on which a client's status depends on stressors and the client's response to them
2. Who is considered the head of the psychiatric treatment team based on the medical model?
   a. Psychiatrist
   b. Clinical psychologist
   c. Psychiatric social worker
   d. Psychiatric clinical nurse specialist

3. What is the role of the LPN/LVN in a psychiatric setting?
   a. Assumes responsibility for intake assessment
   b. Has the same responsibilities as unlicensed personnel
   c. Works under the supervision of the RN
   d. Functions as an independent practitioner
4. What is the effect of reduced lengths of hospital stays on client care?
   a. Clients are stabilized and moved into less restrictive settings
   b. Clients respond with increased enthusiasm to shorter stays
   c. Visitors are discouraged during the acute stay period
   d. Clients show rapid improvement under pressure

5. What is the role of the psychiatric clinical nurse specialist?
   a. Provides psychological testing to assist in client diagnosis
   b. Works as a liaison with client, family members, and community services
   c. Assists the client in evaluating job skills and the need for training
   d. Plans for client care and provides client therapy as needed

References

US Department of Labor, Employment and Training Administration: Dictionary of Occupational Titles, 4th ed, vol 1. Washington, DC, 1991, pp 9, 49, 50, 51.

Foster R: Gentle Self Defense Workshop. Lawrence, Kan, Camelot Behavioral Systems, 1979.

Developing a Therapeutic Milieu

Outline

- Milieu, Milieu Therapy, and Therapeutic Milieu
- Developing a Therapeutic Milieu

- Therapeutic Settings
  Inpatient Treatment
  Outpatient Treatment
  Community Treatment

Key Terms

- JCAHO
- milieu

- milieu therapy
- therapeutic milieu

Objectives

Upon completing this chapter, the student will be able to:

1. Define *milieu, milieu therapy,* and *therapeutic milieu.*
2. Relate Gunderson's five components of a therapeutic milieu to Maslow's hierarchy of needs.
3. Give an example of each type of treatment setting:
   - inpatient
   - outpatient
   - community
4. Discuss the nurse's role in establishing and maintaining a therapeutic milieu.
5. Provide an example of how to establish continuity of care between inpatient, outpatient, and community treatment settings.

Changes in legislation, insurance, and state and local funding have affected mental health care services. The greatest impact has been to decrease the length and availability of services for clients with acute and chronic mental illness. New community facilities and services have emerged to fill the gap. In some areas, these have been well-planned changes with a focus on continuity of care. In other areas, new services have capitalized on the availability of "new pots of money" without including continuity of care as part of the plan. Changes in funding have become an excuse for providers who say "this is all we can do."

The nurses and other psychiatric treatment team members (see Chapter 5) who are meeting the challenge of providing continuity of care view their work as both skill and art. Skill involves learning mental health concepts, knowing their client's psychological and medical needs, and learning about available support systems. Teaching is a primary intervention that involves applying knowledge of behaviors and approaches. The art involves a change in mindset, and includes the following:

- Viewing possibilities in a new way
- Working together to apply knowledge of mental health concepts, client needs, support systems, and behaviors and interventions
- Considering one client at a time whenever a contact occurs

MILIEU, MILIEU THERAPY, AND THERAPEUTIC MILIEU

Milieu means "total environment." This type of environment occurs on any unit and may be therapeutic, nontherapeutic, or neutral (Bonner, 1995, p. 508). It is what happens as a result of staff-to-client, staff-to-staff, and client-to-client interactions. When managed skillfully, milieu becomes a major resource in assisting clients to function at their highest level. Most often, the responsibility to structure the environment in a therapeutic way belongs to the nurse. In most health facilities, the

nurse is the most consistent authority figure and therefore can influence the establishment and maintenance of a therapeutic environment, the consistency of care, and the promotion of open communication between psychiatric treatment team members and clients. The nurse can also serve as primary caregiver and consultant, group leader, and therapist.

Milieu therapy is therapy in which the total environment becomes a therapeutic mechanism. Specific approaches to clients may be assigned by the psychiatrist or psychiatric treatment team. Consistency in approach is intended to influence the client's behavior and thinking in a positive way. Milieu therapy focuses and builds on the client's strengths. Limits are set firmly and without agreeing or disagreeing with the client. Milieu therapy originated in the inpatient setting, and it continues to be a valuable intervention. Staff must, of necessity, be creative in providing consistency and follow-through as the client is moved within the system as a part of treatment.

Changes that started in the 1950s involved the client and staff in decision making on unit responsibilities and activities, using a scheduled community-meeting format. This **therapeutic milieu** focuses on participation of clients and staff at all levels. Therapeutic milieu also highlights the significance of therapeutic communication between the nurse and client as being more than a social exchange. The nurse has become recognized as an agent of change when focusing on goal-directed and client-centered conversation. Sometimes the term *therapeutic milieu* is used interchangeably with *milieu therapy.*

DEVELOPING A THERAPEUTIC MILIEU

J. G. Gunderson offered five key components for milieu therapy in 1978. They are containment, structure, support, validation, and involvement (Carson and Arnold, 1996, pp. 447–448). These components, along with physical environment, open communication, and links with support systems, are of value for both inpatient and outpatient settings. Each of Gunderson's five components is explained below.

Containment is assisting clients to be safe if they are unable to do so for themselves. This includes a variety of methods, such as a one-to-one relationship, seclusion, psychotherapeutic medications, time out, and restraints. Methods vary according to the client's level of need.

Structure involves providing an orderly environment with predictable daily patterns. It provides interaction at both individual and group levels. It can be either formal or informal. Clients are encouraged to choose activities according to their level of need. The structure is more rigid in inpatient settings and more flexible in community settings.

Support involves protection from self if the client is suicidal, homicidal, or self-mutilating. This may involve one-to-one supervision, supervision at 15-minute intervals, or monthly monitoring in the community as the client progresses. Decisions are based on the client's level of need.

Validation is a way of affirming individual worth. In a safe milieu, each client's symptoms are taken seriously. Clients are provided with information and experience on how to cope with symptoms and life events.

Involvement includes interacting with others according to the client's level of need. The purpose is to increase ego strength and modify personality by promoting interpersonal skills and interactions. Methods vary from basic one-to-one interaction to community meetings to outpatient therapies to volunteer work and employment.

Maslow's hierarchy of needs (Fig. 6–1) provides a way to link Gunderson's components of a therapeutic milieu to previous knowledge. Although clients may attain the highest level (self-actualization), only the four basic levels of needs are considered in the diagram. Usually, clients functioning on or above Maslow's third level (love and belongingness) are functioning in the community with minimum supervision. Recall that people frequently function on more than one level at a time. When they have mostly worked through a level successfully, they are ready to tackle the next level.

The physical environment is an important part of any therapeutic milieu. In 1994, the Joint Commission on Accreditation of Healthcare Organizations (**JCAHO**) published criteria for the therapeutic milieu for mental health, chemical dependency, and mental retardation/developmental disabilities services (see Appendix A).

THERAPEUTIC SETTINGS

Therapeutic milieu depends on the attitudes of members of the psychiatric treatment team. It begins during the first contact and involves the willingness of all staff to focus on the greatest good for the client. It involves cooperation instead of competition between staff.

Inpatient Treatment

Inpatient treatment is not limited to dedicated psychiatric facilities. Inpatient services and facilities for clients include those described below. Keep in mind that this is only a partial list.

Locked Inpatient Units

Locked inpatient units are generally useful for involuntary clients who are potentially dangerous to themselves or others. Locked inpatient units may also include clients experiencing an acute episode or crisis. In some hospitals, the admission/complete evaluation unit is also locked.

Emergency Room

Some clients and families use the emergency room for primary care, including treatment for acute episodes for some drug users and others who are mentally ill. Clients who rely on an emergency room for treatment may include those without financial means, a primary care physician, or a well-established plan of community care. Emergency room staff may be exposed to more aggressive behavior than in the past. Some emergency rooms maintain a psychiatric nurse on staff or on

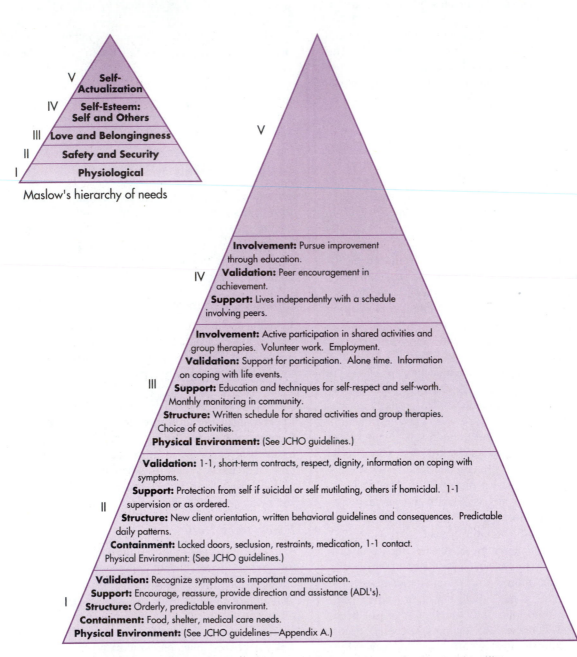

V   **Self-Actualization**
IV   **Self-Esteem: Self and Others**
III   **Love and Belongingness**
II   **Safety and Security**
I   **Physiological**

Maslow's hierarchy of needs

V

IV   **Involvement:** Pursue improvement through education.
Validation: Peer encouragement in achievement.
Support: Lives independently with a schedule involving peers.

III   **Involvement:** Active participation in shared activities and group therapies. Volunteer work. Employment.
Validation: Support for participation. Alone time. Information on coping with life events.
Support: Education and techniques for self-respect and self-worth. Monthly monitoring in community.
Structure: Written schedule for shared activities and group therapies. Choice of activities.
Physical Environment: (See JCHO guidelines.)

II   **Validation:** 1-1, short-term contracts, respect, dignity, information on coping with symptoms.
Support: Protection from self if suicidal or self mutilating, others if homicidal. 1-1 supervision or as ordered.
Structure: New client orientation, written behavioral guidelines and consequences. Predictable daily patterns.
Containment: Locked doors, seclusion, restraints, medication, 1-1 contact.
Physical Environment: (See JCHO guidelines.)

I   **Validation:** Recognize symptoms as important communication.
Support: Encourage, reassure, provide direction and assistance (ADL's).
Structure: Orderly, predictable environment.
Containment: Food, shelter, medical care needs.
Physical Environment: (See JCHO guidelines—Appendix A.)

FIG. 6–1   Using Maslow's model to apply the components of a therapeutic milieu.

call. Some hospitals provide emergency room staff with additional training in areas such as the following:

- Assessing clients with emotional problems
- Assessing suicide potential
- Crisis intervention
- Use of psychotherapeutic medications
- Gentle self-defense
- How and where to refer clients for additional treatment

The attitude of the staff sets the tone for a therapeutic or nontherapeutic client contact.

Psychiatric Unit in a General Hospital

Clients are admitted for stabilization of symptoms, crisis intervention (perhaps a transfer from the emergency room), developing and implementing a care plan, and planning for follow-up. The nurse is focused initially on the first step of the nursing process: collecting data (assessment). A plan of care is developed and implemented based on immediate client needs such as physical and safety/security needs. Actual psychotherapy does occur. Although the stay is generally brief, the essential steps for a therapeutic milieu are continued (if client is a transfer) or established (if client is a direct admission). Direct discharge or transfer to another facility may also occur. In case of a transfer, the client summary of care provides information to future caregivers.

Psychiatric Facility

The stabilized client who needs additional structured care may be transferred to a psychiatric facility. Court-committed clients are also sent to freestanding psychiatric facilities for treatment. Previously collected data and the initial care plan provide the treatment team with a starting point. Through planning, the team at the psychiatric facility can provide continuity and consistency in client care. Ideally, staff from various facilities get to know one another and work with each other as part of the team (see Chapter 5). Data is shared among facilities based on policy and client permission.

Outpatient Treatment

Motivated clients who are not considered dangerous to themselves or others are candidates for outpatient therapy. Some of the more common outpatient facilities are described below.

Outpatient Psychiatric Clinics

Outpatient psychiatric clinics often provide services such as crisis intervention, evaluation, and individual and group therapy. They may also monitor clients' use of psychotherapeutic medications. The therapeutic milieu is an important part of outpatient psychiatric clinics, and includes all the staff who see or speak with the client. The initial greeting a client receives influences his or her comfort level.

Day Treatment (Partial Hospitalization)

As the name implies, day treatment includes treatments and therapy sessions during the day. This arrangement is useful when the client's home situation is such that he or she can go home for the night. Many of these clients are in day treatment for a prolonged period. The relationships that develop between clients and staff are intended to influence the client's thinking and behavior therapeutically. Unfortunately, some excellent day treatment programs have failed because of lack of financial support by insurance companies and others.

Home Visits

Home nursing visits are based on the physician's orders and client consent. The purpose of these visits may include psychotherapy, monitoring medication, monitoring personal care, and so on. The number and frequency of visits is usually determined by client need and the presence of insurance or other means to pay for the visits. Box 6–1 describes the origin of one psychiatric home nursing program.

Community Treatment

Community treatment refers to facilities such as residential homes, half-way houses, and drop-in clinics for emergency care. For some clients, these facilities bridge the gap between hospitalization

BOX 6–1	Origin of Psychiatric Home Nursing

One of the original psychiatric nurse home-visiting programs was piloted in the 1960s by a psychiatric nurse as part of a multicounty outpatient mental health clinic outreach program. Referrals for follow-up were made primarily by the regional psychiatric center, which served half of the state. The psychiatric nurse visited the regional hospital on a regular basis (every 3 months) to become familiar with clients, staff, and plans of care. The psychiatric nurse also sat in on community treatment groups and individual and group therapies when permitted by clients. The social worker at the regional hospital contacted the nurse by phone to set up a client visit during a "pass" home. The purpose was to evaluate the client for discharge. If discharge followed, the client and nurse would set up a schedule for follow-up home visits. Initially, the visits were frequent. Medication evaluation in the home environment helped the nurse identify effects and side effects of the medication. Clinic visits with the psychiatrist for medication changes were scheduled on an as-needed basis. As the client adjusted to the discharge, the nurse lengthened the space between visits, and finally terminated the visits.

The pilot program lasted 3 years and was considered a success by clients and staff involved. Most of the clients involved in the program had repeated hospitalizations during the previous 10 years. Only one client was rehospitalized during the pilot program.

and home. For many others, they provide permanent residence. Staffing varies from a few hours each day to 24-hour coverage.

Overall, residential treatment focuses on activities of daily living. Clients live by house rules, and regular residence meetings deal with issues and resolve disputes. Some clients are able to work part-time in the community and attend activities with a mental health focus. In some states, residential treatment facilities fall under social services. A social worker is assigned to aid in establishing and maintaining a therapeutic climate.

Adult foster homes are another form of community treatment facility. These homes are useful for clients with chronic psychiatric problems that interfere with living more independently. These clients often need assistance and supervision in completing activities of daily living. Because this is a family setting, clients must be reasonably stable and able to accept direction.

Foster parents are screened carefully, usually by social services. The therapeutic milieu is ideally that of a family that supports positive behavior and progress and sets limits on unacceptable behavior. Foster parents are taught how to recognize specific behaviors, how to intervene effectively, and when to seek help.

Reality Check

What is the role of the treatment team in supporting adult foster care? Clue: Think of what is important in promoting consistency and continuity in a therapeutic milieu.

SUMMARY

Creating a therapeutic milieu is both a skill and an art. Shortened inpatient stays with transfers to other facilities and services provide a challenge to the nurse and other team members. Viewing changes through a "new lens" helps nurses see possibilities for continuity and consistency of care. This involves getting to know staff from other facilities and seeing them as an extension of total client services. The attitude of the entire staff affects the milieu of any facility. The milieu can be therapeutic, nontherapeutic, or neutral.

Therapeutic milieu involves Gunderson's five key components: containment, structure, support, validation, and involvement. Other components include physical environment, open communication, and involvement of support systems.

Therapeutic settings include inpatient, outpatient, and community facilities. The type of milieu attained in therapeutic settings begins during the first contact with the client.

Critical Thinking Activities

1. Using the client you were assigned this week as an example, identify how each of Gunderson's five components are used to create a therapeutic milieu for the client. Can you think of additional ways to enhance the client's milieu?
2. Describe the differences in the various milieus you have observed (e.g., colors, smells, sounds).

Review Questions

Multiple Choice—Choose the best answer to each question.

1. What is meant by *milieu?*
   a. Total environment, which can be neutral, therapeutic, or nontherapeutic
   b. Using environment as a therapeutic mechanism
   c. Physical environment and open communication
   d. Protection for self and others if suicidal or homicidal
2. How do Gunderson's components of support apply to the lowest level of Maslow's hierarchy of needs?
   a. Living independently with a schedule involving peers
   b. Protection from self if suicidal or self-mutilative
   c. Education and techniques for self-respect in community
   d. Encouragement, reassurance, direction, and assistance with activities of daily living

3. Why is the nurse's role in establishing and maintaining a therapeutic milieu significant?
   a. Clients are likely to trust the nurse's judgment
   b. Nurses are a consistent authority figure on the unit
   c. Nurses are taught to care as a part of their education
   d. Nurses cross boundaries between personal and professional relationships
4. What is the role of nurses who work in inpatient facilities in continuity of care?
   a. The nurse's roles are limited in scope to the facility in which the nurse is employed
   b. Other treatment team members have more expertise in dealing with continuity of care
   c. Because of confidentiality, nurses choose to limit involvement with community caregivers
   d. The nurses cooperate, not compete, with professionals from outpatient and community agencies
5. Which of the following is a major ingredient of therapeutic milieu?
   a. Level of psychosis
   b. Treatment team's attitude
   c. Length of hospitalization
   d. Changes in funding

References

Bonner JL: Milieu therapy. In: Antai-Otong D (ed): Psychiatric Nursing: Biological and Behavioral Concepts. Philadelphia, WB Saunders Co, 1995.

Carson VB, Arnold EN: Mental Health Nursing. Philadelphia, WB Saunders Co, 1996.

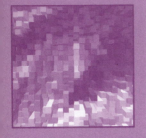

Communication and Mental Health

Outline

- **Understanding Self**
- **Communication Skills**
    - Verbal Communication
    - Nonverbal Communication
    - Active Listening
    - Communication Behaviors
- **Blocks to Effective Communication**
- **Communicating With Other Team Members**
    - Managing Conflict
    - Criticism
- **Communicating With the Client**

Key Terms

- active listening
- aggressive behavior
- assertiveness
- body language
- constructive criticism
- destructive criticism
- nonassertive behavior
- verbal communication

Objectives

Upon completing this chapter, the student will be able to:
1. Describe ways that one person's behavior can affect another's behavior.
2. Discuss the significance of nonverbal communication clues.
3. Describe the techniques of active listening.
4. Explain the differences among assertiveness, aggressiveness, and nonassertiveness.
5. List four blocks to effective communication.
6. List five ways of managing conflict.
7. Describe the difference between constructive and destructive criticism.
8. Identify six aspects of caring.

Communication is a complex process involving many skills. It involves the exchange of attitudes, feelings, and ideas, requiring a full understanding of the other person's position. These messages include the following:

- What you *actually* say
- What you *think* you said
- What the other person actually *hears*
- What the other person *thinks* he hears
- What the other person *says*
- What you *think* the other person said

Source Unknown

UNDERSTANDING SELF

Everything that irritates us about others can lead us to an understanding of ourselves.

Carl Jung

The effectiveness of any communication depends on understanding one's self. It is important for the nurse to get in touch with his or her own feelings and to understand the reactions to those feelings. Most significant of all, the nurse should be aware of how his or her feelings influence other people's behavior.

Reality Check

Before you went to work or school, you had an argument with your spouse, significant other, or child. How might this incident at home affect your behavior and feelings during the day? What effect might lack of sleep have on your behavior and feelings the following day?

Self-awareness is gained by evaluating reactions to specific situations. One person's behavior can affect the whole environment positively or negatively.

COMMUNICATION SKILLS

Communicating an intended message accurately involves more than just using and understanding words. Both verbal and nonverbal communication depend on context and other clues for their meaning.

Verbal Communication

Verbal communication includes the oral and written word. For effective verbal communication to occur, the receiver needs to understand the sender's messages. In addition to understanding the actual words, the receiver must interpret other clues that may have subtle meanings. For example, the tone of voice used affects how the message is received.

It is always helpful to ask the receiver what he or she heard. Clients with certain mental illnesses cannot process abstract ideas and concepts. Therefore the nurse needs to send messages that contain concrete ideas; for example, "exercises will be at 10:00 AM."

Nonverbal Communication

Nonverbal communication is often referred to as **body language.** It includes facial expressions, eye contact, postures, gestures, touch, personal space, and appearance. Sometimes the nonverbal message contradicts the verbal message, which is the source of the well-known cliché, "Actions speak louder than words." For example, when asked how she feels, a person responds, "Just fine." However, her facial expression is drawn and contradicts her verbal message, so she is sending a mixed message.

The following are common forms of nonverbal communication.

- Eye contact is helpful in establishing a relationship. It tells the receiver that you are paying attention. The eyes send many messages: joy, sorrow, happiness, and anger. It is important to be aware of cultural differences when using eye contact. In some cultures, people drop their gaze as a sign of courtesy or politeness.
- Body posture, gestures, and personal space are other nonverbal ways of communicating. When working with clients, the nurse needs to have a relaxed posture at eye level. Hands folded across the chest or clenched fists can communicate an

authoritarian attitude. Touch can be reassuring or threatening (see Chapter 27). Personal space indicates territory, and the nurse needs to respect the client's special boundaries.

- Many messages are conveyed by a person's appearance. An individual's feelings are sometimes reflected by his or her grooming and personal hygiene. Extremely depressed persons frequently lack the interest and energy to take care of themselves.

Reality Check

What is a better greeting than "How are you?" to someone whose body language communicates discomfort and sadness?

Active Listening

In **active listening,** the nurse tries to understand what the client is feeling or what his or her verbal or nonverbal message means. The nurse then *rephrases* this feeling or meaning using the nurse's own words. The nurse *reflects* it back for the client's clarification. The nurse and the client both need to determine whether the return message or feedback was clear. The nurse does not send a new message, such as an evaluation, opinion, advice, logic, or analysis. Instead, the nurse feeds back only what he or she understands the client's message to mean—nothing more, and nothing less. The nurse's goal in active listening is always to keep the door open. For example:

Client to nurse: "I don't know whether to go out and look for a job or get a place to live."

Good response by nurse: "It sounds as though you are having difficulty in deciding which is more important to do first, look for a job or a place to live!" (open response—rephrasing and reflecting)

Poor response by nurse: "If I were you, I would certainly get a job before looking for a place to live." (closed response—nurse's opinion)

Active listening can be risky. This is why understanding one's self is so important. The poem "Listen" in Box 7–1 conveys clearly what active listening is.

BOX 7–1	Listen

When I ask you to listen to me
and you start giving advice,
you have not done what I asked.

When I ask you to listen to me
and you begin to tell me why I shouldn't feel
that way, you are trampling on my feelings.

When I ask you to listen to me
and you feel you have to do something to solve
my problem, you have failed me, strange as
that may seem.

Listen! All I asked was that you listen,
not talk or do—just hear me.
Advice is cheap: 25 cents will get you both Dear
Abby and Billy Graham in the same newspaper.
And I can do for myself; I'm not helpless;
Maybe discouraged and faltering, but not helpless.

When you do something for me that I can and need
to do for myself, you contribute to my fear and
weakness.

But, when you accept as a simple fact that I do feel
what I feel, no matter how irrational, then I can
quit trying to convince you and can get about the
business of understanding what's behind this irrational feeling.
And when that's clear, the answers are obvious and
I don't need advice.
Irrational feelings make sense when we understand
what's behind them.

Perhaps that's why prayer works, sometimes, for
some people because God is mute, and He doesn't
give advice or try to fix things. "They" just listen and let you work it out for yourself.

So, please listen and just hear me. And, if you want
to talk, wait a minute for your turn; and I'll listen
to you.

Anonymous

Communication Behaviors

A person's attitude toward others and method of communicating are related. Nurses can help clients most when they are assertive without being aggressive. This honest, direct approach also helps nurses get along with co-workers. Table 7–1 shows assertive, aggressive, and nonassertive responses.

Assertiveness

Assertiveness includes expressing one's feelings, needs, and ideas without violating the rights of others. The following three rules are helpful in being assertive:

1. Own your own feelings. Do not blame others for the way you feel.
   Effective: "I feel angry because you continue to be late for work without notifying the unit."
   Ineffective: "You make me mad because you're always late."
2. Make your feelings known by being direct. Begin your statements with "I."
   Effective: "I find your habit of referring to the client by diagnosis very annoying."

Ineffective: "You shouldn't call the client by his diagnosis."

3. Be sure that your nonverbal communication matches your verbal message.
   Effective: "I want you to take your hand off my leg" (said in a serious tone of voice and with a serious expression).
   Ineffective: "You shouldn't put your hand there" (accompanied by a smile).

Using "I" messages is a way of owning one's problem. They are clear and honest statements of fact. "You" messages are focused on the receiver. They can make the receiver feel defensive. "You" statements can be made fairly easily because such statements do not involve revelation of self. "I" messages, which are focused on the person who is sending the message, are harder to make but are usually more effective.

Table 7–1	Assertive, Aggressive, and Nonassertive Responses		
Functions	**Assertive Response**	**Aggressive Response**	**Nonassertive Response**
Problem	Faces problem	Attacks person instead of dealing with problem	Avoids problem
Dealing with others	Lets others know what he or she thinks and feels and gains their respect	Takes advantage of others; others fear and avoid him or her	Allows manipulation by others
Rights	Claims rights	Considers own rights superior to those of others	Gives up rights
Decisions	Makes own choices	Chooses activities for others	Lets others choose activities
Goals	Expresses goals and works toward them	Works toward goals	Hopes goals will be accomplished
Confidence	Possesses self-confidence	Exhibits demanding, hostile, egotistical behavior	Lacks confidence
Thinking and behavior	Thinks and behaves in ways that coincide with his or her rights; often able to achieve goals	Behaves verbally or physically in a way that expresses own rights, but at the expense of others	Develops a pattern of self-denial; feels inadequate to express thoughts and feelings; unable to achieve goals

Data from Alberti R, Emmons M: Your Perfect Right: A Guide to Assertive Living, 6th ed. San Luis Obispo, Calif, Impact Publishers, 1990.

Aggressiveness

Outspoken people are often automatically considered assertive when, in reality, their lack of consideration for others is aggressive. **Aggressive behavior** violates the rights of others. It is an attack on the person rather than on the person's behavior. The purpose of aggressive behavior is to dominate or put the other person down. The behavior is self-defeating because it quickly distances the person from others.

Nonassertiveness

Another self-defeating behavior is nonassertiveness. **Nonassertive behavior** is dishonest. The nonassertive person does not express his or her own feelings, and needs are infringed on deliberately or accidentally. By not taking the risk and not being honest, the person typically feels hurt, misunderstood, and often angry.

Reality Check

What would be an assertive response to a co-worker who keeps giving you all of her work to do?

BLOCKS TO EFFECTIVE COMMUNICATION

Growth is fostered through effective communication. This is done by allowing people to solve their own problems. A person is thwarted in his or her effort to own and solve problems if the nurse sends a message such as the following:

- An order or command: "You must . . ."; "You have to . . ."
- A threat: "If you don't, then . . ."
- A moral obligation: "It is your duty to . . ."
- A lecture or judgment: "The facts are . . ."
- A criticism or judgment: "You are not thinking straight"
- An evaluation or compliment: "You've done a good job." If the person has a problem with what he has done, a general compliment does not help him or her deal with it.

- Advice or suggestions: "If I were you, I would . . ."
- An interpretation: "Your problem is that . . ."
- Reassurance: "Everything will be all right."
- A probing question: "Why would you do something like that?"

The most ineffective question is one that begins with "why," because it is usually followed by the word "because." The "why-because" interaction leads into an endless exchange of futile "why" questions and fruitless "because" answers. In such an exchange, those involved move further away from a solution to the problem. Nurses can use "what" questions much more effectively. For example, the nurse might ask, "What seems to be going on inside you?"

COMMUNICATING WITH OTHER TEAM MEMBERS

The mental health setting uses a multidisciplinary team. This team is composed of various health professionals who work together with the client to develop a plan of care. An essential ingredient of a successful relationship with team members is *respect*. A respectful attitude translates into behaviors that make people feel important and worthwhile (Balzer-Riley, 1996, p. 76). Team members are then acknowledged for their contributions to client care. (See Chapter 5 for more information about team members.)

Reality Check

What are factors that prevent you from being as respectful as you would like?

Managing Conflict

The members of the health care team come from diverse backgrounds. They may differ on goals for the client and on the best way of meeting those goals. Conflict can result when there is disagreement. Conflict is normal and, if handled well, can have very creative results (Wisinski, 1993, p. 1). In managing differences, one can gain awareness of certain characteristics that lead to change, such as how one communicates with another. Especially important is to realize how one's behavior affects the behavior of others.

Table 7–2 compares five options for managing conflict. These methods are effective in the nurse's personal life, as well as his or her professional life.

Reality Check

What conflicts have you handled satisfactorily?

Criticism

If criticism is handled correctly, conflict can usually be avoided. Criticism can be constructive or destructive.

- **Constructive criticism** focuses on the issue, not the person. It consists of two parts: the criticism itself and helpful suggestions for improvement (Wisinski, 1993, p. 40).
- **Destructive criticism** attacks a person rather than an issue, and is an aggressive "put-down." The individual being criticized may become defensive and angry. "Sometimes people like to criticize for the sake of starting a conflict" (Wisinski, 1993, p. 44).

COMMUNICATING WITH THE CLIENT

The therapeutic relationship between nurse and client is a helping relationship focused on the needs of the client. It is the basic tool used by the nurse in working with people who are mentally ill. The essence of this helping or interpersonal relationship is *caring*.

Figure 7–1 depicts some of the aspects of caring that are most meaningful in working with people who are mentally ill. The most important tool used to develop a helpful relationship is one's self. Having a knowledge of one's own needs, strengths, and limitations is vital. Such knowledge prevents the nurse from imposing his or her value system on the client. Having gained this knowledge of self, the nurse must then try to understand the client's needs, strengths, and limitations. This information helps the nurse know how to respond to a client and what would be beneficial to the client's growth (Mayeroff, 1990, p. 19).

These basic understandings prepare the nurse for the involvement in and commitment to the treatment of clients in psychiatric and nursing home settings. The nurse uses problem-solving skills to assist the client in exploring alternatives for dealing with the client's situation. The nurse might say, "Look, you have five ways of dealing with this problem. This is the one you took. It didn't work out for you. So let's look at the other four." In this way, the nurse becomes involved in the client's growth process and makes a commitment to caring. This extension of oneself into the unknown, with no certainty of the outcome, is risky, but this is a type of risk that nurses must take. The poem in Box 7–2 makes several good points about the need to take risks.

To take a risk, one must have trust in one's self, have confidence in one's ability to make decisions. If the nurse is continually preoccupied with whether his or her judgment was correct, the nurse becomes indifferent to the client's needs. Once self-trust is established, the nurse can begin to trust others, including clients. This involves letting go and allowing the person to grow in his or her own way (Mayeroff, 1990, p. 27).

The nurse needs other characteristics as well to communicate with clients effectively, including the following:

- *Courage:* It takes courage to trust the other person to grow, allowing that person to make mistakes and learn from them. The direction the nurse must take is sometimes unclear, but knowledge of self and past experience provide guidelines. The nurse's role is to guide the client through the problem-solving process at the client's level of functioning.
- *Honesty:* The word *honesty* means being genuine in caring for another. This aspect of caring is

Table 7–2 Five Methods for Managing Conflict

	Competition (Win–Lose)	Accommodation (Lose–Win)	Avoidance (Lose–Lose, when used nonassertively)	Compromise (Win–Lose/Win–Lose)	Collaboration (Win–Win)
Definition	Attempt at complete dominance Power-based approach	Willing to yield one's position to another person	Unwillingness to cooperate, denial problem exists	Involves negotiation, tradeoffs, and flexibility; get some, also give some Need to set limits on how much one is willing to give away	Involves identifying areas of agreements and differences, evaluating alternatives, and finding solutions that have support of those involved Need atmosphere of trust
Appropriate uses	In emergency when quick, decisive action is needed When unpopular changes need to be made	Can assertively choose to be nonassertive Important to preserve relationship rather than argue Issue is more important to the other person Need to encourage others to express their point of view	When additional time is needed When negative impact of situation may be too damaging to both parties involved	Reach agreement when both sides have equal power Maintain personal objectives while preserving the relationship	Preserving important objectives that can't be compromised Allows creativeness through willingness to explore alternatives together May help solve unresolved problems that may have hindered a relationship

Data from Wisinski J: Resolving Conflicts on the Job. New York, Amacon, a division of American Management Association, 1993, pp 17–21.

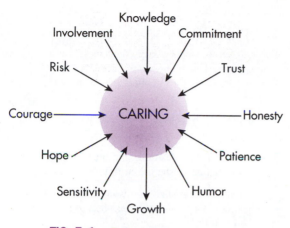

FIG. 7–1   Bauer's aspects of caring.

very significant in working with people who are mentally ill. Because the interpersonal relationship is the therapeutic tool used to facilitate growth in the client, this interaction must "ring true" (Mayeroff, 1990, p. 26). In other words, the nurse's feelings and actions must coincide. Otherwise, the client will not grow as a result of the interaction with the nurse.

- *Hope:* Hope is an important aspect of caring for people with mental illness because of the long-term nature of most illnesses. It is hoped that the client will grow through the nurse's caring. Hope denotes activity, not passivity; it is "an expression of a present alive with possibilities" (Mayeroff, 1990, p. 33). These possibilities consist of very small, realistic, measurable, and attainable goals. Perhaps a goal is simply to get the client to look the nurse in the eye for a second. This tiny goal triggers another goal and thus keeps the fire going. It is like building a house; each small brick is added to another until the house is completed.

- *Patience:* It takes patience to work with people who are mentally ill, and patience involves time and space. Being patient means allowing the other person to grow in his or her own time and way. Patience also includes tolerance for another's confusion and floundering, and the realization that such behaviors also characterize growth. Most importantly, the people who

care are patient with themselves, giving themselves a chance to learn—and a chance to care (Mayeroff, 1990, p. 24).

- *Sensitivity:* Nurses can be sensitive to the needs of the client by letting the client know that they are trying to understand how the client feels. Such sensitivity communicates the message of caring. A sensitivity to the humor inherent in a situation, while having insight enough to understand the serious nature of it, also communicates caring.

- *Humor:* Laughter can sometimes help people gain a better perspective on a problem. This includes being able to laugh at one's self. Humor can be used to facilitate trust in a relationship and establish a bond between people. In reaching out to a client, the nurse shares with the client one of life's essential ingredients: caring. Through caring, the client has the opportunity to experience success and grow.

Box 7–3 lists specific examples of ways to reach out to clients.

BOX 7–2	**Risk Taking Is Free**

To laugh is to risk appearing the fool
To weep is to risk appearing sentimental
To reach out for another is to risk involvement
To expose feeling is to risk exposing your true self
To place your ideas, your dreams before the crowd
   is to risk their loss
To love is to risk not being loved in return
To live is to risk dying
To hope is to risk despair
To try is to risk failure,
But risk must be taken, because the greatest hazard
   in life is to risk nothing.
The person who risks nothing, does nothing, has
   nothing, and is nothing,
He may avoid suffering and sorrow, but he simply
   cannot learn, feel, change, grow, love, live.
Chained by his certitudes, he is a slave, He has
   forfeited freedom.
Only a person who risks . . . is free.

Author Unknown

BOX 7–3	Specific Examples of Reaching Out

Listening to what the client has to say

Example: "You were telling me, Joe, about what you did on the weekend. I would like to hear more about your activities."

Allowing the client to *own* his or her problem

Example:
Client: "What should I do first, take a bath or clean my room?"
Nurse: "It sounds as though you are having difficulty in making a decision."

Being consistent in the care that is given the client

Example: Follow the care plan that has been developed for the client. If you don't agree with the plan of care, do not change it on your own; instead, request a care plan meeting.

Setting limits for the client's benefit, not for the nurse's convenience

Example: "I want you to go to your room. I'll be there in 5 minutes to see if you've gained control of your behavior."

Focusing on the client's strengths and giving credit for positive behavior—simple decisions may be major decisions for the client and represent a strength.

Example: "I'm pleased to see that you made the decision to wash your hair today."

Trusting the client's desire to find more positive behaviors than he or she has at this time

Example: "I know that you want to control your behavior, but right now you need some help from me."

Promising only what you can deliver; determining in advance whether you can follow through on a promise

Example: "I've checked my schedule, and I'll be here tomorrow, so I will take you to the store then."

Holding the client responsible for his or her behavior

Example: "When you made the decision to run away, you knew what the consequences of your actions would be."

SUMMARY

Communication promotes growth. An essential part of the communication process is to understand one's self. Other important factors in transmitting a message include the following:

- Verbal communication: the spoken and written word and tone of voice
- Nonverbal communication: facial expressions, eye contact, body posture, gestures, touch, use of personal space, and appearance.
- Active listening: trying to understand what the sender's message means.
- Assertiveness: expressing feelings, needs, and ideas without violating the rights of others. Aggressiveness and nonassertiveness are both self-defeating behaviors. Aggressiveness puts others down; nonassertiveness is dishonest.

- Blocks to effective communication prevent a person from owning and solving his or her problems.
- Communicating with other team members involves showing respect for each member of the team; it is important to acknowledge each member for his or her contribution to client care.
- Conflict can be managed through competition, accommodation, avoidance, compromise, or collaboration.
- Constructive criticism focuses on the issue, whereas destructive criticism focuses on the person.

The nurse uses the interpersonal relationship as a tool in working with someone who has a mental illness. The essence of this relationship is caring. Caring involves trust, honesty, patience, sensitivity, hope, courage, risk, humor, involvement, and commitment.

Critical Thinking Activities

1. How would you use assertive skills in returning a faulty item to a department store? For example, you bought a shirt. When you took it home, you found a misweave in it.
2. How would you refuse to do a favor for someone because you do not want to do it?
3. Apply the method of collaboration in managing your work schedule, which conflicts with previous plans that you have made.

Review Questions

Multiple Choice—Choose the best answer to each question.

1. Nonverbal communication includes
   a. tone of voice.
   b. facial expressions.
   c. written word.
   d. oral message.
2. Assertiveness
   a. violates the rights of others.
   b. allows manipulation by others.
   c. considers the rights of others.
   d. chooses activities for others.
3. A win–win method of managing conflict is
   a. accommodation.
   b. compromise.
   c. competition.
   d. collaboration.
4. An example of a block to effective communication is
   a. rephrasing a client's feelings.
   b. giving advice or a suggestion to a client.
   c. reflecting a client's communication.
   d. keeping the response open for the client.
5. An example of reaching out to a client is
   a. solving a problem for the client.
   b. focusing on the client's weaknesses.
   c. listening to what the client has to say.
   d. setting limits that are convenient for you.

References

Balzer-Riley JW: Communications in Nursing, 3rd ed. St. Louis, Mosby, 1996.

Mayeroff M: On Caring. New York, Harper Perennial, 1990.

Wisinski J: Resolving Conflicts on the Job. New York, Amacon, a division of American Management Association, 1993.

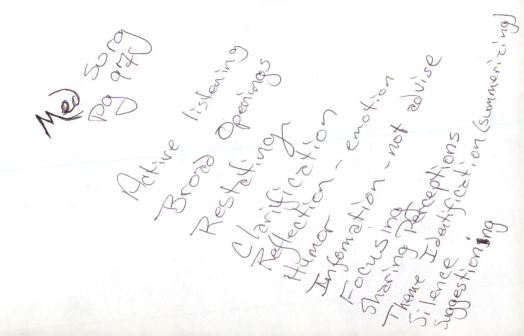

Data Collection

Outline

- **Ways of Thinking**
    - **Influence by Attitude**
    - **Influence by Capability**
- **Prioritizing Critical Thinking**
    - **Integrating Into Practice**
- **Case Study**
    - **Assumption**
    - **Result of Critical Thinking**
    - **Conclusion**

- **NCLEX-PN Guidelines: The Nursing Process**
    - **Data Collection**
    - **Planning**
    - **Implementation**
    - **Evaluation**
    - **Interdisciplinary Plans**

Key Terms

- **data collection**
- **evaluation**
- **hallucination**
- **illusion**

- **implementation**
- **interdisciplinary care plans**
- **planning**

Objectives

Upon completing this chapter, the student will be able to:

1. Define three noncritical thinking styles.
2. Explain in his or her own words what is meant by *critical thinking*.
3. List three components of critical thinking.
4. Discuss how one's attitude influences critical thinking.
5. Explain why prioritizing personal needs assists in developing self-respect.
6. Describe how self-respect and respectfulness toward clients are related.
7. Apply the nursing process in developing a daily plan of care for a client (form included in Instructor's Manual).
8. Discuss the nursing role in interdisciplinary client care plans in a psychiatric facility.

Data collection begins with the initial client contact. The nurse uses four of the five basic senses: sight, hearing, smell, and touch. He or she focuses on the physical aspect plus the client's thinking, feeling, and behavior. Critical thinking skills, observation, and therapeutic communication become the nurse's greatest assets. If it sounds challenging, it is!

Reality Check

Think about how you think. Which statements apply to you?

_____ My thinking has purpose.
_____ My thinking is goal-directed.
_____ I have an organized method of thinking.
_____ I question what I do not understand.
_____ I continually question: What does this mean? Is this useful? Is it fact?
_____ I question the reliability of sources and information available.
_____ I keep an open mind.
_____ My judgments are based on fact.

Count the number of statements that apply to you.

3 = need help!
5 = on your way!
8 = keep up the good work!

WAYS OF THINKING

There are many forms of thinking. Most people indulge in all of them at times. Listed below are examples.

- *Random thoughts:* Thoughts that come and go, as though there were a television set in the head and someone is sitting there surfing the channels. Incomplete thoughts (scenes) come and go with no particular purpose (goal).
- *Ruminative thinking:* The same situation is replayed in the mind over and over again, like an "instant replay" shown over and over on a sports program. Unless there is deliberate intervention, the person will not reach the goal of finding out what else happened during the game.

- *All-or-none thinking:* This kind of thinking is sometimes referred to as "black or white thinking with no grays in between." Additional data will not be considered by this person because the person has already made up his or her mind.
- *Problem-oriented thinking (problem-solving):* The person focuses on a particular problem to find a solution to it. When the goal is reached, no further attention is given to the situation until another problem arises.
- *Critical thinking:* A synonym for critical thinking is "reasoning." The following statement applies to nursing (Alfaro-LeFevre, 1995, p. 9):

Unlike the "mindless" thinking we do when going about our daily routines, critical thinking is purposeful, goal-directed thinking that aims to make judgments based on evidence (fact), rather than conjecture (guesswork). Based on principles of science and the scientific method, (e.g., maintaining a questioning attitude, following an organized approach to discovery, and making sure information is reliable), critical thinking requires developing strategies that maximize human potential (e.g., "the powerful influence of personal perceptions, values, and beliefs").

The nurse must accept that there may be more than one way to achieve a desired outcome.

Influence by Attitude

Critical thinking is an advanced way of thinking. It is a problem-solving method and more. Critical thinking is used to resolve problems and to find ways to improve even when no problem exists.

Attitude influences thinking. During data collection, it makes a critical difference in whether a problem is recognized, missed, or ignored.

Reality Check

Take time to collect data on your attitude.

_____ I am aware of the limitations of my knowledge.
_____ I am aware that my biases may influence my decisions.
_____ I try to be fair.
_____ I am interested in understanding other people's thoughts and feelings.

_____ I check to find out if my statements are clear.

_____ I can be influenced by other people's conclusions, if based on facts.

_____ I question other people's sources of information.

_____ I acknowledge that what I have been thinking can be incorrect.

_____ I question the availability of additional alternatives.

_____ I listen to my intuition and compare it to my reasoning.

_____ I am aware that perfect solutions are not always available.

_____ I am willing to work as a team member.

_____ I attempt to anticipate problems before they occur.

_____ I am continually looking for ways to improve my thinking.

Count the number of items that apply to you.

1–11 = request help

12–14 = good start

The purpose of the reality check on attitude is to gain a baseline for where you are now. The items left unchecked clue you into areas to work on. _Mark this page in your text._ Check from time to time to see how you are doing.

Influence by Capability

Critical thinking is paramount at all levels of nursing. If someone tells an LPN/LVN that it is not necessary to learn to think critically, the LPN/LVN should ask, "What is the implication of this statement? Why should I be less than I can be?"

Reality Check

Which of the following statements reflect your capability to think critically?

_____ I know what my style of thinking is.

_____ I know what my attitude is and how it affects thinking critically.

_____ I am willing to put the work into thinking critically.

_____ I work to understand others before expecting them to understand me.

_____ I am willing to listen and consider ideas and views different from my own.

_____ I use the problem-solving steps to work out problems.

_____ I am able to read with understanding. I can express my thoughts clearly in writing.

_____ I acknowledge the limits of my knowledge and skills.

_____ I have examined my values and can separate them from values held by others.

Count the number of items that apply to you. What areas do you need to focus on? If the unchecked skills include reading with understanding and writing, check out your school learning skills center for possible help.

PRIORITIZING CRITICAL THINKING

Have you ever wondered why, when there are self-help books and courses and workshops available, people continue to stay in the same rut? In _The 7 Habits of Highly Effective People_, Stephen Covey tells the story of a man who has been sawing a tree trunk for hours with a dull saw. The man becomes very tired. When someone suggests to him that he would probably do better if he sharpened his saw, he answered "I don't have time" and kept on sawing. (Covey, 1989, p. 287.)

Reality Check

Apply the lesson to your experience. Think about a time you were on a hospital or nursing home unit when the unit was filled with clients with acute illness and the nursing ratio was low. Did anyone on the staff (including you) engage in similar thinking and "keep on sawing"? What could have been done differently?

Prioritizing personal needs helps people develop self-respect. A starting point is to use critical thinking to determine where and how to prioritize. There is an obvious extension into a nurse's professional life. As the nurse develops self-respect, it becomes easier to use critical thinking to prioritize client care needs. Self-respect also enables the nurse to extend genuine respectfulness to clients and co-workers.

Integrating Into Practice

Nurses need to learn and apply critical thinking skills before they become an integral part of their thinking. They should continue to look for flaws in their thinking and permit errors to become a source of learning. Saying "I'll find out"—and then making the effort to find out—should become a standard procedure. Nurses must keep asking *why, what else,* and *what if* questions.

Reality Check

Work at figuring out what questions your instructor (or client) will ask. Classroom discussions suddenly become far more interesting when you think about the information. Do you understand the information in your own words? Does the information fit with what you already know? If not, what is the difference? What facts underlie the information being discussed? How will you be able to apply what you have just learned?

CASE STUDY

A 56-year-old man requests admission to the psychiatric hospital because he thinks he is mentally ill. He is a single man who has been a farmer all of his life. During the past few months, he has developed symptoms that have become increasingly incapacitating. His memory is playing tricks on him. He has a hard time concentrating and staying focused on his farm tasks. He finds himself staying away from other people. The hallucinations frighten him the most.

The initial intake interview shows signs of psychosis. The admission occurs during the change of shifts. The afternoon RN charge nurse plans to do the physical assessment as soon as report is over.

Assumption

Based on the data available at this point, what is probably going on with this new client? (Remember that this assumption is not based on fact.)

The afternoon charge nurse always walks through the unit with the daytime charge nurse so he can actually see all the clients at the beginning of the shift. This gives him a quick visual overview and an opportunity to ask last-minute questions. The newly admitted client is pointed out to him. To his experienced eye, the client seems psychotic. However, there is something about the way the client walks that raises doubts.

Result of Critical Thinking

■ The charge nurse recognizes an inconsistency. He recalls that there are physical illnesses (e.g., some neurological illnesses) that include mental symptoms. The charge nurse recognizes that doing the physical assessment is a priority and proceeds to do so.

The charge nurse begins to verify the accuracy of the data that accompanies the client and the information obtained during the admission interview.

■ The nurse changes the usual order of the physical assessment. He begins with the neurological portion. The client definitely has problems with his gait. He also has other disturbing signs that seem abnormal.

The nurse begins to identify some abnormal neurological signs using an organized approach. (The approach remains organized even though the sequence of the physical assessment has been changed.)

■ As the charge nurse is doing the assessment, he also asks the client questions about the onset of his signs and symptoms. The client identifies a sensation of pressure in his head, headaches that come and go, confused thinking, memory changes, difficulty doing his work, and visual changes. When asked to explain, he says he "sees things" off and on.

The nurse begins to compare the data he obtained from the assessment with the client's story.

■ Upon completing the assessment, the nurse contacts the doctor on call and reviews the data. The doctor arrives quickly, does a physical exam, and orders an immediate transfer to the neurological unit of the general hospital.

The nurse has identified patterns from the data that arrived with the client and his physical assessment. The doctor on call is his immediate next resource. The doctor's physical examination supports the possibility of neurological involvement.

■ The client is seen by a neurologist, who orders immediate testing to rule out a brain lesion. The client is diagnosed as having an astrocytoma.

Valid conclusions are drawn, with supporting evidence from the neurological examination and tests.

Conclusion

Surgery relieved the psychological symptoms, the sensation of pressure in the head, and the headaches. Initially after surgery, the client needed rehabilitation to walk again. The client returned to his home to put his affairs in order. Because the condition is so advanced, the neurosurgeon predicted that the client will live an additional 6 to 9 months. As a side note, it was interesting to learn that the client was relieved to find out "I'm not crazy after all." This thought overshadowed concerns about his prognosis.

▲

Reality Check

1. Which issue, shared by most cultures, contributed to the client's positive reaction to learning that he was not mentally ill?
2. Which characteristics of noncritical thinking helped delay the client's diagnosis and treatment?

NCLEX-PN GUIDELINES: THE NURSING PROCESS

Nursing process provides nurses with a methodical way of doing the work of nursing. It provides the steps for nursing care. Critical thinking is necessary to use the steps effectively. Currently, unlicensed persons do all the tasks and skills that practical nurses do. It is the nursing process that separates practical nurses from unlicensed persons. The nursing process is as practical in the care of clients with emotional illness as it is in all other areas of nursing.

The four steps of the nursing process for the practical nurse are presented in the 1995 National Council Licensure Examination for Practical Nurses (NCLEX-PN) test plan. The steps are:

1. *Data collection:* The nurse participates in establishing a data base.
2. *Planning:* The nurse plans to set goals to meet client's needs and designs strategies to achieve these goals.
3. *Implementation:* The nurse initiates and completes actions necessary to accomplish the defined goals.
4. *Evaluation:* The nurse participates in determining the extent to which goals have been achieved and interventions have been successful.

The RN has the major responsibility for all five steps of the nursing process. The LPN/LVN works from the established nursing diagnosis written by the RN (the other step of the nursing process). LPN/LVNs take an active part in the four steps of the nursing process listed above according to their skill level. They assist in data collection (assessment), planning, implementation, and evaluation of care. They turn the RN's nursing diagnosis into *nursing problems.* In this way, LPN/LVNs clearly understand the nature of the problem.

Data Collection

Practical/vocational nurses learn to assess (collect data about) the client and the environment during every encounter with a client. **Data collection,** or assessment, includes checking vital signs, checking therapeutic responses to medications and treatment, assessing for symptoms of health problems, and so on. For the LPN/LVN, data collection also involves observing for symptoms of health problems. This includes identifying client perceptions, thoughts, feelings, and behavior. Suggestions for identifying a client's spiritual and cultural needs are offered in Chapter 3.

RNs are taught assessment skills, including performance of the client interview and physical assessment of all body systems, as part of their basic education. Practical/vocational nurses may *choose* to learn complex assessment skills as part of a postgraduate course.

Initial Data Collection

The initial assessment guide in Table 8–1 may be used as it is or adapted to the needs of the psychiatric facility. It is a method of rapidly obtaining information on the client's immediate physical and mental state at the time of admission.

An expanded vocabulary is required in the area of psychiatric nursing. Table 8–2 provides definitions to help new LPN/LVNs get started. The list is based on the "mental assessment" portion of the initial assessment guide. New LPN/LVNs should learn the definitions used to describe the signs and symptoms of mental illness. They should look for examples of the signs and symptoms during client care.

Refer to Table 8–1, the initial assessment guide. The physical assessment is based on those areas discussed in the section on physical care (see Chapter 26). The mental assessment zeroes in on presenting problems, many of which are addressed in Chapters 9 to 20. The initial assessment lends itself to the development of a problem list and initial care plan. In this way, nurses and other staff will almost immediately have guidelines for supporting the client in a united manner. Problems to be addressed immediately will depend on the RN's judgment call.

The initial assessment guide is divided into sections so that it can be completed by nurses with different levels of expertise. Sections I and II, which can be completed by the LPN/LVN, include basic personal information and observations regarding the client's immediate physical condition. Sections III, IV, V, and VI call for judgment based on the RN's evaluation of what he or she sees and hears during the interview. Regional variations may apply. Specific observations leading to the conclusions on the initial assessment form are recorded in the client's admission note. Recognizing subtle clues is of major importance.

A Respectful Approach

The nurse approaches the client in a friendly way, introducing himself or herself by name and title and extending a hand for a handshake. Should the client refuse the hand, the nurse simply withdraws the hand without comment. This provides the nurse with information about the client's social interaction with others. The nurse makes a statement such as, "I am going to ask you some questions in order to understand better how we can help you during your stay at the (name facility). Please answer to the best of your ability. However, if any of the questions make you feel uncomfortable or you do not wish to answer, please feel free to say so." The nurse's primary objective is to observe and listen, rather than talk. The nurse should look for nonverbal clues that may contradict the verbal data. Such nonverbal clues often tell more about the client's thoughts and feelings than the words do.

Using the Initial Assessment Guide

The following outline provides an explanation of the initial assessment guide. It discusses the rationale behind various entries and suggests appropriate ways to conduct each part of the assessment.

I. Personal Data
   A. Although this information may already have been recorded on another form, asking the questions again is a way to test memory and orientation. The nurse may use a lead statement such as "I know that you have been asked these questions before, but I want to make sure I have the correct information." The nurse may also

Table 8–1	Initial Assessment Guide

I. Personal Data

A. Name _____   Admission Date _____

   Address _____   Phone _____

   _____   Social Security # _____

   Birth Date _____   Age _____ Sex _____

   Spiritual Belief _____   Race/Culture _____

   Education _____   Occupation _____

   Next of Kin _____   Phone _____

   Address _____   Prefer to Be Called _____

B. Type of Admission (Voluntary/Involuntary) _____

   Reason for admission (in quotes) _____

   Presenting Problem _____

   Diagnosis _____

C. Allergies _____

II. Physical Assessment

A.

	Good	Fair	Poor	Comments
Nutrition				
Elimination				
Sleep and Rest				
Grooming				
Special Problems				

B. B/P _____ T _____ P _____ R _____ Height _____ Weight _____

C. Coping Habits: Smoking Amt. _____ Alcohol Amt. _____

   Prescribed drugs and dosage _____

   Nonprescribed drugs and dosage _____

   What triggers coping habits? _____

III. Mental Assessment (Check those that apply.)

A. Perceptions:

   _____ Hallucinations

   _____ Illusions

B. Thoughts:

   _____ Bizarre thinking or speech   _____ Irrelevancy

   _____ Confusion   _____ Lack of insight

   _____ Defective judgment   _____ Poor concentration

   _____ Delirium   _____ Pressure of speech

   _____ Delusions   _____ Slowed speech

   _____ Disorientation   _____ Somatic concern

   _____ Flight of ideas   _____ Suicidal thoughts

   _____ Grandiosity   _____ Suspiciousness

   _____ Homicidal ideas   _____ Thought disorganization

   _____ Ideas of persecution   _____ Unusual thoughts

   _____ Incoherence

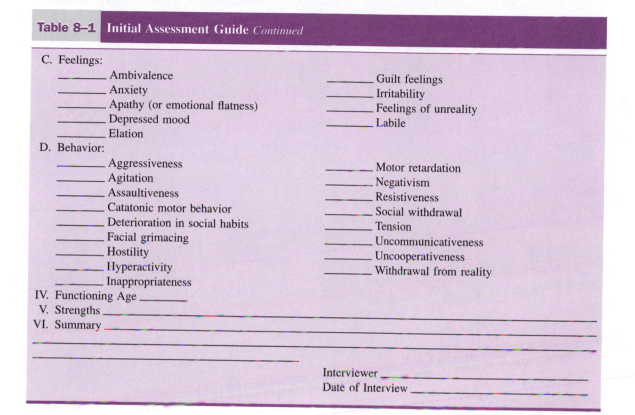

Table 8–1   Initial Assessment Guide *Continued*

C. Feelings:

_____ Ambivalence   _____ Guilt feelings
_____ Anxiety   _____ Irritability
_____ Apathy (or emotional flatness) _____ Feelings of unreality
_____ Depressed mood   _____ Labile
_____ Elation

D. Behavior:

_____ Aggressiveness   _____ Motor retardation
_____ Agitation   _____ Negativism
_____ Assaultiveness   _____ Resistiveness
_____ Catatonic motor behavior   _____ Social withdrawal
_____ Deterioration in social habits _____ Tension
_____ Facial grimacing   _____ Uncommunicativeness
_____ Hostility   _____ Uncooperativeness
_____ Hyperactivity   _____ Withdrawal from reality
_____ Inappropriateness

IV. Functioning Age _____
V. Strengths _____
VI. Summary _____

_____
_____
_____

Interviewer _____
Date of Interview _____

---

have the client spell his or her name. This shows the nurse's interest and also tests memory, as do questions about social security number, address, town, and phone number. A "fill-in-the-blank" statement is an easy way to deal with the date: "Let's see, today's date is ____." Information about spiritual and religious needs indicates whether this is a source of strength and whether the client is involved in a delusional system. Occupation and education offer information about potential strengths and the level of instruction that will be needed to present new information to the client. "Is there a family member you turn to when you need help? Do we have your permission to contact him (her) during your stay here at (name the facil-

ity)?" These questions deal with legal issues of client rights. They may also indicate another source of strength in the client's life.

B. The client's understanding of his or her reason for admission is often best obtained by offering an open-ended statement such as, "Obviously, something was not going right for you at home or at work. Tell me about that."

C. Be especially attentive to allergies. Add a word of explanation if needed.

II. Physical Assessment

A. At this point, basic, overall information is needed, rather than systems information. Is the client in immediate physical distress? Look carefully at all the areas that show— hair, skin, eyes, lips, nails, and personal

Table 8–2   Definitions: Perceptions, Thoughts, Feelings, and Behaviors

Word	Definition
A. Perceptions	
Hallucination	A false sensory perception that is real to the person and cannot changed by logic.
Illusion	A misperception of reality; for example, perceiving lint as a bug.
B. Thoughts	
Bizarre thinking or speech	Thoughts expressed or speech do not make sense.
Confusion	A disturbance in consciousness. Person feels distracted or anxious. Cannot respond correctly to stimuli. May experience altered awareness of person, time, place, or events.
Defective judgment	Inability to make wise decisions.
Delirium	Change of consciousness that occurs over a short period.
Delusions	Belief or idea that is not supported by logic.
Disorientation	Inability to identify person, place, or time.
Flight of ideas	Rapid switches from topic to topic. Ideas are complete as far as they go but are not completed. A common characteristic in manic episodes.
Grandiosity	Unrealistic idea about one's own significance or identity.
Homicidal ideas	Thoughts of killing someone or has attempted to do so or has a strong desire to do so.
Ideas of persecution	Beliefs, not based on reality, that someone is "out to get" the person.
Incoherence	Loose, rambling, disjointed sentences.
Irrelevancy	Not applicable or pertinent.
Lack of insight	Not understanding the reason for one's own thoughts, feelings or actions.
Poor concentration	Lack of ability to focus on the issue at hand.
Pressure of speech	More talkativeness than usual with pressure to keep talking.
Slowed speech	Normal tempo of speech decreased.
Somatic concern	Preoccupation with physical illness or bodily functions, such as constipation.
Suicidal thoughts	Person has thoughts of killing self, has attempted to do so, or has a strong desire to do so.
Suspiciousness	Distrusts thoughts, motives, or behaviors of others.
Thought disorganization	Absence of orderly organization of thinking pattern. Thinking is different from the thinking accepted by society as normal.
Unusual thoughts	Delusions are an example of unusual thought content.
C. Feelings	
Ambivalence	Existence of opposing emotions, such as love and hate for someone at the same time.
Anxiety	A feeling of impending doom accompanied by physical symptoms such as diaphoresis, tachycardia, tremors, gastrointestinal symptoms.
Apathy	Emotional flatness.
Depressed mood	Feelings of sadness, disappointment, and despair. Sense of no hope.
Elation	Emotional excitement marked by acceleration in mental and bodily activity.
Guilt feelings	A subjective feeling of self-blame regarding life experiences.
Irritability	A state of excitement and undue sensitivity.
Feelings of unreality	A sense of not existing or of being in a place other than where you are. Also called *depersonalization*.
Labile	Sudden variations in mood, such as explosive temper outbursts and sudden crying.

Table 8–2	Definitions: Perceptions, Thoughts, Feelings, and Behaviors *Continued*

Word	Definition
D. Behavior	
Aggressiveness	Attacking behavior that occurs in response to frustration and hostile feelings.
Agitation	Disturbed, upset, excited. Apparent in face or movement of involved person.
Assaultiveness	Inflicting verbal or physical harm.
Catatonic motor behavior	Reduction of spontaneous movement or excited motor activity, apparently purposeless and not influenced by external stimuli.
Deterioration in social habits	Change in habits to what is considered less than the social norm.
Facial grimacing	Contortions of the face caused by physical or psychogenic reasons. May also be drug induced.
Hostility	Antagonistic or angry feelings directed toward another.
Hyperactivity	Above-normal increase in activity. May be caused by physical or psychological causes.
Inappropriateness	Unacceptable according to social norms.
Motor retardation	Abnormal decrease in motor activity. Common during severe depression. May also be caused by drugs or physical illness.
Negativism	Resistance in doing what is expected or desirable.
Resistiveness	Opposition to what is suggested or desired by others.
Social withdrawal	Seclusiveness.
Tension	Internal discomfort, uneasiness.
Uncommunicativeness	Because persons communicate nonverbally, this term is limited to lack of verbal communication.
Uncooperativeness	An unwillingness or lack of ability to work together.
Withdrawal from reality	Functioning within one's own created reality that is not a part of the real world.

hygiene. Ask simple, to-the-point questions about change: what the change is, when it began, and what the client thinks is the reason for the change. Remember to ask if the client is on any special diet, either prescribed by the doctor or of his or her own choice.

B. The nurse should check the client's vital signs, height, and weight in accordance with institutional policy.

C. Find out about the client's coping habits, including how much and how often. For example, ask about the client's use of drugs, including prescription, over-the-counter, and street drugs. List each drug name and amount the client takes. Ask what the client does when he or she is anxious, angry, sad, or happy. The LPN/LVN assists in data collection (assessment) on a daily basis. Consequently, it is important for the LPN/LVN to know how the RN conducts the initial mental assessment.

III. Mental Assessment

A. The RN must find out how the client perceives (gathers and interprets) sensory data. A question such as "Do you ever see or hear things that other people cannot see or hear?" may or may not be answered. Again, observation will offer the RN and LPN/LVN additional information.

B. Information about the client's thoughts can be obtained while eliciting personal data from the client.

Reality Check

Why is it critical for the first nurse (LPN/LVN) to share these data with the second nurse (RN) before continuing the interview?

The LPN/LVN may have noted bizarre thoughts or speech, confusion, defective judgment, disorientation, flight of ideas, grandiosity, incoherence, lack of insight, poor concentration, pressure of speech, slowed speech, somatic (bodily) concerns, and thought disorganization. Pointed, simple questions will help the RN obtain the rest of the data. For example, "Have you ever had thoughts of hurting yourself? Tell me about it. When was this? Tell me about your plan. What stopped you? Do you still have these feelings?" A similar set of questions is needed in regard to hurting others. "Do you have any enemies who are trying to hurt you? Tell me about it." The client's response provides information about suspiciousness and ideas of persecution. "Do you have thoughts that others do not understand? Tell me about them." Throughout the session, observing and listening more than speaking, as well as asking additional questions for clarification, are essential.

C. The client's feelings are often easier to evaluate because of the accompanying nonverbal information. "Has anything unpleasant happened to you lately that has changed the way you feel? Tell me about it. Do you sometimes feed sad? Is this more than usual? When did this begin? Do you sometimes feel that you are not really here? Tell me about it. Do you blame yourself for bad things that happen to you or others? Tell me about it." Questions are based on the need for more information and clarification.

D. The RN looks at the client's nonverbal behavior—his or her mannerisms; how he or she sits, stands, walks, and gestures—as well as the accompanying expression for clues that support observations. Suggested questions include "Tell me about things that make you angry. What do you do? Does it help?"

IV. Functioning Age

This is based on an assessment of the overall level of functioning. A review of the growth and development chart in Chapter 2 will be helpful in determining the client's functioning age. As you will recall, it is impossible for the client to comply past the actual functioning age. The nurse and the client will feel less frustrated if this is considered in the client's care plan.

V. Strengths

The client's strengths have already been identified, but additional questions may give clues to other strengths. For example, "What helps you feel better when you get upset? What activities help you relax? Who helps you most when you get upset?" Remember that ability to care for oneself physically is a strength.

After completing the questions on the assessment, the nurse always thanks the client for his or her cooperation. A handshake is offered at the end of each session. The notes recorded will provide an excellent admission note on the client.

VI. Summary

The nurse completes the summary after thanking the client and moving away. The summary identifies what is going on now for the client and the specific characteristics of the present behavior.

Planning

In the **planning** phase, practical/vocational nurses take the nursing diagnosis and state it as a problem, set goals, list interventions, and then list data that has been collected. This process seems to reverse that of the RN, but remember that practical nurses do not have primary responsibility for assessment and rely on the RN for the nursing diagnosis. To understand the nursing diagnosis, the practical nurse states it in objective, specific terms. Problem statements for sensory-perceptual needs are italicized in each of the following examples.

- Perception (illusion): *misperceives that staff members are family members*
- Thoughts (suicidal thoughts): *strong feelings of wanting to kill self*
- Feelings (guilt): *blames self for death of son although there is no basis for this feeling*
- Behavior (motor retardation): *sits motionless on bed for hours*

Goal Setting (Outcomes)

According to Hill and Howlett (1997, p. 31):

Specific goals (outcomes) provide direction for individualizing the care of the client. To be useful, outcomes must be client-centered and be determined by the client and nurse together. Goals must be (1) measurable, (2) realistic, and (3) time referenced. The focus of the outcome is on the client, not the nurse. A goal is thought of as "The client will do this, or that." To get the best results, an outcome must be set for each priority problem or need. Reverse the problem and state it in positive terms.

The example in Table 8–3 shows how a client's care plan might look.

Identifying the Interventions

Interventions focus on the "related to (R/T)" portion of the nursing diagnosis. They tell all nursing personnel who, what, where, when, and how much. Anyone should be able to carry out the interventions. The nurse should check them: Are they objective and specific? Table 8–4 lists client goals and associated nursing interventions that might be identified.

We have focused on developing an individualized care plan. Standardized care plans, based on research of the best possible options for a nursing diagnosis (nursing problem), are available. Standardized plans can be individualized by crossing out interventions that do not apply and adding others.

Implementation

Implementation is the process of initiating the nursing intervention. Remember those client strengths? It is time to build on them to initiate the plan. The nurse should consider the following questions:

- What is the client's level of education?
- Are spiritual beliefs a source of support?
- Is there a family, friend, or spiritual support system?
- Does the client have cultural values and beliefs that support treatment?
- What is the client's occupation and/or level of responsibility?
- Is the responsibility for the interventions within the LPN/LVN role?

These, of course, are only some of the questions that may be addressed.

Documenting and charting the client's response to care, therapy, or teaching is part of the LPN/LVN's expected role in implementation. Regardless of the method of documentation, whether on

Table 8–3	Typical Client Care Plan	
Nursing Diagnosis	**Nursing Problems**	**Client Goals**
Risk of self-inflicted violence related to (R/T) painful feelings of guilt about son's death evidenced by actual suicide attempt	Attempted suicide with medication and alcohol; blames self for death of teenage son; no actual basis	1. The client will remain safe during hospitalization. 2. The client will talk about painful feelings of guilt regarding son's death by [insert date].

Table 8–4	Nursing Interventions for Specific Client Goals

Client Goal	(Sample) Nursing Interventions
1. The client will remain safe during hospitalization.	The nurse will maintain suicide precautions according to unit policy.
2. The client will talk about painful feelings of guilt regarding son's death by [insert date].	The nurse will encourage talking in detail about painful feelings of guilt regarding teenage son's death.

computer or traditional nurse's notes, accuracy is vital. The nurse should use his or her care plan as the basis for recording. Using the initial assessment guidelines form helps ensure that important information is not omitted. Reporting without notes may look smart. It is not.

Evaluation

Evaluation begins as soon as client contact occurs.

(Hill and Howlett, 1997, p. 33).

The nurse evaluates the effectiveness of interventions, rather than nursing behavior. **Evaluation** is a way of measuring client progress toward meeting goals. Continual data collection (assessment) helps make daily evaluation part of the natural flow of good nursing care. The nurse should think of the client's goal and look at daily data collection. If the data collection list is complete, evaluation becomes the result of the data collection.

Table 8–5 shows the result of the entire nursing process for the LPN/LVN. Note that if a goal cannot be evaluated, it probably was not written accurately.

Interdisciplinary Plans

Have you noticed that regardless of changes within a facility, a physician continues to do the work of physicians in a prescribed way? So do the social worker, the psychologist, and other psychiatric team members. Nursing process is a way to do the work of nursing in an organized way. It tells the team members where they are going and lets them know if they get there.

Interdisciplinary care plans are plans developed with an interdisciplinary focus reflecting the specific interventions for each profession (e.g., nurse, social worker, occupational therapist, recre-

Table 8–5	LPN/LVN Nursing Process Results Showing Evaluations

Data Collection (Assessment List)	Nursing Problem	Goals	Evaluation
Suicide precautions: (#1) 1–1 continuously in client's room: no exceptions	Attempted suicide with medication and alcohol. Blames self for death of teenage son; no actual basis.	1. The client will remain safe during hospitalization. 2. Client's verbalization of guilt associated with son's death will decrease by [insert actual date].	Precautions maintained first 2 days: D/C [insert date]. Able to talk for short periods about son's death without sobbing and blaming self.

ational therapist). A separate plan for each profession is considered repetitious. These plans work well in short-term and long-term psychiatric settings. Staff from a variety of professions are involved with the clients. The focus is on client problems, rather than nursing diagnosis. The language used in the plan must be common to all professions represented.

Regardless of the type of plan used in the facility, nursing interventions must be dated and signed. Plans are documented as well and remain part of the client's permanent record. Interdisciplinary care plans generally have the following characteristics:

- The client's medical diagnosis is generally used (instead of nursing diagnosis).
- Observations (data collected) about the client are shared: each profession represented shares observations based on the team member's area of expertise.
- A problem list is developed and prioritized. The client's statement of problem(s) leading to admission is considered. Life-saving/physiological needs are supported by all professions as immediate priorities.
- A shared plan is created, identifying specific and shared responsibilities of all professions represented.
- The plan is discussed with the client (when possible) or client representative. After all, these are client goals based on client needs: the team plays a supportive role during implementation of the plan.
- Documentation of progress is usually on a common form or computer to allow easy access for all team members involved with the client.
- Evaluation is ongoing, with periodic in-depth evaluations on agreed-upon dates. Interventions are deleted, added, and changed as needed.

The interdisciplinary plan is begun during admission. It can be used to provide continuity of care should transfer to another facility be needed. Planning meetings are effective when critical thinking is practiced by all professions involved.

Nurses have excellent guidelines for this: the nursing process (modified).

SUMMARY

Data collection (assessment) is ongoing in the care of the client with emotional problems. All nurses participate in gathering data. The nursing process provides a methodical way to do the work of nursing. The LPN/LVN assists the RN in completing the steps of the process. The 1995 NCLEX-PN provides guidelines for the LPN/LVN role. Postgraduate courses provide knowledge and skill beyond the graduate level.

Critical thinking is a necessary part of nursing. Nursing decisions must not be based on assumptions. They must be based on accurate data, critical thinking, and sound conclusions. A nurse's critical thinking skill varies and is enhanced by experience and knowledge. As the nurse develops critical thinking skills, it becomes less threatening to prioritize and modify client care according to conditions. Nursing has unique contributions and necessary skills to contribute to collecting data, planning, implementing, and evaluating client care. This applies to the nurse's involvement in developing individualized plans, modifying standardized plans, or working as a part of an interdisciplinary team.

An expanded vocabulary is required in the area of psychiatric nursing. The nurse should learn the definitions used to describe the signs and symptoms of mental illness because some commonly used words have a different meaning in this context. It is possible to participate as a member of the team when you know the language. This becomes the basis for data collection.

Critical Thinking Activities

1. Maintain a journal for one day using Table 8–6 as a basis.
2. Make a list of all the ways you collected data on the client to whom you were last assigned. To whom, and how, did you report these data?

Table 8–6	Sample Journal Entries	
What the client said	**My thoughts about what the client said**	**Alternative ways of thinking about what the client said**
Example: "You are the only one who has ever understood me; will you keep a secret if I tell you?"	*Example:* I must be really special. Maybe I can really help him/her.	*Example:* Be careful. Secrets are out! They could cause harm to the client or others. Perhaps I'm being manipulated and need some guidance.

Review Questions

Multiple Choice—Choose the best answer to each question.

1. According to the 1995 NCLEX-PN, what is the role of the LPN/LVN in nursing process?
   a. Assist the RN in data collection, planning, implementation, and evaluation
   b. Write nursing diagnosis in the absence of an RN on duty
   c. Assume responsibility for planning who will be assigned care
   d. Be responsible for client intake evaluations
2. How does critical thinking differ from problem solving?
   a. Incomplete thoughts come and go with no particular goal
   b. Additional data will not be considered because the decision is final
   c. A particular problem is focused on with the purpose of finding a solution
   d. Critical thinking finds ways to improve even when no problem exists
3. Why does the critical thinking concept encourage you to look for flaws in your thinking?
   a. It aims to make judgments based on evidence
   b. It builds self-esteem by "toughening you up"
   c. It assists you in prioritizing your thoughts
   d. It improves your attitude toward others who make errors
4. Why is it important to learn the meaning of words used to describe signs and symptoms of psychiatric illness?
   a. It increases your level of sophistication
   b. It helps you pass the NCLEX-PN
   c. It assists you during data collection
   d. It demonstrates your ability to learn
5. When does data collection begin?
   a. After the client's level of anxiety is reduced
   b. When you have mastered critical thinking
   c. During the psychiatrist's initial client interview
   d. At the time of initial client contact

References

Alfaro-LeFevre R: Critical Thinking in Nursing: A Practical Approach. Philadelphia, WB Saunders Co, 1995.

Covey SR: The 7 Habits of Highly Effective People. New York, Simon and Schuster, 1989.

Hill SS, Howlett HA: Success in Practical Nursing: Personal and Vocational Issues, 3rd ed. Philadelphia, WB Saunders Co, 1997.

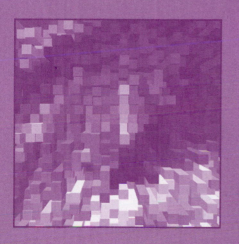

Nursing Responses to Specific Disorders

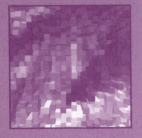

Disorders of Infancy, Childhood, and Adolescence

Outline

Key Terms

- attention-deficit/hyperactivity disorder (ADHD)
- autism
- bipolar disorder
- conduct disorders
- Down syndrome
- dysthymia
- encopresis
- enuresis
- environmental deprivation
- learning disabilities
- normalization
- pica
- regression
- rumination
- schizophrenia
- tic
- Tourette's syndrome

Objectives

Upon completing this chapter, the student will be able to:
1. Define *mental retardation*.
2. Discuss the need to respond to both mental retardation and mental disorders when they occur in the same person.
3. List five general nursing interventions that are helpful in accomplishing Objective 2.
4. Provide a brief explanation of each of the following disorders.
   - attention deficit/hyperactivity disorder
   - conduct disorder
   - Tourette's disorder
   - autistic disorder
5. Explain the differences among pica, rumination, and feeding disorders of infancy or early childhood.
6. Differentiate between encopresis and enuresis.
7. Describe the following adult-like childhood and adolescent disorders.
   - mood disorders
   - anxiety disorders
   - schizophrenia
8. Discuss possible treatments available for infant, childhood, and adolescent disorders.
9. List three statistics regarding the effect of infant, childhood, and adolescent mental disorders.
10. Discuss general nursing interventions for dealing with children and adolescents.

Exciting things are happening in the area of childhood disorders. Extensive studies and research projects involving children have resulted in a new classification of mental health disorders in infancy and early childhood up to age 4. To provide the most complete information possible before planning an appropriate intervention program, all areas relevant to the child's functioning are considered. These areas include the following (Greenspan and Wieder, 1997, p. 584):

- Presenting symptoms and behaviors
- Developmental history: past and current affective, language, cognitive, motor, sensory, family, and interactive functioning
- Family functioning and cultural and community patterns
- Parents as individuals
- Caregiver–infant (child) relationship and interactive patterns
- The infant's constitutional and maturational characteristics

- The family's psychosocial and medical history, the history of the pregnancy and delivery, and current environmental conditions and stressors

Childhood disorders, when not treated successfully, can lead to more severe problems, both during childhood and when the client becomes an adult. The effects of mental disorders that occur during childhood or adolescence are described in Box 9–1.

MENTAL RETARDATION AND MENTAL DISORDERS

Information about mental retardation is included in this chapter because people with mental retardation are at risk for mental disorders of all types. To understand the special needs of the client who is mentally retarded and also emotionally disturbed, a review of some information about mental retardation is important. The definition of mental retarda-

BOX 9–1	The Impact of Childhood Mental Disorders

The statistics shown below are a partial list of those distributed by the National Mental Health Association regarding childhood and adolescent mental disorders.

- 9% to 13% of children in the United States between the ages of 9 and 17 have a serious emotional disturbance. These youths have severe emotional or behavioral problems that significantly interfere with their ability to function socially, academically, and emotionally.
- Anxiety disorders affect an estimated 8 to 10 out of every 100 young people at any given time.[*] 48% of students with serious emotional disorders drop out of grades 9 to 12, and 20% are arrested at least once before leaving school.[†]
- Each year, almost 5000 young people ages 15 to 24 commit suicide.[‡]
- Approximately 60% of teenagers in juvenile detention have behavioral, mental, or emotional disorders.[§]
- Untreated children's needs may grow into more severe problems in adulthood, such as mental illness, homelessness, and incarceration.
- The majority of children with mental disturbances (an estimated two thirds) do not have access to services.

[*]Source: Center for Mental Health Services.
[†]Source: U.S. Department of Education.
[‡]Source: National Mental Health Association Teen Suicide Sheet Index.
[§]Source: U.S. Department of Justice.
From National Mental Health Association: The Impact of Childhood Mental Disorders. Fact Sheet, 1997.

tion offered by the American Association on Mental Retardation (1992) is as follows:

Mental retardation refers to substantial limitations in present functioning. It is characterized by significantly subaverage functioning, existing concurrently with related limitations in two or more of the following applicable adaptive skill areas: communication, self-care, home living, social skills, community use, self-direction, health and safety, functional academics, leisure, and work. Mental retardation manifests by age 18.

The cutoff for IQ for mental retardation is 70 to 75, and people are classified according to the support they need in defined areas of functioning. The American Psychiatric Association's *Diagnostic and Statistical Manual of Mental Disorders, fourth edition* (DSM-IV) definition of retardation is essentially the same, except that the categories of severity are included as follows:

Degree of mental retardation	Approximate IQ range
Mild	50–55 to approximately 70
Moderate	35–40 to approximately 50–55
Severe	20–25 to approximately 35–40
Profound	below 20–25
Undiagnosed	

It is important to understand that the term *mental retardation* is not a medical diagnosis. It does not imply a single cause, course of illness, or prognosis. It defines the person's current intellectual and skill level. This can change with growth in the skill level—a focus of many programs involving people with mental retardation.

Medical Conditions

An important factor in diagnosis is the medical condition that is responsible for the below-normal intellectual level and subsequent functioning. The mental retardation may be part of a syndrome such as **Down syndrome,** the result of an extra chromosome (21) attached to another chromosome (14). The most common and most preventable cause of mental retardation is fetal alcohol syndrome (FAS). FAS is related to maternal alcohol consumption, especially during the first trimester of pregnancy. Malnutrition during infancy and childhood continues to produce mental retardation throughout the world.

Phenylketonuria (PKU) is another problem associated with mental retardation. Fortunately, this issue has been resolved. Infants are now tested for PKU at birth. If affected, the child is begun on a special phenylketone-free diet to prevent retardation.

Other abnormalities are often associated with mental retardation. For example, neurological abnormalities such as seizures or problems with vision and hearing may be present. Mental disorders such as infantile autism and attention deficit disorders with hyperactivity are three to four times greater in children with mental retardation. Behavioral manifestations may occur, such as temper tantrums, aggressiveness, or irritability.

For unknown reasons, more males than females develop mental retardation. The total population with mental retardation is about 1%.

Psychosocial Factors

Psychosocial factors such as the lack of social and intellectual stimulation have also been shown to cause mental retardation. Dr. Marlin Roll's Pine School project at the University of Iowa (late 1950s to early 1960s) identified a number of these children. Dr. Roll showed that appropriate environmental stimulation could help many of them function at a higher level. Stimulation included being read to, talked to, and listened to; drawing; coloring; puzzles; exposure to music; structured and unstructured activities; and so on. If the stimulation was begun early enough during the preschool stage of development (before a series of academic failures), many children functioned within a normal intelligence range. This kind of retardation is often referred to as **environmental deprivation.**

It is important to note that people with mental retardation may experience the same mental disorders as those in the general population. Sometimes it is difficult to determine the basis for the signs and symptoms. For example, limited verbal skills and lack of understanding of questions may result in misinformation. It is also important to discover whether behavioral acting out is an attempt to get needs met. For example, the person with mental retardation may be wanting attention and personal contact. In a busy environment, quiet people may be left to themselves, whereas those who act out receive staff attention. Remember that the mentally retarded person relates to people as a child does to an adult (regardless of chronological age). The focus is on self: getting personal needs met. Interrupting or getting close may be a way of communicating and not necessarily acting out. Limited intellectual ability equals limited social ability.

Nursing Interventions for the Client With Mental Retardation and Mental Disorders

Adequate intervention in the care of the client with mental retardation and a mental disorder is actually dual intervention. It should be based on both the degree of assistance needed with adaptation skills (functions that help a person make it through the day) and the specific pattern(s) of behavior related to the mental disorder.

General Interventions

Some general interventions for children and adolescents who have mental retardation and mental disorders include the following:

- Use adult materials. It is important to know what the client's intellectual level is, meet the client at this level, and proceed at an appropriate pace.
- Avoid using baby talk. Deliver messages simply using the first person. Establish an adult-to-adult relationship, rather than a parent-to-child relationship.
- Avoid mentioning events, days, or weeks too far ahead of time. Because of his or her intellectual limitations, the client with mental retardation sometimes has difficulty understanding time spans.
- Avoid providing attention one day and then withdrawing it the next simply because you do not want to give it. Sometimes a client with mental retardation craves attention and will resort to any means to get it. In seeking the attention, the client may become very possessive. The client needs to receive attention within limits and with a consistent approach. Inconsistency is easily misinterpreted and encourages acting out.
- Always set limits with the client's best interest in mind. Expect the client to behave rationally for his or her level. Keep in mind that clients require more support during mild stress, and

prevalence of other disorders may create behavioral changes.

- Make promises only if they can be granted. Clients may interpret ambiguous answers to mean "yes."

Clients with mental retardation are often anxious to please. It is important that they not be taken advantage of to do the nurse's errands or other tasks unless this is a planned part of care. Tolerance, a consistent approach, understanding, and supervision are most important, with emphasis on normalization. **Normalization** means making available conditions of everyday life that resemble, as closely as possible, the usual patterns of living for the general population. The more competent a person becomes, the more acceptable the distortions. This means that the more skilled the person becomes at following through on activities of daily living on a consistent basis, the less likely it is that differences will stand out.

CASE STUDY

NURSING CARE PLAN

The following case study demonstrates a nursing care plan for an adolescent client with mental retardation and mental disorders. This example describes possible interventions that are appropriate for the 18-year-old client in the case study. Young children may require different interventions, depending on their level of development.

History and Data Collection

Sally DeQuaine—age 18 years, 5 feet tall, 180 pounds—is mentally retarded and emotionally disturbed. She sits in a rocking chair most of the day holding a baby doll. Her speech is difficult to understand and consists mainly of single words. She is very aware of her surroundings and beams when a staff member spends some time with her. However, when she is out of her chair, she wanders into other clients' rooms and goes through their

dresser drawers. She must be reminded repeatedly to comb her hair, brush her teeth, and take a bath. However, she is willing to have staff do these things for her.

As a result of data collection, the LPN/LVN decides that Sally's strengths include an awareness of her surroundings and a pleasant disposition. She can care for herself with encouragement. The nurse then uses the RN's nursing diagnoses to detail nursing problems appropriate for intervention at the LPN/LVN level. Table 9–1 shows the result.

Goals, Interventions, Rationale, and Evaluation

Based on the nursing problems she has defined, the nurse proceeds to list appropriate goals and interventions, along with a rationale for each. These are shown in Table 9–2. With the RN's approval, she implements the interventions.

▲

Table 9–1	Nursing Diagnoses and Nursing Problems for Case Study
Nursing Diagnosis	**Nursing Problem**
1. Knowledge deficit R/T cognitive impairment	1. Sally's knowledge is limited by mental retardation
2. Self care deficit/ bathing and hygiene R/T inability to recognize personal needs	2. Sally needs specific reminders to take a bath or brush her hair or teeth
3. Impaired adjustment R/T inability to recognize inappropriate behavior characterized by wandering into other clients' rooms and going through dresser drawers	3. Sally goes into other clients' rooms and through their dresser drawers without permission

Table 9–2	Goals, Interventions, Rationale, and Evaluation for Case Study	
Goal	**Intervention**	**Rationale**
Sally will maintain her present level of intellectual functioning.	Meet Sally at her level. Proceed slowly at her pace. Remember that Sally thinks and acts like a child but chronologically is an adult. She needs kindness, patience, and interested staff to develop her potential. It is helpful if the same staff person works with Sally and extends to her the affection she needs.	Meet client at her level of functioning.
Sally will brush her own teeth without being reminded by [insert date].	Break down toothbrushing procedure into small steps, and use positive reinforcers such as praise and spending time with her after she accomplishes each step.	Same steps each time reinforce learning.
Sally will respond to cueing "Sally, no." by [insert date].	Provide ongoing close observation during each shift. Collect data on wandering, plus activity before and after wandering. Explain limit and cue to Sally. When she wanders, use the words, "Sally, no." When she responds to the cue, immediately praise her.	Same cue and response by staff reinforces learning.

Evaluation: After the allotted time has passed, the LPN/LVN evaluates the success of the interventions. She documents that Sally appears to have maintained her intellectual functioning. She is able to brush her teeth with limited reminders. She responds to cueing "Sally, no" three out of four times.

LEARNING, MOTOR SKILLS, AND COMMUNICATION DISORDERS

The "world of work" for children and adolescents is school. This is where they need to succeed and practice the skills needed to be successful in their life's work. Their performance in school requires "the integrated interaction of the cognitive, motor, and language functions of the brain" (Silver, 1997, p. 636). DSM-IV defines *related disorders* as follows:

- *Learning disorder:* one in which brain function results in cognitive difficulties
- *Motor skills disorder:* one in which brain function results in motor difficulties
- *Language disorder:* one in which brain function results in language difficulties

The public school system refers to these disorders as **learning disabilities**. Some of the readers of this textbook may choose to work as school nurses. Because of this, the definition of the term *learning disabilities* according to Public Law 101-476, Individuals With Disabilities Education Act, is quoted below.

Specific learning disabilities means a disorder in one or more of the basic psychological processes involved in understanding or in using language, spoken or written, which may manifest itself in an imperfect ability to listen, think, speak, read, write, spell, or to do mathematical calculations. The term includes such conditions as perceptual handicaps, brain injury, minimal brain dysfunction, dyslexia, and developmental aphasia. The term does not include children who have learning problems which are primarily the result of visual, hearing, or motor handicaps, of mental retardation, of emotional disturbance, or of environmental, cultural, or economic disadvantage.

For nurses who are involved in a school system, far more explanation is needed. It is important for these nurses to learn the following:

- How the disorders are classified
- Why parents may decide that it is worthwhile to have a child diagnosed
- What kind of additional help is mandated once a diagnosis is established

Not to be overlooked is the fact that children with learning disabilities may also have a psychiatric disorder. Sometimes, even though the psychiatric disorder has been diagnosed, the learning disability is unrecognized and untreated.

ATTENTION-DEFICIT AND DISRUPTIVE BEHAVIOR DISORDERS

Common examples of psychiatric disorders that may be confused with learning disabilities because of similar symptoms include attention-deficit/hyperactivity disorder (ADHD) and conduct disorder. Both disorders involve maladaptive, age-inappropriate behaviors. Symptoms cause major problems in school or social functioning.

Attention-Deficit/Hyperactivity Disorder

Children, adolescents, and adults may experience attention-deficit disorder. According to DSM-IV (1994, pp. 63–64), **attention-deficit/hyperactivity disorder (ADHD)** for children and adolescents is characterized by developmentally inappropriate degrees of inattention, impulsiveness, and hyperactivity. Core problems include difficulty sustaining attention, underachievement, excessive activity, impulsiveness, noncompliance, other psychiatric disorders, and poor self-concept related to ADHD problems (Stolley, 1995, p. 267). Some of the symptoms are present before age 7 and appear in two or more settings (e.g., home, school, work).

Symptoms of *inattention* may involve lack of attention to detail, carelessness, not listening when spoken to, lack of follow-through even when directions are understood, problems with organization, losing things, distractibility, forgetfulness, forgetting daily activities, an so on. *Hyperactivity* may involve fidgeting, not staying in an assigned place, running and climbing excessively, inability to enjoy quiet activities, always being on the go, talking excessively, etc. *Impulsivity* involves blurting out answers before questions are completed, problems taking turns, interrupting, intruding, etc.

Although ADHD has been studied extensively, many questions remain, including the possibility of a genetic component. Ritalin and Dexedrine (stimulants) reduce symptoms for some children. Cylert and Norpramin have also shown results for select individuals. Psychotherapy is needed to deal with associated individual and family problems. Nursing intervention involves structured behavioral programs and support for both the child and family members in follow-through.

Conduct Disorders

According to DSM-IV (APA, 1994, pp. 66–67), a **conduct disorder** involves a repetitive and persistent pattern of behavior in which basic rights of others or major age-appropriate societal norms/rules are violated. The specific areas involve aggression to people and animals, destruction of property, deceitfulness or theft, or serious violation of rules.

Aggression to people and animals involves behaviors such as the following:

- Bullying, threatening, or intimidating others
- Starting physical fights
- Exhibiting physical cruelty to people
- Using a weapon
- Stealing while confronting a victim
- Forcing sexual activity

Destruction of property includes the following:

- Deliberate fire setting with intent to cause harm
- Other deliberate property destruction

Deceitfulness or theft involves, among other things, the following:

- Breaking into someone else's property
- Telling lies to get goods or favors
- Shoplifting
- Committing forgery

Serious violation of rules involves the following:

- Staying out late past parental guidelines before age 13
- Truancy from school before age 13
- Running away from home

The conduct disorders are a group of behaviors in which overt anger is usually easy to recognize. However, underlying causes of the anger and resulting behavior are not easy to recognize. Questions about possible neurochemical involvement remain unanswered. Nursing intervention, for now, is focused on containment, preventing harm to others, and following through on established behavioral programs.

ADULT-LIKE CHILDHOOD AND ADOLESCENCE DISORDERS

Some of the disorders recognized in children and adolescents are similar to adult disorders. Examples include mood disorders, anxiety disorders, and schizophrenia.

Mood Disorders

Two examples of mood disorders that affect children and adolescents are major depressive disorder and dysthymia. The symptoms may be difficult to separate initially from behaviors related to the child or adolescent's growth stage. Persistence and intensity of a given behavior give clues to a more serious underlying cause, such as a mood disorder.

Major Depressive Disorder

It is now accepted as fact that children develop true depressive disorders that must be treated. Major depression may recur. Without treatment, the interval between remission and exacerbation often is shorter. Some startling statistics that have emerged include the following (Nolen-Hoeksema, 1997):

- 4% to 15% of children under age 16 are clinically depressed at any given time

- 10% to 30% have at least moderate levels of depression
- 25% of adolescents have an episode of major depression by the end of high school
- Average age of onset of depression during high school is 14 years; the course of depression is now lasting longer than it did in the past, and there is a need to intervene with treatment
- The relapse rate for major depression is 72% over 2 years

A statistic of major concern is that teen suicide is the third major cause of death. Each year, almost 5000 young people ages 15 to 24 commit suicide (National Mental Health Association Facts Sheet, 1997).

Reality Check

What are the most common symptoms of depression in a child or an adult? Talk with your peers and share observations.

According to DSM-IV, the criteria for diagnosis of depression in children are the same as those for adults. Irritability is often the outstanding behavior in children and adolescents with depression. Referrals to counselors may be necessary for conduct problems. Additional signs may include physical complaints, clinging behavior, nightmares, slowing down or increasing activity, lack of interest, poor concentration, and drug use.

Some factors thought to be related to childhood depression include the cultural tendency to compress childhood. The rush to instill and perfect skills takes away from the normal tasks of childhood. Other factors include the following (Nolen-Hoeksema, 1997):

- Stressed parents have less energy to respond to and nurture children; children are sensitive to their parents' environment and pick up worries around the house
- Children have less opportunity to talk about what is bothering them
- Children tend to have a pessimistic thinking style and poor social skills; sometimes it is easier

to say "fine, OK, no problems" when asked how they are doing than to explain how they really feel
- Parent problems, including separation, may be involved
- Parental depression and other psychological problems may be involved. For example, mothers with severe depression show more withdrawal and neglect, more hostility and irritability. They have less sophisticated parenting methods, a more negative thinking style, and lead more stressful lives. This does not mean that *all* children of mothers who are severely depressed respond by developing pathology. However, more of them experience depression and anxiety, exhibit conduct disturbances, and have poor problem-solving skills.

Children who do well regardless of extremely stressful life situations share some characteristics. These characteristics include optimism, higher intellect, and a nurturing adult as a constant in their life.

The rate of occurrence of other illnesses along with major depression is high. The most common disorders include dysthymia (described below) and separation anxiety disorder (excessive anxiety related to separation from home or a person to whom the child or adolescent is attached—usually the mother). Children with major depression uncomplicated by another disorder are considered the least impaired.

Childhood and adolescent depression is often difficult to treat. The best method has yet to be identified. Talk therapies have limited value with the exception of those that deal with family problems related to the illness. Dealing with family stressors is often important. Identifying disruptive behavior patterns, practicing new behaviors, and having a therapist assist in evaluating progress can be useful.

Only some of the approximately 40 antidepressant medications are approved by the FDA for use by children. Sometimes medications are necessary as a part of treatment, and sometimes not. Sudden cardiac death with desipramine (Norpramin) has created concerns about the use of tricyclics. Mono-

amine oxidase inhibitors (MAOIs) such as Nardil and Parnate have shown promise, but there is great concern in using them because of possible severe food and drug interactions. Antidepressant medications are discussed further in Chapter 22.

Dysthymia

The major characteristic experienced in **dysthymia** is a chronically depressed mood that is often expressed as irritability. Dysthymic disorder generally occurs earlier than major depression and includes the risk of developing a recurring affective illness. The combination of a dysthymic disorder and major depression is known as "double depression." Recovery from the major depression often stops at the dysthymic level.

Bipolar Disorder

The child or adolescent with **bipolar disorder** experiences depressive and manic (elated) phases. Mixed episodes with both depressive and manic features are more likely to occur in adolescents. Psychotic (out of touch with reality) symptoms are also more common. Bipolar disorder is often confused with schizophrenia in this age group.

Important factors for recovery include previous adjustment and intelligence. The usual treatment includes giving lithium, plus lithium maintenance during a manic phase, and then continuing a lesser dose to prevent relapse. Mood stabilizers such as Depakote and Tegretol are also used. Electroconvulsive therapy (ECT) has been useful in some situations in which adolescents with mania fail to respond to the usual treatments.

For the depressive component of bipolar disorder, selective serotonin reuptake inhibitors (SSRIs) such as Prozac, Paxil, and Zoloft show promise. However, all treatment responses in children and adolescents remain under study.

Anxiety Disorders

Panic disorders, generalized anxiety disorders, obsessive-compulsive disorders, specific phobias, social phobias, and separation anxiety disorders are fairly common. They often occur with other disorders such as major depressive disorder and dysthymia. A correlation seems to exist between these anxiety disorders and a family history of anxiety and inhibited behavior. The anxiety disorder affects how the child functions at school and in social and personal relationships. Sometimes the child's fear of going to school is actually a sign of an anxiety disorder. Table 9–3 summarizes anxiety disorders in children and adolescents.

Schizophrenia

The most common characteristics of **schizophrenia** involve auditory hallucinations, delusions, mood disturbances, and thought disorder. Adolescence is generally considered the age of onset, but schizophrenia also affects younger children. Early-onset schizophrenia is more common in boys and is more frequently preceded by a premorbid schizotypal personality and by a high frequency of neurodevelopmental abnormalities (Koplewicz, Morrissey, and Kutcher, 1997, p. 601). Medication plus psychoeducation involving parents have proved useful in treating this disorder.

OTHER DISORDERS OF CHILDHOOD AND ADOLESCENCE

Several other types of mental disorders affect children and adolescents. These include feeding and eating, elimination, tic, and pervasive developmental disorders.

Feeding and Eating Disorders

Disorders of feeding and eating include pica, rumination, and various feeding and eating disorders of infancy and early childhood.

Pica involves eating substances without nutritional value. This problem is unrelated to developmental age and culture. According to DSM-IV (APA, 1994, p. 69.), pica may occur along with mental retardation or other mental disorders such as pervasive developmental disorders or schizophrenia. However, it can be serious enough by itself to need intervention. Treatment and nursing intervention are behaviorally focused.

During **rumination,** the child regurgitates and rechews food. This, too, may occur with other mental disorders such as those listed with pica. It

may become serious enough to warrant intervention.

Other feeding and eating disorders of infancy and early childhood occur before the age of 6 years. The child has no apparent medical condition, but fails to eat enough to gain weight or loses weight.

Elimination Disorders

Elimination disorders are not generally related to a physical condition. They occur after the age at which children are toilet trained. Elimination disorders include the following:

- **Encopresis** means that the child repeatedly passes feces in inappropriate places such as the clothing or floor, either involuntarily or intentionally. It occurs after age 4 or the developmental equivalent (APA, 1994, p. 73).
- **Enuresis** is a disorder in which the child voluntarily or involuntarily urinates in the bed or clothes. It occurs at age 5 (or equivalent) and causes impairment in social, school, and other important functioning areas. Some success has been attained with treatment by medication such as Tofranil. An awakening method such as the bell and pad system uses an alarm triggered by the child voiding. This system needs motivation and cooperation by both the parents and the child (APA, 1994, p. 74).

Tic Disorders

Tic disorders are sometimes confused with a learning disability because the symptoms are similar. "A **tic** is a sudden, rapid, recurrent, nonrhythmic, stereotyped motor movement or vocalization" (Walkup and Riddle, 1997, p. 703) bold added.

One example of a tic disorder that affects children and adolescents is Tourette's syndrome. **Tourette's syndrome** causes significant difficulties with social, school, and other areas of functioning. According to DSM-IV (APA, 1994, p. 71), both motor and vocal tics are involved, although not necessarily at the same time. The tics occur in bouts many times a day, and the person has never been free of tics for more than 3 continuous months. The onset of this disorder occurs before age 18.

Table 9–3 Anxiety Disorders in Children and Adolescents

Disorder	Characteristics of Disorder	Related Factors	Comorbidity*	Intervention
Panic disorder	Recurrent, unexpected panic attack; may or may not include agoraphobia (fear of open places)	Increases during prepuberty; peaks in early childhood and adolescence	Depression, separation anxiety disorder	Limited studies Medication: clonazepam
Generalized anxiety disorder (GAD)	Excessive worry about things such as personal safety, social interactions, past and future events; physical symptoms such as headaches and stomach aches are common; onset in childhood; affects females more often than males	Often-repeated visits to medical doctor in an attempt to diagnose physical problems		Self control and relaxation training Medication: low dose of benzodiazepines and SSRIs More study needed
Obsessive-compulsive disorder (OCD)	Persistent thoughts and feelings that result in repetitive acts to relieve anxiety; common thoughts (obsession) include fear of contamination, harm to self or others (usually parent); common acts (compulsion) include washing, cleaning, checking, counting; onset in childhood or adolescence	Question genetic or physical cause	Other anxiety disorders, major depression, tic disorders, some developmental disorders, ADHD, Tourette's syndrome	Cognitive behavioral therapy with medication: SSRIs

Specific phobia	Excessive fear (more than normal for age); examples include fear of heights, water, animals, planes, elevators, loud sounds, vomiting blood, injection injury	Fear must interfere with educational or social functioning; client shows less self-competence and temperamental flexibility; may be expressed as crying, tantrums, clinging, freezing		Behavioral: systematic desensitization and progressive relaxation
Social phobia	Persistent fear of social or performance situations; examples: refuse group play; hang around edge of group or stay near adults they are comfortable with; avoid speaking in front of class, writing on board, eating with other children, etc.	Crying, tantrums, freezing, shrinking from social contact	Simple phobia, agoraphobia, alcohol abuse, major depression, drug abuse, dysthymia	Medication, cognitive behavioral therapy with social skills, retraining
Separation anxiety disorder (SAD)	Excessive anxiety when separated from home or from someone to whom child is attached (usually parent); onset 7–9 years	Tantrums, avoiding going to bed, refusing to go to school; sometimes family pattern with other siblings	Other anxiety disorders, major depressive disorder	Behavioral therapy, family therapy, sometimes medication; limited studies

*Comorbidity: other diagnosis that may occur along with primary disorder.

Questions remain about the origin and treatment of Tourette's syndrome. Psychotherapeutic medication has proved useful for some clients. Psychoeducation, which focuses on learning how to suppress tics, is one of the goals of treatment. Psychiatrists, nurses, parents, and teachers all need to be involved in planning and follow-through with behavioral programs.

Pervasive Developmental Disorders

Disorders that occur during childhood and adolescence that relate specifically to developmental tasks and interfere with most or all aspects of the client's life are known as *pervasive developmental disorders.*

Characteristics of Developmental Disorders

Delays or abnormal development are known to occur before age 3. According to DSM-IV (APA, 1994, pp. 57–58), they occur in the areas of social interaction, social language, or symbolic or imaginative play.

Lack of quality of social interaction may be identified by impairment in eye-to-eye gaze, facial expressions, body postures, and gestures. Other characteristics include the following:

- Failure to develop age-related relationships
- Lack of sharing enjoyment, activities, or achievements with others
- Lack of social or emotional response to others

Lack of quality in communication (social language) may be shown by the following:

- Delay in speaking
- Impairment in starting or continuing a conversation
- Stereotyped or repetitive use of language
- Lack of spontaneous make-believe play according to age level

Restricted, repetitive, and stereotyped patterns of behavior may indicate developmental problems in symbolic or imaginative play. These patterns may include the following:

- Preoccupation with stereotyped or restricted patterns of interests that are abnormal or inflexible routines
- Repetitious motor mannerisms such as hand or finger flapping or twisting
- Complex whole body movements
- Preoccupation with parts of objects

Autism

The most common pervasive developmental disorder is **autism.** Typical characteristics of autism include self-absorption, often morbid in nature, and poor perception of reality. Like other physical disorders, autism may mask the presence of learning disorders. Autism is poorly understood and is surrounded by myths such as the one about an intelligent child being trapped in the disorder and awaiting release.

NURSING INTERVENTIONS FOR DISORDERS OF CHILDHOOD AND ADOLESCENCE

Planned interventions for the child or adolescent with a mental disorder are based on assessment by a skilled practitioner. The practitioner must have excellent knowledge of growth and development levels and the associated needs for each level. The child or adolescent may be functioning at several different levels of growth and development at the same time.

The depth of **regression** (return to earlier levels of development) must be identified, and the needs of the level to which the child has regressed must be clarified. For example, the 8-year-old who has temper tantrums may be functioning at a preschool level of emotional development. Intellectually, however, the child may be functioning at or above his or her chronological age.

Interventions depend on the client's level of growth and development. Some suggested interventions are listed in Box 9–2. The goal in working with children and adolescents is to teach them responsibility for their behavior and meeting their own needs. Ultimately, no one else can do it for them.

Reality Check

Carrie Sanders, age 16, frequently cuts herself. "When I feel pain, I know I'm alive." She seemed to do well until the beginning of the ninth grade. Change of school, new friends, a faster crowd, and experimentation with alcohol began the cycle of depression. Her parents tried to help, but they felt trapped by the depression and suicide threats. They never knew when "that call" saying she had made a serious attempt would come.

1. What options would you suggest to the parents in order to help Carrie?
2. Is there an urgency to seek outside help?
3. How do you determine whether this is a growth stage or a serious emotional problem?

BOX 9–2	Suggested Interventions for Child and Adolescent Disorders

- *Communication:* Communicate at the child or adolescent's level of comprehension. To be sure the intended message is understood, have him or her repeat what you said.
- *Limit setting:* Use a direct statement rather than a question, which offers choice. For example, say "I know you are angry, but you cannot hit me," rather than "Why did you hit me?" Follow the statement with information on what the client *can* do. For example, "You can hit the pillow in your room." When the negative behavior has subsided, talk to the client about what has occurred.
- *A structured plan:* Develop a structured plan for the child or adolescent. Create the plan on a daily basis if necessary. Talk about things the client needs to improve. Explain that the client's commitment to change is essential. After the client accepts responsibility for change, excuses are not acceptable. Go through the plan with the client and give him or her a copy of the plan. Provide positive reinforcement for what the child or adolescent achieves. Focus on what has been done correctly. Use the client's strengths to deal with the weaknesses.

SUMMARY

The impact of childhood mental disorders is important because of effects during infancy, childhood, adolescence, *and* adulthood. Clients who experience both mental retardation and mental disorders need attention to both conditions when they occur simultaneously. Meeting the client at his or her level of functioning and using strengths as a way to deal with weaknesses is an effective general rule.

Learning disorders and learning disabilities that are further complicated by psychiatric disorders get in the way of a child or adolescent's successful school career. Skillful intervention is needed as early as possible to assist the child. Some common psychiatric disorders include attention-deficit/hyperactivity disorder, conduct disorder, Tourette's syndrome, and autism.

Infants and young children may experience life-threatening eating disorders including pica, rumination, and lack of sufficient nutritive intake to sustain life.

Encopresis and enuresis are considered disorders when they occur after the usual developmental age for toilet training.

Children also experience adult-like childhood and adolescent disorders. These include mood disorders, anxiety disorders, and schizophrenia. Treatment with psychotherapies and medication needs further study in all areas of infant, childhood, and adolescent disorders.

Critical Thinking Activities

1. Think back to a time during grade school or high school when you were very sad for a number of days.
   a. How did you act toward your parents, teachers, and peers?

b. Who, if anyone, noticed and tried to reach out to you?

c. What was your response?

d. Could someone have reached out to you more effectively? If so, how?

2. Think about the self-talk you engage in when dealing with an irritable child.

a. What are some of the things you say to yourself?

b. How do you deal effectively with an irritable child (or adolescent)?

c. Who was your model for learning to do this?

d. Do you approve of what you do during these circumstances?

e. If not, how can you do it differently?

Review Questions

Multiple Choice—Choose the best answer to each question.

1. Which of the following guidelines is useful when dealing with a client who has both mental retardation and a psychiatric disorder?

a. Vary limits to assist in developing flexibility

b. Establish a parent-child relationship to provide security

c. Avoid mentioning events that are days or weeks away too far ahead of time

d. Use children's materials to support the intellectual level

2. What are the major areas of involvement for the child with an attention-deficit/hyperactivity disorder?

a. Inattention, overactive, impulsiveness

b. Aggression, destruction, deceitfulness

c. Sudden rapid, recurrent motor movement or vocalization

d. Social interaction, language, imaginative play

3. Which of the following is a possible example of pica?

a. Regurgitating and rechewing

b. Failing to eat enough to thrive

c. Eating beyond caloric requirements

d. Eating non-nutritive substances

4. Which of the following is an outstanding behavior of depression in children and adolescents?

a. Anxiety

b. Irritability

c. Delusions

d. Obsessions

5. Which of the following is a guideline for nursing intervention with children and adolescents?

a. Identify the level of regression

b. Treat the person as an adult

c. Modify limits on an as-needed basis

d. Above all else, be a friend

References

American Association on Mental Retardation: Mental Retardation: Definition, Classification and Systems of Support. Washington, DC, American Association on Mental Retardation, 1992.

American Psychiatric Association: Diagnostic and Statistical Manual of Mental Disorders, 4th ed. Washington, DC, American Psychiatric Association, 1994.

Greenspan S, Wieder S: Diagnostic classification in infancy and childhood. In: Tasman A, Kay J, Lieberman J (eds): Psychiatry, vol I. Philadelphia, WB Saunders Co, 1997.

Koplewicz H, Morrissey R, Kutcher S: Childhood and adolescent manifestations of adult disorders. In: Tasman A, Kay J, Lieberman J (eds): Psychiatry, vol I. Philadelphia, WB Saunders Co, 1997.

National Mental Health Association: Facts Sheet "The Impact of Childhood Mental Disorders," 1997.

Nolen-Hoeksema S: Understanding Depression: A Seminar for Health Professionals, Duluth, Minn, 1997.

Silver L: Learning skills and motor disorders. In Tasman A, Kay J, Lieberman J (eds): Psychiatry vol. I. Philadelphia, WB Saunders Co, 1997.

Stolley JM, Garand L, Pries CL, et al: Clients with delirium, dementia, amnestic disorders and other cognitive disorders. In Antai-Otong D (ed): Psychiatric Nursing Biological and Behavioral Concepts. Philadelphia, WB Saunders Co, 1995.

Walkup JT, Riddle MA: Tic disorders. In: Tasman A, Kay J, Lieberman J (eds): Psychiatry, vol I. Philadelphia, WB Saunders Co, 1997.

TEN

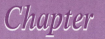
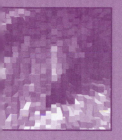

Cognitive Disorders

Outline

- **Delirium**
  Causes
  Symptoms
  Nursing Interventions
- **Dementia**
  Types of Dementia
  Alzheimer's Disease

  **Goals for Nursing Care for a Client
  With a Cognitive Disorder**
- **Case Study: Nursing Care Plan**
  History and Data Collection
  **Goals, Interventions, Rationale, and
  Evaluation**

Key Terms

- agnosia
- aphasia
- apraxia
- delirium

- dementia
- rummaging
- sundowning

Objectives

Upon completing this chapter, the student will be able to:
1. Describe the difference between delirium and dementia.
2. List two nursing interventions for a client with delirium.
3. Describe three symptoms that a nurse might observe in a client with Alzheimer's disease.
4. Differentiate between dementia and cognitively impaired depression.
5. Describe the stages of Alzheimer's disease.
6. List five challenging behaviors of a client with Alzheimer's disease and possible interventions for these behaviors.
7. Give specific examples of goals for a client with a cognitive disorder.

Cognitive disorders are temporary or permanent impairments of the brain that influence perception, thinking, and memory. They are classified in the American Psychiatric Association's *Diagnostic and Statistical Manual of Mental Disorders, fourth edition* (DSM-IV) as delirium, dementia, amnestic, and other cognitive disorders (APA, 1994, p. 123). This chapter will focus on delirium and dementia because they are the most commonly encountered cognitive disorders. Table 10–1 is a comparison of delirium and dementia.

DELIRIUM

Causes

Delirium is a mental disturbance of usually short duration. Causes of this condition include postoperative states, medication effect, infection, head injury, substance intoxication, metabolic disturbances, cerebrovascular insufficiency, sleep depri-

vation, and environmental factors (Frierson, 1997, p. 920).

Symptoms

The nurse usually encounters a client with delirium in the emergency room or in the intensive care unit. The onset of delirium is sudden. The client exhibits fluctuating levels of awareness with confusion and disorientation. Perceptual disturbances such as illusions and hallucinations may occur. Short-term memory is impaired (APA, 1994, pp. 124, 125). If the underlying cause is treated, the condition is usually reversible. However, if delirium is not treated or is untreatable, it may lead to dementia, irreversible coma, and death.

Nursing Interventions

A client experiencing delirium is in an acute stage of physical and psychological distress. The nurse needs to note the client's orientation and perceptual

Table 10–1	Comparison of Delirium and Dementia	
Feature	**Delirium**	**Dementia**
Onset	Usually rapid impairment of memory, orientation, intellectual function; fluctuating levels of awareness	Slow, insidious deterioration in cognitive functioning
Main characteristic	Clouded state of consciousness	Progressive deterioration in orientation, memory, judgment
Cause	Syndrome secondary to underlying disorders that cause temporary disturbance of brain function	Syndrome may be primary (e.g., Alzheimer's disease) or secondary (e.g., Parkinson's disease)
Duration	Usually hours to weeks	Progresses over months or years
Orientation	Disoriented	Often impaired
Memory	Short-term memory impaired	Recent and remote memory impaired
Perception	Illusions and hallucinations, visual and tactile	Usually intact or mildly affected
Thinking process	Markedly altered	Decreased intellectual ability
Speech	May be slurred, incoherent	Slowed; has difficulty finding words
Mood	Fear and anxiety are common	Labile; previous personality traits become exaggerated (e.g., paranoia)
Sleep–wake cycle	Disrupted	Fragmented sleep

Data from Frierson RL: Dementia, delirium, and other cognitive disorders. In: Tasman A, Kay J, Lieberman JA (eds): Psychiatry, vol I. Philadelphia, WB Saunders Co, 1997; and Varcarolis EM: Cognitive disorders. In: Varcarolis EM (ed): Foundation's of Psychiatric Mental Health Nursing, 3rd ed. Philadelphia, WB Saunders Co, 1998, p 694.

disturbances, physical needs, and mood and behavior. Specific interventions include the following:

- *Protecting the client from self-harm:* The client may require one-to-one supervision from a single caregiver. From time to time the nurse should reorient the client to the surroundings using short, simple, concrete phrases spoken in a calm, low voice.
- *Stabilizing the level of sensory input:* Environmental noises often increase agitation. It is best to have the client in a quiet room, apart from the mainstream of activity (Arnold, 1996, p. 986).
- *Providing a well-lit room with a window, clock, and visible wall calendar:* These things provide visual clues that help decrease perceptual distortions. Objects from the client's home environment, such as a stuffed animal and pictures, are concrete objects that may help calm and orient the client (Frierson, 1997, p. 921).
- *Ensuring adequate nutrition and hydration:* Providing these basic needs reduces the probability that delirium symptoms related to these factors will continue.
- *Administering the prescribed medication:* The medication helps in the management of delirium, including sleep deprivation caused by restlessness.
- *Reassuring the client:* Clients may feel guilt or shame for behavior that occurred during their confused state (Frierson, 1997, p. 921).

Reality Check

Joseph is a 46-year-old man who was admitted to the emergency room as the result of an industrial accident. A saw severed his right hand at the wrist. He immediately went to surgery for an attempted reattachment of his hand. No one had informed the medical staff of his long history of drinking. During recovery in the hospital, he was confused and disoriented. He complained about bugs crawling on his arms, and thought the chain on the side of the window blind was a snake. He continually talked about driving a Cadillac. Medication was administered to help manage his behavior. Before Joseph left the hospital, he told the nurse that he had borrowed his friend's Cadillac that day to go to work. He was worried about returning the car safely to his friend.

1. What could you do to reorient Joseph?
2. What would be your response to Joseph when he complained about bugs crawling on him and a snake along the window?
3. How might you handle Joseph's comment about why he was driving a Cadillac during his confused state?

DEMENTIA

Dementia is a progressive deterioration in intellectual functioning of sufficient severity to interfere with a person's daily performance. Areas of thinking, remembering, and reasoning are affected. Dementia is not a disease in itself, but a group of symptoms that may accompany certain diseases or physical conditions (ADRDA Fact Sheet, 1990).

Types of Dementia

Some well-known diseases that produce dementia include Alzheimer's disease (AD) and vascular dementia (formerly multi-infarct dementia). These conditions are irreversible. Dementias can also result from general medical conditions, including HIV (human immunodeficiency virus), head trauma, Parkinson's disease, Huntington's disease, Pick's disease, and Creutzfeldt-Jakob disease (APA, 1994, p. 133).

Alzheimer's Disease

Dementia of the Alzheimer's type is the most common of the dementias, affecting as many as 4 million Americans (Alzheimer's Association brochure, 1996). This section focuses on AD because it is prevalent in the aging population.

Cause

The cause of AD is unknown. Research has focused on possible genetic transmission, toxin causes, and neurochemical and pathological changes. Currently, however, diagnosis can be positively confirmed only by brain autopsy. Characteristic changes include senile plaques and neurofibrillary tangles (Alzheimer's Association autopsy brochure, 1996).

Symptoms

AD is characterized by the development of multiple cognitive defects as manifested by memory impairment and one or more of the following disturbances:

- **Aphasia** (language disturbance)
- **Apraxia** (impaired ability to carry out motor activities despite intact motor function)
- **Agnosia** (failure to recognize or identify objects despite intact sensory function)
- Disturbances in executive functioning (i.e., planning, organizing, sequencing, abstracting)

The course of AD is characterized by gradual onset and continuing cognitive decline. This results in significant impairment in social and occupational functioning (APA, 1994, p. 142). A person with a depressive disorder may be mistaken for someone with AD in its early stage. Table 10–2 differentiates cognitive impairment in depression from dementia.

Stages of Alzheimer's Disease

The number of stages a person goes through may vary. In most clients, three distinct periods present a recognizable pattern of symptom progression. These stages provide a framework for understanding the disease. It is important to remember that every client with AD is different; not everyone will have all of the symptoms, and some of the stages may overlap. Table 10–3 shows the progression of AD through each stage. In each stage of AD, the nurse is challenged with difficult behaviors. Table 10–4 lists some of these behaviors with suggested interventions.

Goals for Nursing Care for a Client With a Cognitive Disorder

Arnold (1996, p. 994) describes the goals for care of a client with cognitive disorders as the "3 Ps (protecting, preserving, promoting)." These goals can be achieved in many ways. Some appropriate methods are listed below.

1. The dignity of the client needs to be *protected.*

   - Recognize the client as a person by acknowledging his or her presence.

Table 10–2	**Characteristics of Dementia and Cognitive Impairment in Depression**	
Feature	**Dementia**	**Cognitive Impairment in Depression**
Cognitive functioning	Slow, insidious deterioration	Impairment fluctuates greatly
Awareness	In early stages, person tries to conceal cognitive losses	Person highlights disabilities
Symptoms	Insidious and indeterminate onset	Rapid onset
Duration	Symptoms usually of long duration	Symptoms usually of short duration
Mood (affect)	Mood and behavior fluctuate	Mood is consistently depressed
Responses	Approximate answers typical	"Don't know" answers typical

Data from Frierson RL: Dementia, delirium, and other cognitive disorders. In: Tasman A, Kay J, Lieberman JA (eds): Psychiatry, vol I. Philadelphia, WB Saunders Co, 1997, pp 899–900; and Varcarolis EM: Cognitive disorders. In: Varcarolis EM (ed): Foundations of Psychiatric Mental Health Nursing, 3rd ed. Philadelphia, WB Saunders Co, 1998, p 694.

Table 10–3	Stages of Alzheimer's Disease	

Stage	Symptoms	Examples
Early	Recent memory loss begins to affect daily living experiences; forgetfulness	Cannot remember phone number; loses things (keys, tools, etc.); gets lost on familiar routes; takes money out of bank and opens new accounts
	Trouble coping with everyday events, especially unstructured	Children notice change in parent: "She is not the same Mom I had."
	Change in personality: becomes anxious about symptoms, irritable, apathetic	Hits head with hand; says "I don't know what's going on."
	Makes bad decisions	Went through a stop light and told police officer it was not there the day before
	Trouble concentrating; attention span is limited	Looks at a magazine for a short period and then gets up and moves around
Middle	Increasing memory loss and confusion	Talks about going home to her mother; client is 80 years old and mother is not living
	Problems recognizing friends and/or family	Misidentifies nurse as daughter
	Repetitive statements or movements	Keeps asking to go to the bathroom over and over after just returning from it
	Pacing and agitation	Keeps walking up and down hallway and does not sit down
	Wandering, especially late afternoon and at night	Dozes off and on during day and then is awake at night and wanders
	Perceptual motor problems	Has difficulty getting into a chair; does not seem to know where the chair is
	Meaningless words and actions; rambles on with words that do not connect	Tries to pick up things from the floor that are not there
	Inability to perform activities of daily living without assistance	Has bowel and bladder incontinence
	Mood is labile; may be suspicious, irritable, teary, or silly	Accuses spouse of hiding things
	Loss of impulse control	Takes off clothes at inappropriate times; needs supervision
Late	Loss of long-term memory as well as short-term memory	Cannot recognize family or image of self; looks in mirror and talks to own image
	Significant weight loss even with good diet	Seems to be wasting away
	Loss of voluntary bladder and bowel control	Needs to be bathed, dressed, fed, and taken to the toilet
	Verbal communication is limited	May groan, scream, or make grunting sounds
	May put everything in mouth or touch everything	May try to eat anything small
	May experience difficulty with swallowing, contractures, skin infections, etc.	Sleeps more; can choke on food and also vomit after eating

Data from Arnold EN: The journey clouded by cognitive disorders. In: Carson VB, Arnold EN (eds): Mental Health Nursing: The Nurse-Patient Journey. Philadelphia, WB Saunders Co, 1996, pp 998, 1005, 1010.

Table 10–4   Challenging Behaviors, Possible Causes, and Interventions

Behavior	Possible Causes	Interventions
Angry, agitated, combative	Frustration over dressing, bathing, eating	Avoid changes and surprises; speak slowly and clearly; use repetition
		Break each task into small steps and allow client to complete one step at a time; keep daily routine as consistent as possible
		Distraction and avoidance are useful approaches
	Overstimulated by loud noises; feeling lost, insecure, unfamiliar surroundings	Simplify environment; be aware that shift changes are often stressful times
	Tired because of inadequate sleep	Plan more difficult tasks for time of day when client is at his or her best; try music, quiet readings to calm client
	Negative response to caregiver's impatience, stress, irritability	Give client adequate time to respond to directions or requests
	Physical discomfort such as pain, constipation, etc.; side effects of medication	Medical evaluation
Hallucinations	Sensory deficits, medications, malnutrition, physical illness	Medical evaluation
	Brain damage	Don't argue with client about what client hears or sees
		If behavior does not cause problems, ignore it
	Unrecognized environment	Reassure client with kind words and gentle touch (if client is willing to accept physical touch)
	Misinterpretation of things in the environment	Look for reasons or feelings behind hallucination and what it means to the client
	Disruption in routines	Use distractions: music, looking at pictures, "Let's go for a walk"
Incontinence	May no longer be able to express need to urinate	Watch for visible cues that client needs to use bathroom, such as pacing, pulling at clothes, etc.
	Task may be too complicated	Observe toileting pattern of client during both day and night; have client use toilet before and after meals and before going to bed at night

Table 10–4	Challenging Behaviors, Possible Causes, and Interventions *Continued*	

Behavior	Possible Causes	Interventions
	May not remember what to do once in the bathroom	Make sure client actually urinates before getting off toilet Simplify clothing: elastic waistbands for pants, protective undergarments, etc.
Repetitive actions	Memory loss caused by dementia; client does not remember what he or she is repeating Separation from loved ones may lead to repetitive talk about going home	Distract client with favorite activity; ignore behavior or question Use memory aids: signs, clocks, calendars, etc. Use calm voice when responding to repeated questions
Rummaging (searching for something familiar, security)	Confused about environment	Distract client; offer a glass of juice or take client on a walk; give client something to do
Sundowning (confusion and restlessness occur because brain can no longer sort out cues in the environment; often worse in dim light)	Cannot see well in dim light and becomes confused Tired at end of day and less able to deal with stress Involved in activities all day long; grows restless if nothing to do in evening May have a hormone imbalance or a disturbance in "biological clock"	Keep rooms adequately lit; good lighting may reduce client's confusion Make afternoon and evening hours less hectic; control client's diet; reduce foods and beverages with caffeine Discourage napping during day if sleeplessness is a problem; help client use up extra energy through exercise Medical evaluation; may need medication
Wandering	Direct results of physical changes in brain Searching for home or people from the past Feels closed in; desire to leave triggered by seeing coat, hat, etc.	Allow client to wander if environment is safe Distract with conversation, food, drink, activity Involve client in activities: folding laundry, setting table Remove items that may trigger desire to go out Develop areas where client can wander independently Keep wanderer safe with ID bracelet
	Need to use bathroom Reaction to medication	 Medical evaluation

Data from Alzheimer's Disease and Related Disorders, Inc: Fact sheets on sundowning and wandering, 1992; Robinson A, Spencer B, White L: Understanding Difficult Behaviors: Some Practical Suggestions for Coping With Alzheimer's Disease and Related Illnesses, Ypsilanti, Mich, Eastern Michigan Press, 1994, pp A–1 to I–3; and Arnold EN: The journey clouded by cognitive disorders. In: Carson VB, Arnold EN (eds): Mental Health Nursing: The Nurse-Patient Journey. Philadelphia, WB Saunders Co, 1996, p 1006.

- Use the client's name when addressing him or her.
- Avoid talking about the client to others when the client is present.
- Assume that the client understands everything that you are saying.
- Speak slowly and in simple sentences. Slow down your rate of speech and lower the pitch of your voice.
- Keep communication on an adult-to-adult level.
- Provide the client with privacy.
- Think of the client as someone who lives in a world that is strange to him or her.

2. It is important to *preserve* the client's functional status.

- Use the client's personal strengths and preferences.
- Be positive, optimistic, and reassuring to the client.
- Give praise for the simplest achievements by making such comments as "You were a great help in folding the laundry."
- Prepare the client for what is about to happen. For example, "It's time to take a bath."
- Allow the client to remain as independent as possible. Use cues to help the client stay involved, such as date boards and clocks.
- Focus on consistency. Keep things in the same place as much as possible.
- Repetitive activities and exercise help distract the client from feeling agitated.
- Reminisce with the client about old memories; allow him or her to tell the same story over and over. Sometimes the nurse can vary this by picking out a part of the repetitive story and asking for more information.

3. Try to continually *promote* the client's quality of life. Throughout the illness, professional and family caregivers can provide for the patient's quality of life by anticipating and responding to patient distress in a compassionate, knowledgeable manner (Arnold, 1996, p. 996).

- It is important for the nurse to educate and provide emotional support for family members. They need to be informed of financial and legal planning before the client is unable to communicate or perform these tasks.
- Hospice services are available during the terminal stages of illness and can be a source of support for the family.

Reality Check

A client states that her mother is waiting for her. You are aware that the mother is no longer living. What type of response and action might you take with this client if she insists on going home to see her mother?

Caring for the client who is cognitively impaired presents a challenge. The rewards from establishing a relationship with such a person, however, cannot be measured.

CASE STUDY

NURSING CARE PLAN

The following case study demonstrates a nursing care plan for a client with a cognitive disorder. The example describes appropriate interventions for this client. Other interventions may also be appropriate, depending on the client and the specific cognitive disorder.

History and Data Collection

Mr. Colter is an 80-year-old man who is disoriented in regard to time and place. His thoughts and conversations relate to the past, especially to his rock collection. He picks up small objects such as buttons and chunks of bread and calls them rocks. He feels alone, unwanted, and helpless. He is impatient and tends to be bossy (like a parent).

As a result of data collection, the LPN/LVN decides that Mr. Colter's strength is his interest in his rock collection. The nurse then uses the RN's nursing diagnoses to detail nursing problems appropriate for intervention at the LPN/LVN level. Table 10–5 shows the result.

Table 10–5	Nursing Diagnosis and Nursing Problem for Case Study

Nursing Diagnosis	Nursing Problem
Altered thought processes related to effects of dementia as evidenced by disorientation of time and place.	Client is disoriented as to time and place; is lonely

Goals, Interventions, Rationale, and Evaluation

Based on the nursing problems she has defined, the nurse proceeds to list appropriate goals and interventions, along with a rationale for each. With the RN's approval, she implements the interventions and evaluates the results. These are shown in Table 10–6.

▲

SUMMARY

Cognitive disorders involve temporary or permanent impairment of the brain. Delirium and dementia are two of the most common and important cognitive disorders.

Delirium has a sudden onset but is secondary to underlying disorders that cause temporary disturbances of the brain. Characteristics include disorientation, short-term memory impairment, illusions, and hallucinations. Nursing care needs to focus on protecting the client from self-harm, decreasing

Table 10–6	Goals, Interventions, Rationale, and Evaluation for Case Study		

Goals	Interventions	Rationale
Mr. Colter will be able to repeat the current time and place when it is reviewed with him daily	Place a calendar and a clock with numbers in a convenient place; orient Mr. Colter daily to month, day, time, and place	Keep Mr. Colter in contact with reality
Mr. Colter will become involved with other clients on the unit by displaying his rock collection at the hobby show in 2 weeks	Refer to Mr. Colter by title and last name; provide links with Mr. Colter's past (relatives or friends)	This is one way of protecting the dignity of the client
	Provide a small bag for his possessions	This provides a container for what he picks up
	Show interest in what he carries around; ask him to share with you some of his experiences	Will make him feel needed
	Provide a consistent routine; try not to move his bed, possessions, or place of eating	Will help orient him to place
	Write letters for Mr. Colter or offer him writing materials; encourage him to make friends with other clients and to do as much as possible for himself	Will help with Mr. Colter's feelings of being alone and unwanted
	Use his special interests (rock collecting) to stimulate his participation in unit activities	Utilizes Mr. Colter's strengths

Evaluation: Mr. Colter was able to identify day and time when a calendar and a clock were in front of him. He did not remember these when the cues were removed. Mr. Colter, with encouragement, began to show interest in activities on the unit. By the end of 2 weeks he shared his rock collection during the hobby show.

environmental noises, maintaining adequate nutrition and hydration, and reorienting and reassuring the client.

Dementia is a slow, progressive deterioration in intellectual functioning that is irreversible. AD is the most common of the dementias.

There are usually three periods in AD that show a recognizable progression of symptoms. In the early stage of dementia, it is possible to confuse the symptoms of cognitive impairment in depression with those of dementia. The client with AD presents many challenging behaviors. Some of these include anger, hallucinations, incontinence, repetitive actions, **rummaging, sundowning,** and wandering.

Goals for nursing care for a client with a cognitive disorder include protecting the client's dignity, preserving his or her functional status, and continually promoting his or her quality of life.

Critical Thinking Activities

1. Evaluate the pros and cons of resources available in the community for people with dementia.
2. Develop a variety of activities that can be used with a client who has dementia.

Review Questions

Multiple Choice—Choose the best answer to each question.

1. Dementia is
   a. temporary impairment of the brain.
   b. caused by environmental factors.
   c. an acute stage of distress.
   d. permanent impairment of the brain.

2. Nursing interventions for a client with delirium include
   a. allowing the client to be independent.
   b. reminiscing with the client.
   c. stabilizing the level of sensory input.
   d. initiating repetitive activities and exercises.
3. A possible intervention for wandering is
   a. involving the client in activities.
   b. reducing food and beverages with caffeine.
   c. keeping daily routine as consistent as possible.
   d. providing the client with privacy.
4. The dignity of the client is protected by
   a. talking about the client in the presence of others.
   b. keeping communication on an adult-to-child level.
   c. referring to the client as "the confused patient."
   d. providing the client with privacy.
5. A client in the last stages of Alzheimer's disease
   a. makes bad decisions.
   b. has a short attention span.
   c. has loss of long-term memory.
   d. keeps pacing and is agitated.

References

Alzheimer's Association, Inc. brochure, 1996.

Alzheimer's Association autopsy brochure, 1996.

American Psychiatric Association: Diagnostic and Statistical Manual of Mental Disorders, 4th ed. Washington, DC, American Psychiatric Association, 1994.

Arnold EN: The journey clouded by cognitive disorders. In: Carson VB, Arnold EN (eds): Mental Health Nursing: The Nurse-Patient Journey. Philadelphia, WB Saunders Co, 1996.

Frierson RL: Dementia, delirium, and other cognitive disorders. In: Tasman A, Kay J, Lieberman JA (eds): Psychiatry, vol I. Philadelphia, WB Saunders Co, 1997.

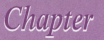

ELEVEN

Substance-Related Disorders

Outline

- **General Definitions**
  - **Substance Abuse**
  - **Substance Dependence**
  - **Substance Intoxication**
  - **Substance Withdrawal**
- **Substance-Abuse Categories**
- **Alcohol**
  - **Psychological Reactions**
  - **Common Physical Effects**

- **Intervention**
- **Detoxification**
- **Rehabilitation and Treatment**
- **Case Study: Nursing Care Plan**
  - **History and Data Collection**
  - **Goals, Interventions, Rationale, and Evaluation**

Key Terms

- **Alcoholics Anonymous (AA) model**
- **alcohol withdrawal delirium (delirium tremens)**
- **CAGE questionnaire**
- **denial**
- **detoxification**
- **MINDS**
- **Moderation Management**
- **projection**

- **rationalization**
- **repression**
- **substance abuse**
- **substance dependence**
- **substance intoxication**
- **substance withdrawal**
- **suppression**
- **volatile substances**

Objectives

Upon completing this chapter, the student will be able to:

1. Explain the differences among:
   - substance abuse
   - substance dependence
   - substance intoxication
   - substance withdrawal
2. Differentiate between alcohol abuse and alcohol dependence.
3. List two of the four questions on the CAGE questionnaire.
4. Discuss the purpose of the MINDS.

Objectives—cont'd

5. Provide an example of a drug that is a
   - central nervous system depressant
   - central nervous system stimulant
   - hallucinogen
   - narcotic, analgesic

The term *substance use* refers to the intake of any drug or nonfood item that alters the way the mind or body functions or changes a person's perception of reality. The substances people use in these ways are often collectively called *drugs*. Illegal drugs and alcohol are the most obvious examples, but other substances also fall into this category. For example, glue becomes a "substance" when a person sniffs it to get "high."

Consumption of these mind-altering substances has been with us through the centuries. Various substances have been used for rights of passage, religious ceremonies, finalizing treaties/agreements, family and community celebrations, treatment of medical ailments, and the list goes on. Cultural standards set the norm for what is acceptable and what is not acceptable.

Today, most people who use these substances begin in their teens. The highest rate of use occurs during ages 18 to 24 years. Symptoms of physical dependence, if they occur, take longer, usually occurring when the person is in the 20s and early 30s. Although the rate of substance-related disorders is higher in men, the rate for women is increasing. Nurses are at high risk for substance abuse. Peer assistance programs are available to nurses and have proved helpful.

Substance-related disorders are considered medical disorders. For example, alcoholism was officially labeled as a medical disease by the American Medical Association in 1956. The treatment remains primarily psychosocial. Intervention is primarily based on self-help groups and peer support. This approach is moderately successful, but the rate of relapse is high.

The legal system helps control use, possession, and distribution of these substances and deals with adverse secondary effects. Overwhelming numbers of people are housed in prisons for possession or selling of drugs illegally and for drug-related crimes. The rate of relapse for graduates of prison drug-rehabilitation programs continues to be high.

GENERAL DEFINITIONS

The American Psychiatric Association's *Diagnostic and Statistical Manual of Mental Disorders, fourth edition* (DSM-IV) has combined diagnostic criteria for alcohol and other drugs (not including caffeine or nicotine) into categories of substance abuse, dependence, intoxication, and withdrawal. Although specific substance categories are discussed later in this chapter, understanding the definitions of abuse categories makes it easier to understand the differences.

Substance Abuse

The term **substance abuse** refers to a maladaptive pattern of substance use that leads to significant impairment or distress. Abuse involves one or more of the following criteria, on a continuing or recurrent basis, within a 12-month period (APA, 1994, pp. 182–183):

- Failure to fulfill major role obligations at work, school, or home. Examples include poor work performance, absences, suspensions, expulsions, and neglect of children or household.
- Involvement in physically hazardous situations. Examples include driving an automobile or operating machinery while intoxicated.
- Legal problems related to recurrent substance abuse. Examples include arguments with a spouse about consequences of intoxication, and physical fights.

Substance Dependence

Substance dependence is also a maladaptive pattern that leads to significant impairment or stress. A person is said to be dependent on a substance if three or more of the following criteria occur in the same 12-month period (APA, 1994, p. 181):

- Tolerance: The person needs more of a substance to get the desired effect or gets less of an effect with the current amount.
- Withdrawal: A syndrome specific to the substance involved or consumption of the substance to avoid withdrawal. For example, a person who is dependent on alcohol consumes alcohol the morning after a heavy drinking bout to avoid withdrawal symptoms.
- The substance is taken in larger amounts or for a longer period than intended.
- The person desires to, but is unsuccessful in, cutting down or controlling use.
- The person spends a lot of time getting, using, or recovering from the effects of the substance. Examples include visits to multiple doctors, driving great distances, and chain smoking.
- Social, occupational, and recreational activities that were formerly important to the person are reduced or discontinued.
- Use continues even with awareness of related physical or psychological problems.

Substance Intoxication

With **substance intoxication,** the syndrome specific to the substance involved is reversible. The maladaptive behaviors or psychological changes develop during or shortly after substance use. Examples include belligerence, mood lability, cognitive impairment, impaired judgment, and impaired social or occupational functioning. The symptoms are not due to a general medical condition or other mental disorder (APA, 1994, p. 184).

Substance Withdrawal

Substance withdrawal occurs when a person stops using the substance or reduces the amount used after heavy or prolonged use. The effects of substance withdrawal are substance-specific. The significant distress or impairment affects social, occupational, and other important areas of functioning. The symptoms are not caused by a general medical or other mental disorder (APA, 1994, p. 185).

Reality Check

Mr. Joe Nippe, age 29, admitted himself for treatment of heroin addiction. His motivation is a 2-year-old son. "I don't want him to have a father who's a junkie. I've tried treatment five times before. It never works. My old buddies begin to drop in at work—I work nights—and finally I join them in a hit. That's all it takes. If I don't make it this time, there's no use going on."

1. When you attempt to change a pattern of behavior, does external motivation work for you? (Mr. Nippe's external motivation is his son.)
2. Give an example of when external motivation did or did not work for you.
3. Describe the self-talk you engaged in during this time.

SUBSTANCE-ABUSE CATEGORIES

Currently four major classifications and two minor classifications cover most illicit drugs involved in substance abuse. The major classifications include sedatives, hypnotics, and anxiolytics; hallucinogens and psychedelics; narcotic analgesics and opiates; and central nervous system (CNS) stimulants. The minor classifications include over-the-counter drugs and volatile substances (Carson and Arnold, 1996, p. 805).

- *Sedatives, hypnotics, and anxiolytics (CNS depressants):* Includes alcohol, barbiturates, and benzodiazepines. Table 11–1 describes these substances, their effects, and withdrawal symptoms.

Table 11–1	Sedatives, Hypnotics, and Anxiolytics

Alcohol
Use: Legal (age 19–21 years, depending on state)
Toxicity: Blood alcohol level 0.4–0.7 results in coma, respiratory failure, and/or death.

Withdrawal	Special Features
Alcohol abuse ("problem drinkers"): No physical withdrawal	**Treatment:** Alternative adversive therapy • Disulphiram (Antabuse) taken daily; results in severe reaction when alcohol is consumed; remains in body for days • Naltrexone (ReVia) reduces craving, decreases the pleasure of drinking; it is a narcotic antagonist: for example, it cannot be given to anyone who is also on codeine (person goes into withdrawal)* • Alcohol-abuse programs limit number of drinks per day and per week, encourage persons to never drink and drive; DrinkWise and Moderation Management programs are examples
Alcohol dependent (alcoholic): Physical withdrawal possible. Delirium tremens (DTs—late-stage withdrawal) occasionally leads to death, especially in the past when people were jailed in a "drunk tank"	Alcohol dependence—detoxification; rehabilitation based on Alcoholics Anonymous (AA) model with abstinence as goal

Barbiturates (Luminal, Amytal, Nembutal, Seconal, Pentothal)
Use: Legally used for medical treatment of insomnia or minor anxiety; illegally used with other drugs to enhance effect or reduce withdrawal; often combined with alcohol for potentiating effect in adult suicides
Toxicity: Overdose is a medical emergency; toxic level depends on individual drug or combination used; gradually decreased doses of drug administered during treatment

Withdrawal	Special Features
Severe physical reaction: agitation, tremors, delirium, convulsions, possible death	Barbiturates are often the drugs of choice for the middle class; dependence or use may be hidden by prescriptions; person uses several physicians in different locations **Treatment:** Gradual withdrawal according to medical protocol

Benzodiazepines (Librium, Valium, Xanax, Halcion, Dalmane, Ativan, Serax)
Use: Used medically for short-term treatment of anxiety, to promote sleep; Librium, Valium, and Ativan are also used for alcohol withdrawal
Toxicity: Lethal, especially in combination with other psychoactive drugs; toxic level depends on individual drug or combination used; common contributor to psychiatric emergency and unintentional death; in the elderly, the liver no longer detoxifies as well (the amount of drug in the body builds up and may reach toxic levels) and respiratory depression may occur

Table 11–1	Sedatives, Hypnotics, and Anxiolytics *Continued*

Withdrawal	Special Features
Short-acting: Halcion, Xanax, Ativan, Serax; severe withdrawal (if heavy dose) soon after drug is stopped **Moderate- to long-acting:** Librium, Valium, Dalmane; withdrawal within 3–5 days	**Treatment:** Gradual withdrawal according to medical protocol; psychotherapy with focus on learning effective coping skills helpful to client; benzodiazepines have few side effects, thereby encouraging consumption; tolerance may develop

*From O'Malley SS, Jaffe AJ, Chang G, et al: Naltrexone and coping skills therapy for alcohol dependence: a controlled study. Arch Gen Psychiatry 49:881–886, 1992.

- *Hallucinogens and psychedelics:* Includes hallucinogens and psychedelics such as marijuana, mescaline, and LSD. Table 11–2 describes typical examples of these drugs in further detail.
- *Narcotic analgesics and opiates:* Common examples of these drugs include heroin, morphine, codeine, and Darvon, among others. Table 11–3 describes narcotic analgesics and opiates in further detail.
- *CNS stimulants:* Includes drugs such as amphetamines and cocaine. Table 11–4 describes selected drugs in this category in further detail.
- *Over-the-counter drugs:* This category includes drugs that are commonly used for medical

Table 11–2	Hallucinogens and Psychedelics

Mescaline, Peyote, LSD, PCP (Synthetic Forms)
Use: Used by some cultures during religious ceremonies
Toxicity: Overdose is a medical or psychiatric emergency; possible violent impulsive behavior, may result in permanent neurological and cognitive changes

Withdrawal	Special Features
No physical withdrawal	Perceptual changes, out-of-body and intense emotional experiences

Marijuana, Hashish
Use: Most commonly used illegal drugs
Toxicity: Functional psychosis (hours to days)

Withdrawal	Special Features
No physical withdrawal	Amotivational syndrome (lack of motivation)

Table 11–3	Narcotic Analgesics and Opiates

Heroine, Morphine, Fentanyl, Codeine, Methadone, Dilaudid, Percodan, Darvon, Talwin, Demerol (Synthetic Forms)
Use: All except heroin used medically for pain; codeine also used for cough suppression; all the narcotic analgesics and opiates also suppress emotional tension
Toxicity: Overdose is a medical emergency; pinpoint pupils, depressed respirations, cardiac dysrhythmia, convulsions, coma, death caused by pulmonary edema; naloxone (Narcan) is used to reverse symptoms; naltrexone (ReVia), an opioid antagonist, is used to treat opioid addiction

Withdrawal	Special Features
Uncomfortable, not a medical emergency	Heroin is the most widely misused drug. **Treatment:** Symptoms can be reversed by using tapered doses of methadone

Table 11–4	Central Nervous System Stimulants

Amphetamines (Benzedrine, Ritalin, Dexedrine, Methamphetamine [Crank or Ice])
Use: Used medically to treat depression (Dexedrine), attention-deficit disorders (Ritalin, Dexedrine), asthma (Benzedrine inhalers), weight loss; methamphetamine (crank or ice) produced and used illegally
Toxicity: Possible psychotic-like behavior while drug is in system

Withdrawal	Special Features
Intense emotional low after use	Increases energy, reduces fatigue; used by truck drivers and athletes, others illegally; crank and ice are extremely addictive (made cheaply in home laboratories)

Cocaine (Crack: Cheaper Form, More Available, Quicker Effect; Highly Addictive)
Use: Illegal, often used with other drugs; for white-collar users, binge use is most common
Toxicity: Overdose may cause respiratory failure and sudden death related to cardiac arrest

Withdrawal	Special Features
Uncomfortable but not a medical emergency; no physical dependence; psychological dependence may be related to intense low that follows use; "cocaine blues" include severe depression and suicidal ideation	Cocaine is a stimulant; it produces euphoria, increased energy, improved performance, loss of fatigue, freedom from boredom, increased sex drive, heightened sense of competency; it also numbs emotional pain Impurities make dose difficult to gauge; it is easy to overdose accidentally Difficult to treat because of reinforcing effect of drug itself, no drug antagonist is available to prevent death from overdose; second most frequent cause of death*

*From American Association of Poison Centers, 1998.

treatment but do not require a prescription for use. Examples include antihistamines and drugs containing scopolamine or atropine. Table 11–5 describes these drugs in further detail.

- *Volatile substances:* **Volatile substances** are nonfood items that are not ordinarily used in medical treatment. They include aerosol sprays, glue, and paint thinners, among others. When introduced into the body, the chemicals in these substances have an adverse effect. Table 11–6 lists volatile substances and describes their toxic effects.

ALCOHOL

Currently, alcohol is the most-abused drug in our society. Because of its enormous public health impact, alcohol is discussed separately in this text. Alcohol abuse and dependence have been viewed in many ways. In the nineteenth century, alcohol use was seen as a moral issue. The person who drank was considered a sinner. Today, some people still cling to this belief. Others view alcoholism as

Table 11–5	Over-the-Counter (OTC) Drugs

Drugs Containing Antihistamine, Scopolamine, or Atropine (Dimetane, Chlor-Trimeton, Benedryl, Claritin, Seldane)
Use: Reduce secretions; symptomatic relief of upper respiratory allergic disorders, urticaria, or motion sickness; some are also used as sleep aids
Toxicity: CNS overstimulation or depression, convulsions, hallucinations

Withdrawal	Special Features
No physical withdrawal	Children are especially susceptible to overdosage; the drug may be assumed safe because of availability; therefore client may lack medical supervision for monitoring use with other drugs and with client's physical condition(s)

Table 11–6	Volatile Substances

Aerosol Sprays, Glue, Gasoline, Paint Thinners, Nail Polish Remover
Use: Inhaled or sprayed from can into nose or mouth for immediate effect
Toxicity: Overdose may cause cirrhosis of the liver or renal failure; some solvents can freeze the larynx and can cause respiratory and cardiac depression and permanent brain damage

Withdrawal	Special Features
No physical withdrawal	These solvents are toxic to body systems; the only known way to manage solvent use effectively is to encourage abstinence

a medical disease, a learned behavior, a psychosocial condition, or a cultural trait. Still others think the origins may be genetic. The common denominator in all alcohol-related disorders is the serious psychological and physical reactions that occur with heavy and/or prolonged drinking.

Psychological Reactions

Psychological reactions involve overuse of alcohol plus defense mechanisms to defend its use. People who abuse alcohol have a variety of psychological reactions, depending on their individual personalities and other factors.

Denial, the major defense mechanism, permits a person to say "alcohol is not a problem for me." It also perpetuates a continuous cycle of low self-concept, drinking to improve self-concept, guilt over behavior connected with drinking, and drinking again to deal with the guilty feelings.

Projection permits the person to deal with drinking as though the overuse and resulting behaviors belong to someone else. **Rationalization** involves excuses that sound possible but are not the real reason, such as "if you had a husband like mine, you'd drink too!"

Repression pushes the memory of drinking-associated behaviors beyond consciousness so that a person might say, "What do you mean? I never said that to you." Repression is not to be confused with actual psychological blackouts. **Suppression** is used as a conscious effort to forget; for example, a person might say "I won't think about what happened last night ever again." Other psychological factors related to alcohol dependency involve manipulation, dependency, depression, loneliness, and suicide.

Reality Check

Provide an example of each of the following defense mechanisms based on people you know who drink too much alcohol.

- Denial projection
- Rationalization
- Repression
- Suppression

Common Physical Effects

Alcohol is high in calories, but it has no food value. Alcohol provides 7% to 10% of total calories in an average American's diet. It may even provide a much larger percentage of calories in the diet long before a person is considered an alcohol abuser or alcohol dependent. A male consuming 2500 calories per day and drinking four or five beers a day receives about 25% of his calories from alcohol. This is not an uncommon practice. The person frequently drinks instead of eating a balanced diet.

Nutritional Effects

Alcohol can also increase excretion of nutrients and decrease their use in the body. This, in turn, leads to decreased levels of nutrients in body tissues. Abnormalities develop if the levels of nutrients are not in the proper concentration for adequate tissue function. Malnutritional diseases may result. Alcohol is an irritant to all cells of the body. Consequently, all systems of the body are affected in some way. Included are esophageal varices, cardiomyopathy, chronic gastritis, cirrhosis, decreased resistance to infection, increased cancer (especially of the mouth, esophagus, pharynx, larynx, liver, and pancreas), permanent brain damage, and polyneuropathy. Alcohol ranks as the third leading cause of death in the United States.

Effects on Body Systems

After a person takes a drink, alcohol is absorbed almost completely from the stomach and intestine into the bloodstream. The body identifies it as a toxin that must be removed from the bloodstream. Most of the alcohol is metabolized in the liver, but the small quantity that remains unmetabolized permits alcohol concentration to be measured in breath and urine (National Institute on Alcohol Abuse and Alchoholism, 1997, p. AA-35).

The products of alcohol breakdown can interfere with normal function of the liver. This can cause problems with bile formation, storage of vitamins and minerals, and proper use of proteins and fats. Fatty liver can result from the liver's inability to utilize fats. Chronic alcohol consumption and malnutrition may cause toxic liver damage. Both cirrhosis of the liver and pancreatitis are common complications. Alcohol stimulates the pancreas to make pancreatic juice and enzymes, but blocks passage of this juice into the small intestine. Chronic alcohol use can cause enzymes to digest the pancreas. The pancreas also produces insulin; lack of enzymes and insulin can cause severe malnutrition and diabetes. Other chronic nutritional affects of alcohol include decreased ability of the blood to clot because of lack of vitamin K, and brittle bones caused by lack of calcium.

Korsakoff's disease, also known as *alcohol amnestic disorder,* is caused by thiamin deficiency associated with prolonged, heavy alcohol use. It is characterized by memory loss and thought disorder and often follows an acute episode of Wernicke's encephalopathy. Wernicke's is a neurologic disease manifested by confusion, ataxia, eye movement abnormalities, and other neurological symptoms. If Wernicke's encephalopathy is treated early with large doses of thiamin, Korsakoff's disease may not develop.

In most states, a person is considered legally drunk with a blood alcohol level (BAL) >100 mg/dl (0.1%). Approximately 15 states use a 0.08% limit. The body can metabolize approximately one drink per hour. One drink equals a 12-oz can of beer or a 5-oz glass of wine or 1.5 oz of 80-proof liquor. The number of drinks per hour that it takes to reach impaired BALs differs based on gender, presence of food and type of food, body weight, muscle, and body fat content. A BAL of 400 to 700 dl (0.4% to 0.7%) results in coma, respiratory failure, and death.

Intervention

The nurse plays a major role in the intervention process. Data-collection assignments vary according to the nurse's skill and education. A number of assessment tools exist for determining if a person has a problem with alcohol use. Two common tools are the MAST (Michigan Alcohol Screening Test) and the CAGE questionnaire. The MAST is made up of 25 questions and is considered fairly reliable in identifying an alcohol habit. The **CAGE questionnaire** has four questions. Key words in the questions make up the acronym *CAGE.*

- Have you felt the need to **c**ut down on your drinking?
- Have you been **a**nnoyed by criticism of your drinking?
- Have you felt **g**uilty about your drinking?
- Have you ever had a morning **e**ye-opener after a night of drinking?

Answering two of the questions positively indicates a substance-use disorder. Three or four positive answers confirm it.

Detoxification

The period of abstinence from alcohol (or another substance) that follows a period of intoxication is known as **detoxification.** Within hours after reduction or discontinuation of alcohol, a person who has been drinking heavily for years may develop

alcohol withdrawal. Major symptoms include the following:

- Coarse tremors of hands, tongue, and eyelids
- Nausea and vomiting
- Malaise or weakness
- Tachycardia
- Diaphoresis
- Hypertension
- Anxiety
- Depressed mood
- Irritability
- Orthostatic hypotension
- Grand mal seizures

Sometimes the symptoms show up unexpectedly. For example, a client may have withdrawal symptoms on a surgical unit when the client's drinking history was not disclosed. Usually these symptoms disappear in 5 to 7 days unless **alcohol withdrawal delirium** develops. This syndrome, known as *delirium tremens (DTs)* may develop on the second or third day after drinking has stopped or been slowed down. Major symptoms include the following:

- Clouding of consciousness, including difficulty in focusing attention and distractibility
- Tachycardia
- Diaphoresis
- Hypertension
- Delusions
- Vivid visual hallucinations
- Agitated behavior

The syndrome subsides in 2 to 3 days unless complicated by another illness. The client needs close monitoring and skilled care. Monitoring is based on protocol agreed on within the agency. An example is the Minneapolis Detoxification Scale **(MINDS),** developed at the Minneapolis Veterans Affairs Medical Center (Dillon and Willenbring, 1995). A set scale is used to evaluate the client's pulse, blood pressure (diastolic), tremors, sweating, hallucinations (auditory, visual and/or tactile), orientation, agitation, delusions, and seizures. A score >10 generally indicates that further treatment is required. Other monitoring protocols are also available.

An additional challenge is provided by a common practice of polydrug abuse. Depending on the drug(s) involved, withdrawal symptoms may show up some days later, often after the client has completed alcohol withdrawal.

Rehabilitation and Treatment

The rehabilitation and treatment phase of intervention continues to be an area of limited hard science. In the United States, people who abuse alcohol (problem drinkers) and those who are alcohol-dependent (alcoholics) are often offered the same treatment: lifelong abstinence. The programs are based on an **Alcoholics Anonymous (AA) model**, which is a carefully developed 12-step program. There is little doubt that when AA works, it works exceptionally well.

Some people who are alcohol abusers say the AA model is not for them. They point to Europe, Britain, Canada, Australia, and other countries who years ago developed moderation-in-drinking programs to reduce alcohol's harm. These people focus on the "reducing harm" issue.

Problem drinkers (alcohol abusers) are approximately four times more prevalent than those who are alcoholic. They are also the ones who reject abstinence as a solution. They do not drink steadily, nor do they experience symptoms of physical withdrawal when they decrease or stop drinking. They are, however, out and about and probably account for a majority of alcohol-related social ills for which the alcohol-dependent (alcoholic) person is blamed. Alcohol figures in 41% of automobile accident fatalities and is a factor in 50% of homicides, 30% of suicides, and 30% of accidental deaths.

Heavy drinking also increases the risk of cancer, heart disease, and stroke long before people have to worry about liver or brain damage. A 1990 report by the Institute of Medicine, an arm of the National Academy of Sciences, concluded that the harmful consequences of alcohol abuse could not be reduced significantly unless more op-

tions were offered to people with only "mild to moderate" alcohol problems (Shute and Tangley, 1997, p. 58).

Effectiveness of Treatment Programs

Psychologists Hester and Miller completed a comprehensive review of the effectiveness of treatment programs. They concluded that "even for people with severe drinking problems, behavioral treatments (such as brief interventions, contracts, governing drinker's conduct and coping-skills training) worked significantly better than the fare routinely offered by 12-step programs: Group therapy, educational lectures, confrontational counseling and referral to AA." (Shute and Tangley, 1997, p. 61.) The researchers did not see their conclusions as absolute because the studies were of uneven quality. Other researchers and practitioners involved in prescribing and studying moderation in drinking are hopeful. They all stress the huge public health impact possible with having persons who abuse alcohol reduce the number of drinks they consume. **Moderation Management,** for example, sets limits for the number of drinks per day (maximum 3) and the number per week (maximum 9 for women, 14 for men) and mandates that the person should never drink when driving (Kishline, 1994).

Successful treatment seems to be related to matching the program to the specific needs of the client. There is limited hard data to show that one treatment program is better than another. Any treatment is thought to be better than no treatment. About two thirds of participants show improvement.

Effect of Bias on Nursing Care

Personal bias can get in the way of providing ethical care for the client. For example, questions and objective information on some alcohol-related treatment protocols can be manipulated by bias. More often than not, the client with alcoholism is hospitalized for physical complaints when withdrawal symptoms become apparent. These physical manifestations must be handled by nursing personnel in a nonjudgmental manner. Bias could keep an individual from receiving the medication he or she needs.

Reality Check

List your personal reactions to people who abuse substances (2 to 3 reactions). Will any of these reactions interfere with your professional responsibility in providing care?

CASE STUDY

NURSING CARE PLAN

The following case study demonstrates a nursing care plan for a client with a substance-related disorder. The example describes appropriate interventions for this client. Other interventions may also be appropriate, depending on the client and the specific substance involved.

History and Data Collection

Mr. David Morgan, age 37, was brought to the chemical dependency unit by police. He appears to be intoxicated. Neighbors called police when he hit a newspaper boy on a bike. The bike was damaged, but the boy was okay.

Mrs. Morgan accompanied him. She was visibly upset. "Either shape up this time or I'm leaving you. No more covering, no more lies, no more taking back. I've finally learned that love is a behavior, not a feeling. It's about how you treat me and the kids."

Staff recognized Mr. Morgan from previous admission. He has a history of delirium tremens (DTs), including seizures during one of three previous admissions.

An initial MINDS assessment was performed on Mr. Morgan. As shown in Table 11–7, his score of 8 (<10) confirmed that he is in the early stages of withdrawal.

The LPN/LVN then used the RN's nursing diagnoses to detail nursing problems appropriate

Table 11–7	MINDS Assessment Score for Case Study	
	Mr. Morgan's Score	**Highest Possible Score**
Pulse	1	(2)
BP (diastolic)	1	(2)
Tremor	2	(6)
Sweating	2	(6)
Hallucinations	0	(6)
Orientation	0	(6)
Agitation	2	(6)
Delusions	0	(4)
Seizures	0	(6)
TOTAL	8	(44)

for intervention at the LPN/LVN level. Table 11–8 shows the result.

Goals, Interventions, Rationale, and Evaluation

Based on the nursing problems she has defined, the nurse proceeds to list appropriate goals and interventions, along with a rationale for each. These are shown in Table 11–9. With the RN's approval, she implements the interventions.

If Mr. Morgan's condition continues to deteriorate as shown by further MINDS testing, further in-

Table 11–8	Nursing Diagnosis and Nursing Problem for Case Study
Nursing Diagnosis	**Nursing Problem**
Sensory: perceptual alterations related to withdrawal from alcohol	Mr. Morgan is in the beginning stages of withdrawal; he will need careful monitoring according to established protocol

Table 11–9	Goals, Interventions, Rationale, and Evaluation for Case Study	

Goals	Interventions	Rationale
Stabilize and prevent progression to next level (MINDS score <10)	Admit to detoxification room (well-lighted, uncluttered, easy observation, quiet)	Decrease stimulation: loud noises may cause overreaction
	Complete MINDS q4h × 24h (or other protocol); rate according to scale and total score (pulse, BP, tremors, sweating, hallucinations, orientation, agitation, delusions, seizures)	A score of >10 generally indicates that further treatment is required
	Administer medications as ordered by physician	Common orders; thiamin may be ordered to prevent Wernicke's encephalopathy; prophylactic Dilantin may be ordered if client has a history of seizures
	Offer one cup juice (such as grape or cranberry) every hour; assist with feeding if needed	Maintain adequate hydration and nutrition
	Offer frequent supportive contacts; be aware of personal attitude	Reduce fearfulness; Mr. Morgan tends to exaggerate signs of rejection, responds to one-to-one contacts and reassurances
	Assist with personal hygiene as needed	Meet physical care needs, maintain skin integrity

Evaluation: Mr. Morgan attained a MINDS of 14. Benzodiazepines were given as prescribed by the MD. No seizures occurred. Mrs. Morgan was put in touch with an Alcoholics Anonymous member for assistance.

terventions become necessary. Table 11–10 shows appropriate goals and interventions, as well as the nurse's evaluation.

SUMMARY

Substance-related disorders are classified as medical disorders in the DSM-IV. Treatment is primarily psychosocial except during detoxification. Most substance use begins in the teens, with the highest rate in the age group 18 to 24 years.

Substance abuse is a maladaptive pattern of use that can involve failure to fulfill major role obli-

gations, involvement in hazardous situations (such as drinking and driving), and/or legal problems related to the substance abuse. Substance dependence is a maladaptive behavior that can include developing tolerance to the substance and a substance-specific withdrawal syndrome. People who are psychologically addicted experience uncomfortable withdrawal that is not a medical emergency. Those who are physically addicted because of the nature of the substance (alcohol for example) may find themselves in a medical emergency. People who are dependent have probably tried to stop substance use unsuccessfully and/or find that substance use replaces the social, occupa-

Table 11–10	Goals and Interventions for Advanced Cases		
MINDS Score	**Goals**	**Nursing Interventions**	**Medical Interventions**
10–20	Return to score <10; prevent delirium	Increase MINDS interval to q2h until score is <10; raise side rails; meet skin care needs; make sure room is well lighted (non-shadowy lighting increases orientation and decreases hallucinations); check with physician for further orders	Use of diazepam (Valium) or lorazepam (Ativan); IV; other medications as necessary
>20	Prevent complications; provide life-sustaining measures; return to score <10; prevent delirium if not already present	Immediate contact with physician; seizure precautions; maintain adequate respirations; turn client on side; reassure client; orient client to reality; use restraints only if necessary; possible transfer to monitored bed; medication according to orders	Increase in diazepam (Valium) or lorazepam (Ativan); rule out co-existing conditions and complications such as infection, subdural hematoma; IV; consults; transfer to ICU; order constant nurse supervision

Data from Dillon N, Willenbring M: MINDS (Minneapolis Detoxification Scale), private communication, January 1995. Minneapolis Veterans Affairs Medical Center, One Veterans Drive, Minneapolis, MN 55417.

tional, and recreational activities they formerly held important.

Alcohol continues to be the most abused drug in many countries. The public health toll is considerable because of its relationship to physical health, accidents, homicides, suicides, violence, etc. The usual model for treatment for people that are alcohol abusers and those who are alcohol-dependent is based on the AA model of abstinence.

Critical Thinking Activities

1. Think of convincing arguments for following the traditional AA model of treatment for alcohol abuse and alcohol dependence.
2. Think of convincing arguments for following a modification model of treatment for problem drinkers (alcohol abusers).

Review Questions

Multiple Choice—Choose the best answer to each question.

1. Which of the following is specific to substance dependence?
   a. Client fails to fulfill major role obligations at work, school, and home
   b. Maladaptive behaviors or psychological changes develop during or after use
   c. Withdrawal symptoms occur when drug is discontinued
   d. Client shows belligerence, mood lability, cognitive impairment
2. What is the purpose of the MINDS protocol?
   a. Determine if the client has a drinking problem

b. Monitor the client's condition during detoxification

c. Differentiate between problem drinkers and alcoholics

d. Moderation management program for alcohol abusers

3. What are the four key words included in the CAGE questionnaire?

a. Crave, alcohol, guilty, eye

b. Coarse, anxious, guts, eager

c. Consciousness, attention, guilt, energy

d. Cut, annoyed, guilty, eye

4. Why are the methamphetamines crank and ice of major concern?

a. They are used by some cultures during religious ceremonies

b. They can freeze the larynx, causing respiratory and cardiac depression

c. They are used medically to treat psychotic depression

d. They are extremely addictive, cheap, and produced in home labs

5. Why is cocaine and crank addiction difficult to treat?

a. The reinforcing effect of the drugs themselves

b. They are lethal, especially in combination with psychoactive drugs

c. Onset is with prescription use with several physicians prescribing

d. They are used for treatment of severe asthma

References

American Psychiatric Association: Diagnostic and Statistical Manual of Mental Disorders, 4th ed. Washington, DC, American Psychiatric Association, 1994.

Carson VB, Arnold EN: The journey anesthetized by substance abuse. In: Carson VB, Arnold EN (eds): Mental Health Nursing: The Nurse-Patient Journey. Philadelphia, WB Saunders Co, 1996.

Dillon N, Willenbring M: MINDS (Minneapolis Detoxification Scale), private communication, January 1995. Minneapolis Veterans Affairs Medical Center, One Veterans Drive, Minneapolis, MN 55417.

Kishline A: Moderate Drinking: The Moderation Management Guide. New York, Three Rivers Press, 1994.

National Institute on Alcohol Abuse and Alcoholism: Alcohol Alert No. 35, PH371, January 1997.

O'Malley SS, Jaffe AJ, Chang G, et al: Naltrexone and coping skills therapy for alcohol dependence: a controlled study. Arch Gen Psychiatry 49:881–886, 1992.

Shute N, Tangley L: The Drinking Dilemma. US News & World Report, pp. 55–65, Sept. 8, 1997.

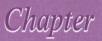

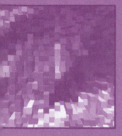

TWELVE

Schizophrenia and Other Psychotic Disorders

Outline

- Theories of Schizophrenia
  Biological Theories
  Environmental and Social Theories
- Symptoms
- Diagnostic Criteria
- Types of Schizophrenia
  Paranoid Type
  Disorganized Type
  Catatonic Type

Undifferentiated Type
Residual Type
Schizoaffective Disorder
- Nursing Care of Clients With
  Schizophrenia
- Case Study: Nursing Care Plan
  History and Data Collection
  Goals, Interventions, Rationale, and
  Evaluation

Key Terms

- alogia
- affect
- ambivalence
- anhedonia
- associative looseness
- autism
- avolition

- delusion
- echolalia
- echopraxia
- ideas of reference
- psychotic
- regression

Objectives

Upon completing this chapter, the student will be able to:
1. Discuss biological, environmental, and social theories of the cause of schizophrenia.
2. Differentiate between the positive and negative symptoms of schizophrenia.
3. List the subtypes of schizophrenia.
4. Name two ideas that the nurse tries to convey to a client who is delusional.
5. Describe the approach needed to establish a trusting relationship with a client who has schizophrenia.

Schizophrenia comprises a large group of disorders that constitute a major health problem. The illness is highly complex, and few generalizations hold true for all people diagnosed with it. Eugen Bleuler coined the term *schizophrenia*. It comes from two Greek words—one that means *split*, and one that means *mind*. Bleuler used the term to describe the division between the intellectual and emotional aspects of the personality. There is confusion about this term because the general public uses the word to describe people with dissociative identity disorder (formerly multiple personality disorder) (Kaplan, Sadock, and Grebb, 1994, p. 457).

Most people with schizophrenia initially develop the symptoms during adolescence or early adulthood. Schizophrenia affects about one person in a hundred and affects men and women about equally (Lichtenstein Creative Media, p. 4).

THEORIES OF SCHIZOPHRENIA

Numerous theories relating to the cause of schizophrenia exist. Biological theories have been the focus of considerable research during the "decade of the brain" (see Chapter 1).

Biological Theories

Biological theories of schizophrenia include neurochemical changes, genetic factors, and structural changes in the brain. Studies have found that certain chemical messengers called *neurotransmitters* are affected in schizophrenia. Neurotransmitters allow nerve cells to send messages to each other. The neurotransmitter dopamine was found in excess in people with schizophrenia. When medications were used to block dopamine receptors, the symptoms of schizophrenia were reduced. These medications had undesirable side effects, however, so newer, atypical antipsychotic drugs were developed. These drugs have fewer side effects and have been shown to cause a remission of symptoms, especially in people with long-term illness (Marder, 1997, p. 1583).

Genetic research by E. Fuller Torrey and colleagues (1994) involved the largest study done on pairs of identical twins in which one suffered from schizophrenia or manic-depressive disorder and the other did not. He discovered that the twin with schizophrenia or manic-depressive disorder almost always had structural and functional changes in the brain. He states that "despite the knowledge of multiple measures of brain structural pathology and brain dysfunction in schizophrenia, it is not yet possible to use these measures diagnostically to say whether any given individual is or will become affected." (Torrey et al., 1994, p. 213).

Modern techniques such as computed tomography (CT), magnetic resonance imaging (MRI), and positron emission tomography (PET) have shown that some people with schizophrenia have changes in the size and shape of certain brain structures. Certain tests revealed less activity in the prefrontal cortex, the part of the brain that governs thought and higher mental functions (NARSAD, 1996).

Environmental and Social Theories

Studies have shown that the symptoms of schizophrenia have not only a biological component but also an environmental aspect (Pinals and Breier, 1997, p. 958). Environmental conditions such as stress, viral illness, or head injury are considered significant contributors to schizophrenia for someone who has a genetic factor.

Harry Stack Sullivan's interpersonal theory of psychiatry proposed that when an infant grows up in a warm and caring environment with minimal anxiety, the child develops a sense of trust. But if a child grows up with fear and rejection, the child sees the environment as a frightening place. The child's ability to test reality is impaired and might result in a personality deficit or schizophrenia. There has been little data to support Sullivan's theory and its relationship to schizophrenia.

At one time, theorists emphasized family relationships. Often parents were blamed when their children developed the illness, especially the mother. These beliefs are considered less important today. Nevertheless, in working with a person who has schizophrenia, it is important to consider the environmental and social concerns along with the biological factors.

SYMPTOMS

A specific characteristic of schizophrenia is deterioration from a previous level of functioning. Family or friends may note that the person is "not the same." The person with schizophrenia experiences disturbances in thinking, feeling, and behavior. Noticeable distortions occur in each of these areas. During the active phase of the illness, the person is usually **psychotic** (out of touch with reality).

Bleuler is well-known for describing the symptoms of schizophrenia as the "four As." They include the following:

- **Ambivalence:** the existence of opposing emotions, such as love and hate, at the same time
- **Autism:** preoccupation with self
- **Associative looseness:** words and thoughts shift from one subject to another in an unrelated manner
- **Affect:** blunting or dulling of mood in a manner that is incongruous with what is going on at the time

Pinals and Breier (1997, p. 928) saw the influence of Bleuler's descriptions in the American Psychiatric Association's *Diagnostic and Statistical Manual of Mental Disorders, fourth edition* (DSM-IV).

DIAGNOSTIC CRITERIA

The DSM-IV includes a mixture of characteristic signs and symptoms, both positive and negative (APA, 1994, p. 274, 275). Positive symptoms reflect excess or distortion of normal functioning. They include the following:

- *Delusions:* persistent false beliefs that are not supported by logic
- *Hallucinations:* false sensory perceptions (seeing, hearing, tasting, smelling, or touching) for which there are no external stimuli; hearing voices and/or seeing things are the most common types of hallucinations
- Disorganized speech
- Grossly disorganized or catatonic behavior

Negative symptoms are a diminution or loss of normal functions. They include the following:

- **Affective flattening**
- **Alogia:** restriction in the fluency and productivity of thought and speech
- **Avolition:** restriction in the initiation of goal-directed behavior
- **Anhedonia:** total loss of feeling of pleasure in acts that normally give pleasure

According to the DSM-IV (APA, 1994, p. 274), at least two of the positive or negative signs and symptoms need to be present for a significant portion of time during a 1-month period, with some signs persisting for at least 6 months, to justify a diagnosis of schizophrenia. This in itself characterizes schizophrenia as a long-term serious illness. Clients with schizophrenia also display a noticeable change in functioning in the areas of work, interpersonal relations, or self-care.

TYPES OF SCHIZOPHRENIA

Several types of schizophrenia exist. The diagnosis is defined by the predominant symptoms evident at evaluation.

Paranoid Type

Cognitive functioning and affect are fairly well preserved in paranoid schizophrenia (APA, 1994, p. 287). The essential feature of this type of schizophrenia is the presence of delusions or auditory hallucinations ("hearing voices"). The delusions are usually grandiose or persecutory. Someone with a grandiose delusion might think that he or she is God and therefore can do anything. A person with a persecutory delusion feels that people are trying to harm or destroy him or her.

Disorganized Type

In disorganized schizophrenia, behavior is regressive and primitive. There is an inappropriate affect that includes silliness, giggling, and facial grimaces, with extreme social withdrawal. Communication is incoherent (Townsend, 1994, p. 141).

Catatonic Type

The clinical picture for catatonic schizophrenia is dominated by at least two of the following characteristics (APA, 1994, p. 289):

- Marked psychomotor disturbance as evidenced by diminished responsiveness; usually takes the form of trance-like states or stupor or excessive motor activity not influenced by external stimuli
- Extreme negativism, such as resistance to instructions or maintenance of a rigid posture against attempts to be moved, and mutism (inability or refusal to speak)
- Voluntary assumption of inappropriate or bizarre postures
- **Echolalia:** the person repeats words spoken to him or her
- **Echopraxia:** the spasmodic and involuntary imitation of the movements of another person

The client who has catatonic schizophrenia is also very lonely and fearful. He or she copes with these feelings by withdrawing from reality and retreating to a simpler form of existence in a private world (**regression**). In this world, the client turns attention inward and relates to an imaginary environment as if it were real.

Such a client has a pronounced difficulty in relating to other people in a meaningful way. The client sets up barriers that make it difficult to establish contact. For the nurse, these barriers are obstacles to establishing a trusting relationship.

Below the surface is a person who desperately wants someone to care for him or her. The client's loneliness and fear are evident in distorted thoughts, feelings, and actions. The distortions vary and may include delusions, hallucinations, flat or inappropriate affect, socially unacceptable behavior, and ambivalence. Ambivalence in particular presents many problems because the client experiences, at the same time, opposing feelings toward the same object, person, or idea. These opposing feelings interfere with decision making.

When working with a client who is withdrawn, the nurse first needs to initiate contact on a one-to-one basis, then meet the client at his or her level of functioning. The nurse should be sensitive to the clues that the client provides, such as the need for personal space or an inability to engage in meaningful conversation. For example, it may be helpful to say, "If you would rather not talk, I'll just sit here for 10 minutes." The client develops trust when observing the nurse doing what was promised.

The nurse must be patient when working with the client who is withdrawn. A rejection from such a client is often a clue that the nurse has been allowed to enter the client's private world. However, the entrance may have made the client uncomfortable; the nurse needs to move more slowly. Developing a relationship is a slow but rewarding process. This client needs a supportive nurse who will make no demands. It is most important that the nurse focus on the client and not the symptoms.

Reality Check

Miss Shari Hall, age 20, has good features, fair skin, and long ash-blond hair. She spends the day sitting on the floor in the corner of the dayroom with her arms clasped about her knees. When she is alone, she sometimes laughs for no apparent reason, turns her head to the side as though listening to someone, and responds with lengthy conversations that seem meaningless but indicate a good vocabulary. Because she is so preoccupied, she neglects her physical care. She can be distracted from her preoccupation if approached in a warm and casual way.

1. What would be your goals for working with Shari?
2. What approaches might you use to help Shari stay in contact with reality?
3. How might you encourage Shari to eat and care for her personal needs?
4. How might you use Shari's strengths to increase her self-esteem?

Undifferentiated Type

A person with undifferentiated schizophrenia has prominent delusions and hallucinations. The person is incoherent. His or her behavior is grossly disorganized but lacks the criteria necessary for a paranoid, disorganized, or catatonic type of disorder (APA, 1994, p. 289).

Residual Type

Residual schizophrenia meets the following criteria (APA, 1994, p. 290):

- Absence of prominent delusions, hallucinations, or disorganized or catatonic behavior
- Continuing evidence of the disturbance, as indicated by the presence of negative symptoms or two or more symptoms listed for schizophrenia but present in a weakened form (e.g., odd beliefs, unusual perceptual experiences)

Schizoaffective Disorder

Another type of schizophrenia is known as *schizoaffective disorder*. This type sometimes includes a major depressive episode, a manic episode, or a mixed episode concurrent with symptoms of schizophrenia. During the absence of prominent mood symptoms, a person with schizoaffective disorder has delusions or hallucinations for at least 2 weeks (APA, 1994, p. 292).

NURSING CARE OF CLIENTS WITH SCHIZOPHRENIA

The most challenging behaviors to work with are those exhibited by a client diagnosed with paranoid schizophrenia. This client exhibits an overly suspicious pattern of behavior, setting up obstacles for care by displaying attitudes of superiority, ridicule, and sarcasm. These attitudes are a way of coping with feelings of inadequacy. Basically, the client is a lonely person. As anxiety increases, he or she manifests ideas of persecution. Statements such as "You don't like me" reflect the use of the projection defense mechanism. The client is actually revealing distrust of himself or herself. These ideas are fixed and cannot be changed because they meet the client's basic need to feel significant. The distorted ideas will remain until the client finds a more constructive way to meet this need.

The goal of the nurse is to help the client find constructive ways to meet these needs. This client irritates and arouses aggressive feelings in others. Consequently, the nurse must deal with these feelings before working with the client. Tact and courtesy are necessary in responding to the client's negative behavior and emotions. Ridicule and sarcasm from the client must never be met with retaliation. The following suggestions provide guidelines for working with clients who have paranoid schizophrenia:

- Never speak sharply to the client or make fun of the client's ideas
- Listen to the client's story, but neither agree nor disagree
- Respond to the client's direct questions about his or her ideas calmly and matter-of-factly: the exact words will vary, but two ideas to be conveyed are the nurse's understanding and the fact that the client's beliefs do not reflect reality; a suggested response might be, "I know this is real to you, but I do not see it that way, and it is not reality"
- It is important to speak in a noncritical, well-modulated tone of voice
- Whenever possible, praise the client for accomplishments; give honest, specific praise rather than overall compliments
- If the client is hearing voices (having auditory hallucinations), suggest positive ways to help the client deal with the voices; Box 12–1 offers suggestions that the nurse can make to accomplish this

The nurse must be professional at all times and sensitive to the client's need for space. In addition, the nurse must proceed slowly, taking cues from the client. The client is best approached on a one-to-one basis. Clients with paranoid schizophrenia do not function well in groups or in competitive situations. The client who is suspicious often identifies others' behavior as referring to him or her (**ideas of reference**). Whispering or

BOX 12–1	**Suggestions for Dealing With Voices**

When a client with paranoid schizophrenia is having auditory hallucinations, the nurse may be able to help the client deal with the voices by instructing the client to do the following:

- Turn the voice's statements into "I statements." If the voice says "you are no good," say out loud, "Right now I feel I am no good." If you recognize the thought as your own, the voices quiet down.
- Keep a record of the time, place, and circumstances of hearing voices. Eventually you might notice a pattern and be able to avoid certain situations and thereby eliminate voices related to those situations.

telling secrets may arouse further suspicion. Before a client can learn to trust another person, the client must learn to trust himself or herself. Within a one-to-one relationship, a nurse can help by identifying moments when the client exhibits trusting behavior. For example, when the client makes a positive decision about his or her life, the nurse can respond by saying, "That was a positive choice you made. See, you can trust your decisions."

Being honest with the client is essential. Frequently, the client will give the nurse clues as to when a sense of trust has been established by allowing the nurse into his or her space.

Overly suspicious clients are potentially dangerous to themselves and others. The client needs constructive outlets for anger and aggressive drives. The nurse should be alert for early behavior clues (e.g., angry facial expression, flushed face, tremulous voice, limited attention span). By actively intervening, the nurse can help prevent later violent outbursts. Noncompetitive solitary tasks such as puzzles, ceramics, using a punching bag, and running are therapeutic. All require some concentration, yet do not require the client to compete or cooperate with others.

As the client finds alternatives for dealing with strong feelings and develops trust in self and the environment, he or she can begin to move into group situations. After experiencing success in group relations, the client is well on the way to a healthier state of being. Box 12–2 tells the story of one patient who is beginning to experience success.

CASE STUDY

NURSING CARE PLAN

The following case study demonstrates a nursing care plan for a client with paranoid schizophrenia. The example describes appropriate interventions for this client. Other interventions may be more appropriate for other types of schizophrenia.

History and Data Collection

Mr. Harry Stone is 40 years old, about 6 feet tall, and has black hair. He is a lawyer who constantly quotes legal statutes that personnel have supposedly violated while giving him care. He insists that the bank owes him $50,000, which it doesn't, and he wants to leave the hospital to get the money. He feels superior to the other clients and refuses all medications because he feels the staff are trying to change him. He is well-informed on current events.

As a result of data collection, the LPN/LVN decides that Mr. Stone's strength is that he is well-informed on current events. The nurse then uses the RN's nursing diagnoses and the data collected to detail nursing problems appropriate for intervention at the LPN/LVN level. Table 12–1 shows the result.

Goals, Interventions, Rationale, and Evaluation

Based on the nursing problems she has defined, the nurse proceeds to list appropriate goals and interventions, along with a rationale for each. These are shown in Table 12–2. With the RN's approval, she implements the interventions. ▲

BOX 12–2 | **Virginia's Story (as told in her own words)**

My diagnosis is paranoid schizophrenia. From time to time, I get upset about my diagnosis. I feel like I have been cheated out of a normal life and I blame God. I have been categorized as mentally ill for 20 years. I wouldn't say I like my condition, but age and experience have taught me that "I" am not totally defined by my diagnosis. Other people sometimes defined me by it but I have decided to be "in my corner"—to be on my side and to support and take care of me and believe I am just as "OK" as anybody else.

I try these days to see who I can be and what I can do, illness and all. The thing I am proudest of is my ability to be a friend. I work at being a friend actively. I contact people on a regular basis if I think they might become my friend. I make time to listen when my friends want to talk to me. I schedule activities with friends regularly. I try to put myself in the other person's shoes and not judge others. I try to accept that I won't be liked by everybody and pursue only those friendships where there is mutual positive regard. I realize that people with mental illnesses need support and friendship as much as anybody, but we sometimes drive others away by our "problem" behavior and eccentricities. But if we can forgive each other's problem behaviors, we can come a long way toward having satisfying relationships. Something else I try to do is become involved in meaningful work. I volunteer. I have been a lit-

eracy tutor for several years, volunteered at a hospital and at community social service agencies, and I have become involved in the mental health consumer movement. I think that the more involved I become in the community, the less I wallow in my problems. It gives me satisfaction to work with other consumers on voicing our opinions to the governmental bodies who have so much say in how we live our lives. I like to think that my experience could help somebody else in a similar situation to mine.

I like also to tackle the stigma that surrounds "mental illness." Just the act of gathering in a restaurant with three friends who struggle with the same situation is a blow to the stigma we face. We talk openly, we laugh. We may talk about our doctors and say the word schizophrenia and people may hear us, but we don't cower and we don't stop having fun. We may show others that we are not all dangerous, evil people, but just normal in most ways.

I guess more important than blaming God is believing there is some organization to life, which I have no control over. I am a tiny, small part. I want to be as happy as possible and avoid suffering as much as possible. I was given a unique life with negatives and positives and it's up to me to make it work for me by balancing out the give and take. Once I figured that out, I was on my way.

Table 12–1 | **Nursing Diagnosis and Nursing Problem for Case Study**

Nursing Diagnosis	Nursing Problem
Altered thought processes related to delusions evidenced by inability to evaluate reality	Mr. Stone has a false belief that the bank owes him money; he also believes the staff are trying to change him by giving him medication

SUMMARY

Schizophrenia is a serious, long-term illness. It includes a mixture of characteristic signs and symptoms. Normal perceptions of reality become distorted. Some of these distortions include hallucinations, delusions, ideas of reference, disorganized speech, and flat affect.

There is no one theory at present that explains all the characteristics and symptoms of schizophrenia. Biological, environmental, and social theories contribute to an understanding of schizophrenia. There are five basic types of schizo-

Table 12–2 Goals, Interventions, Rationale, and Evaluation for Case Study

Goal	Intervention	Rationale
Will take medication orally or by injection within 3 days	Use client's proper name and title (e.g., Mr. Stone) when requesting that he take medication	Use of proper name shows respect
	Offer medication orally; if he refuses, calmly state that it will be given intramuscularly because his medications are court-ordered	Nonpunitive attitude is essential; be professional at all times
Will limit his delusional verbalizations to sessions with his case manager twice daily within 1 week	Do not argue or disagree with client's delusional ideas; remind him that he is to speak of these to his case manager only	Client's ideas are fixed; by limiting expression of them to one person, trust can be developed
Will write a feature article for the hospital newspaper within 2½ weeks	Praise client for his real ability and accomplishments	Contributes a realistic sense of importance and trust in self; provides outlet for aggressive drives

Evaluation: With medication, Mr. Stone's delusional ideas began to subside. Upon discharge, he no longer believed that the bank owed him money. He agreed to see his case manager on a regular basis for medication evaluation and environmental and social support.

phrenia: paranoid type, disorganized type, catatonic type, undifferentiated type, and residual type. Schizoaffective disorder is a related disorder.

Nursing care of clients with schizophrenia presents many challenges. The nurse's goal is to help find constructive ways to meet the client's needs. The two ideas to convey to the client are (1) understanding and (2) that the client's beliefs do not reflect reality. Tact, courtesy, sensitivity, and patience are needed to establish a trusting relationship. This relationship is best achieved on a one-to-one basis.

Critical Thinking Activities

1. Evaluate the resources in your community that support the person who has schizophrenia and his or her family.

2. Describe how new knowledge about the chemistry of the brain has affected the general public's description of the illness. How does the public define *schizophrenia?*
3. You are sitting in a booth in a restaurant. Behind you is a single young man who is actively talking to himself. What are your feelings about being in a public place with someone who is exhibiting this behavior?

Review Questions

Multiple Choice—Choose the best answer to each question.

1. Negative symptoms of schizophrenia include
   a. delusions.
   b. affective flattening.
   c. disorganized speech.
   d. hallucinations.

2. A nursing intervention for a client who is delusional is to
   a. disagree with the client's delusion.
   b. make fun of the client's ideas.
   c. respond calmly and matter-of-factly.
   d. agree with the client's delusion.
3. The type of schizophrenia that involves an overly suspicious pattern of behavior is
   a. residual.
   b. paranoid.
   c. catatonic.
   d. disorganized.
4. Biological theories of schizophrenia focus on
   a. neurochemical changes in the brain.
   b. interpersonal relationships with peers.
   c. environmental changes that affect children.
   d. parental relationships with children.
5. The best way to establish a trusting relationship with a client who has schizophrenia is to
   a. involve the client in a group activity.
   b. correct the client's distorted thinking.
   c. establish a one-to-one relationship.
   d. engage the client in a game of volleyball.

References

American Psychiatric Association: Diagnostic and Statistical Manual of Mental Disorders, 4th ed. Washington, DC, American Psychiatric Association, 1994.

Kaplan HI, Sadock BJ, Grebb JA: Synopsis of Psychiatry, 7th ed. Baltimore, Williams & Wilkins, 1994, p. 457.

Lichtenstein Creative Media, Inc: Schizophrenia: Voices of an Illness, Education Kit. New York, Lichtenstein Creative Media, Inc., 1994, p 4. (Audiotape plus educational material, 60 min. Available from Burrell's Transcripts, PO Box 7, Livingston, NY 07039-0007, (800) 777-8398, cost $21).

Marder SR: Antipsychotic drugs. In: Tasman A, Kay J, Lieberman JA (eds): Psychiatry, vol 2. Philadelphia, WB Saunders Co, 1997.

NARSAD Research: Understanding Schizophrenia: A Guide for People with Schizophrenia and Their Families. Great Neck, NY, NARSAD, 1996.

Pinals DA, Breier A: Schizophrenia. In: Tasman A, Kay J, Lieberman JA (eds.): Psychiatry, vol 2. Philadelphia, WB Saunders Co, 1997.

Torrey EF, Bowler AE, Taylor EH, et al: Schizophrenia and Manic-Depressive Disorder: The Biological Roots of Mental Illness as Revealed by the Landmark Study of Identical Twins, New York, Basic Books, 1994. p. 213.

Townsend MC: Nursing Diagnoses in Psychiatric Nursing: A Pocket Guide for Care Plan Construction. Philadelphia, FA Davis Co, 1994.

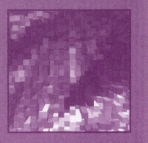

Chapter THIRTEEN

Depressive Mood Disorders

Outline

- **Types of Depressive Disorders**
    Major Depression
    Melancholic Depression
    Unipolar Depression
    Dysthymic Depression
    Double Depression
    Seasonal Affective Depression
        Disorder
- **Gender Differences**
    Serotonin
    Internal Versus External Disorders
    Sexual Harassment, Discrimination,
        and Abuse

  Psychological Differences
  Coping Style
  Special Female Issues
  Special Male Issues
- **Treatment Options**
  Physical/Medical Treatments
  Psychosocial Therapies
- **Nursing Interventions**
- **Case Study: Nursing Care Plan**
  History and Data Collection
  Goals, Intervention, Rationale, and
      Evaluation

Key Terms

- **affect**
- **egocentrism**
- **hypersomnia**
- **insomnia**
- **intra-aggression**

- **mood**
- **psychomotor agitation**
- **psychomotor retardation**
- **serotonin**

Objectives

Upon completing this chapter, the student will be able to:
1. Differentiate among:
    - major depression
    - melancholic depression
    - unipolar depression
    - dysthymic depression
    - double depression
2. Discuss responses to depression based on gender differences.

Objectives—cont'd

3. Describe two types of treatments available for depressive disorders.
4. Give an example of the type of suicidal feelings common with depression.
5. Discuss nursing interventions that may be helpful when dealing with clients experiencing depression.

Mood disorders, also known as *affective disorders,* refer to depressive and bipolar disorders. **Mood,** in this context, refers to a prolonged, exaggerated emotion that overwhelms a person's psychic life. Terms such as *joy, grief, elation,* and *sadness* are used to describe a particular mood (Varcarolis, 1998, p. 552). **Affect** describes how a person expresses an emotion that accompanies an idea verbally or nonverbally.

People of all ages are vulnerable to mood disorders. The highest rate occurs in people who are 25 to 44 years of age. The age of onset continues to become earlier and is now in the teens. Mood disorders continue to be among the most common treatable disorders; yet the diagnosis is often missed, or the problem is diagnosed as something else.

Mood disorders affect the way people feel about themselves and their world. People with depression experience feelings of unbearable sadness or irritability, despair, and hopelessness. They frequently desire death. Their ability to think, feel, and function, as well as their physical and spiritual health, are all affected.

Reality Check

If someone tells you he or she is feeling depressed, how can you determine if the person is truly depressed or "feeling bad"?

Numerous theories attempt to explain why a person becomes seriously (clinically) depressed. Some of these include the following:

- The inability to deal with angry feelings in a positive way, causing anger to be turned in on oneself (introjection)
- Flawed thinking (cognitive theory)
- Neurotransmitter irregularities (biological theory)

It is widely accepted that, as with many physical illnesses, people may be biologically predisposed to depression and that environmental factors are needed to trigger the illness. Despite the cause, the basic characteristic in all types of depression is low self-esteem.

TYPES OF DEPRESSIVE DISORDERS

The American Psychiatric Association's *Diagnostic and Statistical Manual of Mental Disorders, fourth edition* (DSM-IV) identifies features that define and differentiate the various forms of depression. Depending on the features, depression is labeled as major, melancholic, unipolar, dysthymic, and double depression. Researchers are only now beginning to study double depression (APA, pp. 317–391).

Major Depression

The distinguishing feature of major depression is a depressed mood (extreme sadness that influences functioning). Other characteristics include loss of interest or pleasure in activities (anhedonia) and at least four of the following:

- Weight gain or loss
- **Insomnia** or **hypersomnia** (sleeping too little or too much without a satisfying rest)
- **Psychomotor agitation** (constant motion, person may be prone to accidents)
- **Psychomotor retardation** (all physical activity slowed, including speech; speech is often monotone or a whisper; constipation is common)
- Fatigue (unrelated to work or rest)

- Sense of worthlessness or guilt (no logical reason involved)
- Problems concentrating or indecisiveness (these symptoms bring people into treatment)
- Suicidal ideation or attempts (most consider a passive way such as "I wouldn't mind if a truck hit me." Suicide is more common in mania or schizophrenia disorders than in depression (Nolen-Hoeksema, 1997).

Symptoms must last continuously for at least 2 weeks and be severe enough to interfere with activities of daily living. All depressions share similar symptoms. Diagnostic difference is based on severity, length of time, effect on activities of daily living, and response to treatment. Although the DSM-IV does not include loss of sexual interest as a criteria for depression, it is common. Even after recovery, with or without medication, it is the slowest to return.

Reality Check

Think of an example, other than the ones provided, for each of the symptoms of major depression: depressed mood, anhedonia, weight gain or loss, sleep disturbance, psychomotor retardation, fatigue, problems of concentration or indecisiveness, and suicide ideation.

Melancholic Depression

Melancolic depression is a severe form of major depression. Symptoms are worse in the morning. The person tends to awaken early and feels terrible. This is an especially at-risk time for suicide attempts. Guilty thoughts may be of psychotic proportions. Clients with melancholic depression are especially responsive to antidepressive medication. Therefore the illness is considered biological in nature.

Unipolar Depression

Major depression can occur separately or as part of a bipolar (manic-depressive) disorder. *Unipolar*

depression is a major depression that is not part of a bipolar disorder. (The "uni" prefix in the word *unipolar* means "one.")

Dysthymic Depression

A less severe, but more chronic, low-grade form of depression is known as *dysthymic depression (dysthymia)*. The client has a depressed mood most of the day for more days than not. Onset can be in childhood (see Chapter 9). Clients who experience a major depression usually return to the dysthymic state when they recover from the major depression.

Double Depression

When a person has both dysthymia and a major depression, he or she is said to have *double depression*. This type of depression appears more resistive to treatment than other types of depression. Recovery, when it occurs, is to the dysthymic level only. This means that the person maintains a low level of depressive symptoms as a part of his or her ongoing thinking, feeling, and doing (Nolen-Hoeksema, 1997).

Seasonal Affective Depressive Disorder

Some people experience depression during the fall to spring season if there is less sunlight. This form of depression is known as *seasonal affective depressive disorder (SADD or SAD)*. The depressive symptoms are similar to those of other depressions. Use of light therapy has been shown to be effective with some people.

GENDER DIFFERENCES

Women are twice as likely to become depressed as are men. Current studies are disputing earlier gender-related findings, providing new information and raising numerous questions. Some issues that are being studied in regard to their relationship to depression follow.

Serotonin

One small study on healthy adults used new imaging techniques to measure the level of **sero-**

tonin, a mood-regulating hormone and neurotransmitter that is secreted in the brain. The men in the study produced an average of 52% more of the neurotransmitter than women. Researchers wonder if this means that women have less reserve of the neurotransmitter and therefore go into depression more quickly. However, more studies are needed before conclusions can be drawn. Researchers need to confirm that the serotonin was measured accurately, for example. They also need to determine whether women have less serotonin, but use it more efficiently. Although the number of people in the study was small (15 people), it shows the effort to begin to measure scientifically the amount of neurotransmitters in the brains of live males and females.

Internal Versus External Disorders

Women in general are more prone to internal disorders (depression, anxiety, eating disorders) but not to other psychopathology. Men are more prone to develop external disorders (conduct disorders, antisocial disorders).

Sexual Harassment, Discrimination, and Abuse

The rate of depression for women is significantly greater than it is for men when sexual harassment, sexual discrimination, or physical or sexual abuse is present. (Nolen-Hoeksema, 1997.) However, depression in these circumstances may be underreported by men.

Psychological Differences

Nolen-Hoeksema's 1990 study of gender differences in depression provided interesting information about psychological differences in women. Women tend to define themselves by relationships (wife, mother, daughter, friend). They generally have a larger, broader, and deeper social network than men. Although the broader network gives women a larger support system, it also gives them more people to be depressed about. Men tend to focus on the whole picture, whereas women often focus on details.

Coping Style

Ruminative coping is more common for women than men. Rumination is a way of going through the same thoughts again and again without determining a course of positive action to solve the problem (see Chapter 8). The passive thoughts focus attention on the depressed mood, its causes, and its consequences. This increases the depressive thinking and interferes with problem solving. Furthermore, women generally choose activities that focus on the issue(s). Men choose activities that get their mind off the issue(s). This is often played out in relationships where she says "I've been going over what happened again and again" and he says "I really haven't given it any thought" (Nolen-Hoeksema, 1997).

Reality Check

Think of an example of ruminative thinking from real life.

Special Female Issues

Some problems, by definition, are associated more with women than men. These include issues surrounding menstruation, childbirth, and role overload.

Premenstrual Period

Contrary to conclusions drawn from earlier studies, current studies show that the premenstrual period is not a major time of depression for most women. A small subgroup of women (1% to 3%) who do become depressed share a personal and/or family history of depression (Nolen-Hoeksema, 1997).

Reality Check

What was your belief before reading this section about the premenstrual period and its relationship to depression?

Postpartum Blues

About 50% of women experience emotional lability (mood swings) after childbirth. This is commonly known as the *postpartum blues*. The mood swings are thought to be related to hormonal changes and sleep deprivation. New fathers may experience similar symptoms. The common thread for both mother and father is sleep deprivation.

Postpartum Depression

Postpartum depression is a true depression that needs intervention. It affects one in four women. A clue to assist in predicting its possible occurrence: whatever depression was present during pregnancy will only get worse. Other contributing factors include marital problems, obstetric complications, child-care problems, lack of a social support system, pessimistic thinking style, and/or other current life stressors perceived as severe.

Premenopause and Postmenopause

Premenopause and postmenopause are not considered a high-risk time for depression unless the woman has a history of previous depression.

Role Overload

Although frequently a subject of cartoons, role overload is not an important contributor to depression. In fact, women with more roles are less likely to get depressed. A varied social support system contributes to positive mental health. Multiple roles act as a buffer to stress.

Special Male Issues

Issues specific to men emerge in childhood as emotions are externalized. A common male practice is to translate negative emotions into anger and act them out (for example, the fast-driving teen). Irritability often substitutes for a sad mood. The number of men incarcerated is sometimes compared to the number of women in pain (internalized emotion).

Suicide is the number five killer of males between ages 25 and 44 years. (The top four are accidents, AIDS, heart disease, and cancer.)

Whereas the rates of depression in women have decreased by approximately 33%, rates for men have shown a 26% increase in the last 20 years. Caucasian men over age 65 have the highest suicide rate in the United States. Men over 85 years kill themselves at a rate 13 times greater than women in general. Roughly 24,000 men commit suicide each year. Although no one knows exactly why, some of the reasons suggested include the following:

- Single and divorced men have higher rates of depression and suicide than married men.
- Unemployed men (related to job loss) are twice as likely to commit suicide than those who are employed. Women's rates are not affected by job status. It is thought that men bottle their emotions and kill themselves quietly.
- The typical male suicide victim is a middle-class, well-educated man who knows how to hide his emotions.
- The nomadic family lifestyle that is so common today disrupts long-lasting relationships and support systems. Men tend to be more isolated.
- Loneliness that is eased by drinking alcohol and other substance abuse increases suicide risk fivefold.
- Fear of exposure of secrets men wish to take to the grave may prompt suicide (e.g., affairs).
- Chemical/biological differences yet to be clearly defined may provide clues.
- An unexpected reason for increasing male suicide may be success. The easier life becomes, the harder men are on themselves. Suicide is usually farthest from the mind when struggling to survive. One study found that both men and soldiers in the general population have an increased suicide rate during peacetime, not war (Gutfield, 1996, pp. 136–163).

TREATMENT OPTIONS

It was initially thought that depression was time-limited and would go away without treatment. It appears now that, even after a year, only about half of those people diagnosed with depression have recovered. Furthermore, the relapse rate is higher than was originally recognized. The more episodes a person experiences, the more frequently the episodes reappear. The earlier the onset in life, the earlier the relapse. Current thinking is that intervention must be both early and aggressive with both adults and children. Comorbidity (mixed diagnosis) is common with depression and is considered as part of the treatment decision. Common coexisting diagnoses include substance abuse, anxiety, and traumatic stress syndrome. The combined diagnosis of depression and anxiety poses the greatest suicidal risk.

Physical/Medical Treatments

Physical and medical treatments that are currently available include psychotherapeutic medications, light therapy (for people with SADD) and electroconvulsive therapy. Additional information about these treatment forms is found in Chapter 23.

Psychosocial Therapies

Psychosocial therapies are also known as *talk therapies*. The purpose is to deal with underlying issues causing the problems and to help the client learn and practice more effective ways of coping. Psychosocial therapies include psychoanalysis, cognitive-behavioral therapy, and interpersonal therapy, among others.

Psychosocial therapy is often used with psychotherapeutic medications. When these methods are used together, the medication is meant to take the edge off the symptoms and permit the client to explore underlying issues. Enough discomfort remains to provide motivation for change. Additional information is provided in Chapter 24.

NURSING INTERVENTIONS

Nursing interventions include attention to physical health issues: eating, sleeping, elimination, and personal hygiene. To intervene effectively, the nurse must understand something about the client. The client who is depressed may deal with his or her anger using **intra-aggression**—turning the anger inward so that it no longer poses an exter-

nal threat to the individual. However, the client feels guilty about the anger and verbalizes these feelings through self-depreciation. Statements such as "Why do you waste your time on me?" or "Why don't you talk to someone more deserving?" are repeated over and over. The client's entire conversation centers around himself or herself. This is known as **egocentrism** (me, myself, and I). The client's relationships are immature and dependent.

The appearance of the client who is depressed is also distinctive. The face appears deeply sad and hopeless; posture is usually stooped. All of the body movements are slow, even though the client may pace back and forth. The pacing is a way of dealing with anxiety and is sometimes referred to as *agitated depression*.

The nurse feels the client's depression; it is usually obvious. The nurse should remember that the client needs to feel this way, at this time, to deal with the guilt and ultimate anger. Therefore it is useless to reassure the client that he or she is worthy and that there is no need to feel unworthy.

Reality Check

Explain why it is important for the nurse to separate his or her feelings from those of the client.

The client's ability to process information is decreased. Sometimes just being with the client without trying to carry on a conversation is the most reassuring thing a nurse can do. For example, it may be helpful to tell the client "You do not need to talk; I just want to sit with you for awhile." When the nurse leaves, he or she might say, "I'm leaving now. I'll be back before I leave work at 3:00 PM." It is then important to be there as promised.

All of the client's internal body functions are slowed down, so elimination, eating, and sleeping can become problems. The nurse must evaluate and provide for the client's physical care.

When depression is severe, it is important to keep the client's life simple and to make minimal demands. Menial tasks or hard work may be a way of dealing constructively with the client's covert anger and need for self-punishment. Asking the client to do something for himself or herself is usually unsuccessful because the client feels unworthy. However, the client may be receptive to doing something for the nurse if it is a sincere request. For example, "I am pressed for time. I would appreciate it if you would straighten out the magazines, books, and newspapers in the day room." When the client has completed the task, the nurse should thank the client sincerely, but without overdoing it: the "thank you" should be simple and task-related.

If the client expresses hostility outwardly in a positive way, this is a good sign. The nurse can use this opportunity to support the client, sharing with him or her the benefits of dealing with anger constructively. For example, "I am glad you told me that you do not want to straighten the magazines, books, and newspapers." The nurse should remember that although he or she is able to pick up on the client's feeling tone, the comments are not personally directed toward the nurse.

Early morning hours are difficult for the client who is severely depressed. Regardless of the number of hours slept, the sleep has been disrupted and unsatisfying. Sometimes sleep involves nightmares or bad dreams. The client tends to awaken early and feels terrible. The promise of a refreshing sleep has not been delivered. Clients who are suicidal and have improved enough to make a plan and carry it out may attempt suicide at this time. Sometimes they pretend to be sleeping during early morning bed checks. It is a good idea for the nurse to check on these clients more frequently and at unexpected times. The client is aware of what lies ahead to get his or her life back together. It may seem overwhelming, especially if the client has been through a depression before. The suicide attempt may be an effort to avoid the emotional pain that lies ahead.

It is often difficult to engage clients with depression in activities. There is a period in the late afternoon or early evening when the depression lifts slightly. The nurse can take advantage of this period to reach the client and possibly share simple activities with him or her.

When giving the client oral medication, the nurse should check to be sure the client has actually swallowed the medication. "Cheeking," that is, storing the medication in the cheek to pretend it was swallowed, is a common practice. The client may save the pills until he or she has saved enough to attempt suicide. The nurse should check inside the cheeks, the roof of the mouth, and along the top and bottom gum lines for hidden medication.

CASE STUDY

NURSING CARE PLAN

The following case study demonstrates a nursing care plan for a client with major depression. The example describes appropriate interventions for this client. Other interventions may be more appropriate for clients with other personal characteristics and other types of depression.

History and Data Collection

Mrs. Motley is a 50-year-old woman with gray hair who moves very slowly about the area. Her face is haggard, and her head is bent low. She repeatedly states that she is unworthy to have any care and wonders why nurses bother with her. She says "I wish I were dead." She neglects her personal appearance because she says she doesn't deserve to look nice. When her children were home, she was very neat and meticulous about her housekeeping. At present, her appetite is poor, and she insists that she does not sleep much at night.

The LPN/LVN doing the assessment Mrs. Motley identifies psychomotor retardation and self-depreciation, neglect of personal hygiene, decrease in appetite, and sleep disturbance. He further identifies a previous history of adequate functioning as Mrs. Motley's major strength.

Table 13–1	Nursing Diagnosis and Nursing Problem for Case Study

Nursing Diagnosis	Nursing Problem
Ineffective individual coping R/T overwhelming feelings of depression evidenced by statements of unworthiness; inadequate personal hygiene, eating, and sleeping	Mrs. Motley does not take care of her personal needs (hygiene, eating, sleeping) because she feels unworthy

The nurse then uses the RN's nursing diagnoses and the data collected to detail nursing problems appropriate for intervention at the LPN/LVN level. Table 13–1 shows the result.

Goals, Interventions, Rationale, and Evaluation

Based on the nursing problems he has defined, the nurse proceeds to list appropriate goals and interventions, along with a rationale for each. These are shown in Table 13–2. With the RN's approval, he implements the interventions and evaluates their effectiveness. Table 13–2 shows the goals, interventions, and rationales, along with the nurse's evaluation.

Table 13–2	Goals, Interventions, Rationale, and Evaluation for Case Study	

Goal	Intervention	Rationale
Will take medication as prescribed	Give medication as ordered; check to see that she has swallowed it	The medication is a mood elevator
	Offer simple explanation of how soon the medication is expected to work and of side effects, if they occur	Most are effective in 1–4 weeks, depending on the drug; side effects show up before the desired effect
	Sit with the client; avoid being overly cheerful; tell her she does not have to respond; let her know when you are going to leave and when you will return	Support without being annoying Develop trust
	Do not try to convince her that her ideas about herself are wrong	Client needs her symptoms at this time
Will care for her personal needs with minimum supervision; will accept warm milk to help her sleep at night	Initially perform all care for her; gradually withdraw assistance as she is able to care for herself, offer positive reinforcement for what she accomplishes; be specific; avoid gushing	Meet physical needs while encouraging self-care; support self-worth

Evaluation: Day 2—Mrs. Motley is taking medications, recognizes that dry mouth is a side effect, and accepts mouth care and additional liquids. Takes bath and shampoos with minimal help. Eating about half of food at meals and all of snacks. Beginning to respond with single words to nurse.

SUMMARY

People of all ages are vulnerable to depression. Twice the number of women experience depression as do men. Men, however, are more likely to commit suicide. Depression continues to be underdiagnosed, incorrectly diagnosed, and untreated. Effective treatments, including antidepressive medications, light therapy, and psychotherapy, are available.

Depressive disorders are labeled as major, melancholic, unipolar, and dysthymic according to DSM-IV criteria. Double depression is the occurrence of major depression and dysthymia concurrently.

Nursing interventions include attention to physical health issues: eating, sleeping, elimination, and personal hygiene. Monitoring medication effects and side effects and being sure medication is actually consumed are important responsibilities for the nurse.

Critical Thinking Activities

1. When you feel down, what do you do to change your mood?
2. Be aware of how your mood is affected when you are with someone who is feeling down.

Review Questions

Multiple Choice—Choose the best answer to each question.

1. What is a differentiating factor in melancholic depression?
   a. It is part of a bipolar disorder
   b. Clients are especially responsive to antidepressive medication
   c. It is a less severe, but more chronic form of depression
   d. Clients maintain a low level of depressive symptoms
2. Which of the following is a gender factor related to depression?
   a. Ruminative coping is more common for women than men
   b. Men define themselves by relationships such as father, husband, son
   c. Women are more prone to develop external disorders such as conduct disorders
   d. Men experience more depression as a result of sexual harassment
3. Which of the following treatments is effective for clients who experience SADD?
   a. Psychosocial therapy
   b. ECT
   c. Psychotherapeutic drugs
   d. Light therapy
4. Which is an example of common suicidal feelings experienced by a client with major depression?
   a. "I'm going to take my radio in the bathtub with me"
   b. "My husband's gun will work just fine to kill myself"
   c. "I wouldn't mind if a truck would hit me"
   d. "I can't wait to get out and kill myself"
5. What nursing intervention may be most helpful with a client who is seriously depressed?
   a. Expect participation in group games
   b. Sit with the client without making demands
   c. Leave the client alone so he or she can experience the depression
   d. Avoid touching the client because of sexual interpretation

References

American Psychiatric Association: Diagnostic and Statistical Manual of Mental Disorders. 4th ed. Washington, DC, American Psychiatric Association, 1994.

Gutfeld G: Suicide squeeze. Men's Health, April 1996, p 136–163.

Nolen-Hoeksema S: Understanding Depression: A Seminar For Health Professionals. Duluth, Minnesota, April 1997.

Varcarolis EM: Depressive disorders. In: Varcarolis EM (ed): Foundations of Psychiatric Mental Health Nursing, 3rd ed. Philadelphia, WB Saunders Co, 1998.

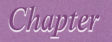

Chapter

FOURTEEN

Bipolar Mood Disorders

Outline

- Characteristics of Mood Episodes
- Classification of Bipolar Disorders
- Treatment Options
    Physical Treatments
    Psychotherapies

- Nursing Interventions
- Case Study: Nursing Care Plan
    History and Data Collection
    Goals, Interventions, Rationale, and
    Evaluation

Key Terms

- delusions of grandeur
- distractibility
- episodes

- flight of ideas
- mania
- reaction formation

Objectives

Upon completing this chapter, the student will be able to:

1. Differentiate between episodes and disorders of bipolar mood disorders.
2. Discuss the range of elated moods.
   - normal
   - hypomanic
   - manic
3. Explain the coping mechanism of reaction formation as it appears in the client with mania.
4. Differentiate among bipolar I, bipolar II, and cyclothymic disorders.
5. Discuss physical and psychotherapeutic treatment options.
6. Describe the kind of physical environment needed as part of nursing intervention for the client during a manic episode.
7. List the usual areas of focus in the physical care of the client.
8. Give an example of using the client's symptom of distractibility to redirect behavior.

dentification of individual mood **episodes,** or occurrences, is used as the basis for diagnosing bipolar disorders (Bauer, 1997, p. 967.) The prefix *bi* reflects that the person has experienced both depressive and elated mood episodes.

Bipolar disorders are distributed fairly equally between both sexes. They tend to occur more in individuals of higher socioeconomic means. The incidence of bipolar disorder has continued to increase since the 1940s. Reasons are unclear. Families with a history of bipolar disorders experience an earlier onset of the illness. The most common comorbidity factors involved are alcohol abuse, drug abuse, and drug dependency. They may be related to the client's effort to self-medicate.

CHARACTERISTICS OF MOOD EPISODES

Elated moods can range from normal highs to hypomania to mania. The person is in touch with reality and is able to continue work and social functioning. People with **mania** experience feelings of excitement, elation, or extreme irritability. Clients with all types of bipolar disease experience elevated, irritable moods. Other symptoms involved may include the following:

- **Delusions of grandeur:** This presents as self-inflated self-esteem, being more talkative than usual. The client experiences a pressure to keep talking.
- **Flight of ideas:** The mind races from one thought to another without completing a thought. The idea is complete, as far as it is expressed.
- **Distractibility:** Attention is easily diverted to unimportant or outside stimuli. Someone walking into the room can trigger an entirely different conversation.
- Increase in goal-directed activity: This may involve socialization, work, sexual activity, etc. The client rarely completes a project before initiating a new project.
- Increased involvement in pleasurable activities that have a high potential for undesired conse-

quences: This may involve unrestrained buying sprees, sexual indiscretions, unwise business investments, and so on.

The symptoms experienced by the client are similar in hypomania and mania. They vary in degree and the amount of time the symptoms last. The person with hypomania experiences a lower level of manic symptoms, is in touch with reality, and is able to continue work and social functioning. As with depression, the person's thinking, feeling, doing, and physical and spiritual health are affected. According to Nolen-Hoeksema (1997), suicide is more common for the client with mania than for the client with depression. Thoughts of suicide are active rather than passive.

Reaction formation is a major coping mechanism during a manic episode. The person acts as though he or she is happy and on top of the world. However, as the nurse may note with careful observation, manic episodes result from underlying depression. It is as though all of the constant physical activity, rapid speech, racing thoughts, and superior attitude are a cover for the feelings of helplessness and low self-esteem. The closer the feelings of depression are to the surface, the more rapidly the person attempts to run from the feeling. Sometimes the mania reaches a psychotic state. The mania can last from weeks to months or cycle rapidly from mania to depression to mania as it does in a mixed episode (both manic and depressive symptoms within the same episode).

CLASSIFICATION OF BIPOLAR DISORDERS

Bipolar disorders are classified as bipolar type I, bipolar type II, and cyclothymic disorders (APA, 1994, pp. 317–391).

- *Bipolar type I* indicates that the person has experienced a major depressive episode plus a manic/mixed episode that has lasted at least a week.
- *Bipolar type II* involves a major depressive episode plus a hypomanic episode lasting at least 4 days.

• *Cyclothymic disorder* involves chronic fluctuations between depressive symptoms and hypomanic symptoms that do not meet the criteria for major depression. Symptoms must have been present for at least 2 years in adults.

TREATMENT OPTIONS

The specific treatment for the client experiencing a bipolar disorder depends on the type of episode. Preventing exacerbation (recurrence of symptoms) is a long-term goal. A therapeutic relationship and cooperation among the client, the psychiatrist, and select staff are essential to make this goal a reality. The client enjoys some of the symptoms: the inflated self-esteem or grandiosity and the decreased need for sleep. When the medication begins to work, it often leaves clients feeling comparatively "low." Approximately 60% discontinue taking the medication on their own.

Physical Treatments

Physical treatments for bipolar disorders are usually based on medication. Lithium, a mood-stabilizing agent, is one widely used medication. Others include antidepressants, anticonvulsants, neuroleptics, benzodiazepines, and various experimental medications (Bauer, 1997, p. 989). The type of medication depends on the needs of the individual client. See Chapter 22 for a discussion on psychotherapeutic medications.

Psychotherapies

Psychotherapeutic treatments are not well defined for clients with bipolar disorders. Symptoms and difficult defensive techniques get in the way of incorporating clients into traditional psychotherapies. Clients do, however, need to learn about the illness and how to participate in long-term management. Treatment must also address the client's family and other interpersonal relationships, behavior and thinking patterns, and becoming involved with community support systems.

One approach to psychotherapeutic treatment for bipolar disorders is a two-phase program developed by Bauer and McBride. The first phase of this program educates the client and family about the course of the disease and addresses disease management issues. Disease management teaches the client to take responsibility for taking medication, stabilizing his or her diet and exercise, and identifying first signs and symptoms of drug side effects and/or recurrence of mania.

The second phase of this program addresses functional deficits such as behavior and interpersonal relationships. It takes a cognitive-behavioral approach, looking at faulty patterns of thought and functioning. It introduces the client to new ways of thinking and doing (Bauer, 1977, p. 983).

NURSING INTERVENTIONS

The client experiencing a manic episode needs a nonchallenging atmosphere and protection from overstimulation. A quiet area removed from the center of activity is often helpful. He or she also needs a nurse who can accept the client's demeaning and challenging verbalizations calmly and matter-of-factly. Any other response tends to increase the client's guilt feelings. Limit setting is also necessary. The nurse should set limits on behavior that is harmful to the client or others, as well as on behavior that interferes with the rights of others. The client's attempts to belittle staff, as well as vulgar conversation and speech, should be ignored. While doing this, it is important that the nurse accept the client as an individual, but not approve of the client's behavior. Anyone with disturbed feelings is sensitive to the nurse's nonverbal communication.

The client has a short attention span and is easily distracted. The nurse should use this distractibility to avoid difficult situations whenever possible. The flight of ideas permits the nurse to introduce a new, nonstimulating idea without waiting for the client to stop talking. As long as the topics introduced do not excite the client, the nurse can help the client stay in control. Overstimulation may result in the client being out of control to the point of needing additional medication and even seclusion. With practice, the nurse can become skilled in assisting the client to avoid out-of-control behavior most of the time.

To distract successfully, the nurse must have constructive outlets and activities in mind. Depending on the client's physical health, a punching bag, jogging, tearing rags, housekeeping, talks, and volleyball may provide outlets for excessive energy. For some clients, these activities may be overstimulating. The nurse must know the client's needs. Finger and brush painting are often a good medium for expressing feelings without overstimulating the client.

The client needs constant reassurance that he or she is a worthy human being. The elevated mood and overactivity may appear humorous. However, the nurse must take care not to encourage this type of behavior and should laugh with, not at, the client. Overstimulating the client is far easier than quieting him or her down. Furthermore, the nurse is responsible for preventing the client from humiliating himself or herself in front of others (e.g., a "decorative" style of dressing, like undershorts over the jeans). Neglect of personal and physical needs is common. The client is too busy to eat, sleep, go to the bathroom, or take a bath. The nurse should provide physical care as needed and try to anticipate what will be needed. For example, the nurse may provide finger foods and fluids while the client is in the manic phase. Dehydration can be a serious problem.

The nurse is an important part of the client's treatment team. Distributing medications and monitoring both effects and side effects of medications is one of those responsibilities. A subtle clue, such as confusion, is an important toxic side effect of lithium that is often missed. Clients treated with antidepressants for bipolar depression may recycle rapidly. The nurse should review effects and side effects of medications over again even if he or she has given medications for years.

Two clients experiencing mania will increase each other's behavior when in the same area. However, a single client with mania is sometimes an asset in the company of withdrawn and depressed clients. The client may be able to stimulate activity even though his or her distractibility will not permit follow-through. The client often assumes too many responsibilities without completing any of them. Be alert to this and control the number of functions the client assumes.

Reality Check

Mrs. Clara Hopper, age 30, was previously hospitalized during a depressive episode. This time, the staff found it difficult to recognize her. The low-cut, short, red, velvet dress decorated with bows; blonde, moussed hair; and multiple necklaces, bracelets, and rings were a contrast to the dark-haired lady in the baggy sweats and slippers during the previous admission. During the current admission, Mrs. Hopper talked continuously in incomplete sentences that were only loosely connected with previous thoughts. Much of the conversation was about her singing career, three-piece band, one-night stands, the numerous men in her life, and living in a van while touring the country. All of this was a stark contrast from the stay-at-home mother of two boys, ages 3 and 5, that had been admitted during the depressive episode.

Explain how Mrs. Hopper is using reaction-formation as her coping mechanism.

CASE STUDY

NURSING CARE PLAN

The following case study demonstrates a nursing care plan for a client with mania. The example describes appropriate interventions for this client. Other interventions may be more appropriate for clients with bipolar disorders and/or other personal characteristics.

History and Data Collection

Mr. Rally is a salesman, rather short and bald, who looks younger than his 45 years. He is dressed in garish clothes trying to emulate his favorite movie star, saying "I'm his right-hand man." He is constantly in motion, calls everyone "darling," and attempts to hug and kiss everyone on the cheek. He talks endlessly in incomplete sentences strung together. Mr. Rally makes sexual remarks and gestures to female clients and staff. He is highly critical of how the unit is run. "I've run hundreds of businesses." However, he recently lost his money and home in a get-rich-quick deal he devised. He is too busy to eat or drink properly. Personal hygiene is long overdue. He reports sleeping 3 to 4 hours per night.

The LPN/LVN who is collecting data on (assessing) Mr. Rally identifies psychomotor agitation, inflated self-esteem, flight of ideas, as well as inappropriate sexual comments and clothing. She further identifies neglect of physical health and hygiene.

The nurse uses the RN's nursing diagnoses and the data collected to detail nursing problems appropriate for intervention at the LPN/LVN level. Table 14–1 shows the result.

Goals, Interventions, Rationale, and Evaluation

Based on the nursing problems she has defined, the nurse proceeds to list appropriate goals and inter-

Table 14–1	Nursing Diagnosis and Nursing Problem for Case Study
Nursing Diagnosis	**Nursing Problem**
Self-care deficit related to overactivity evidenced by poor eating habits, sleep deficit, and inadequate personal hygiene and grooming	Mr. Rally is too busy to eat, sleep, bathe, and groom properly

ventions, along with a rationale for each. With the RN's approval, she implements the interventions and evaluates their effect. Goals, interventions, rationales, and the nurse's evaluation are shown in Table 14–2.

▲

SUMMARY

Mood disorders refer to both bipolar and depressive disorders (Chapters 13–14). People of all ages are vulnerable to mood disorders. Gender differences do not exist in bipolar disorders in the way they do for depression. However, a family history of bipolar disorders is significant.

The American Psychiatric Association's *Diagnostic and Statistical Manual of Mental Disorders, fourth edition* (DSM-IV) uses identification of individual mood episodes for diagnosing bipolar disorder. Classifications include bipolar type I, bipolar type II, and cyclothymic disorders. Each diagnosis implies that the client has experienced forms of both depression and mania.

Treatment options include lithium, antidepressants, and anticonvulsants because of their mood-stabilizing properties. Electroconvulsive therapy (ECT) is used occasionally. Adjunctive medications such as antipsychotics and benzodiazepines are used as needed. Maintenance treatment to prevent relapse into either manic or depressive episodes is a long-term goal. Lithium is often the drug of choice. Education regarding the course of illness and its medical management is essential to attain compliance. Comorbidity may exist.

Nursing intervention includes assisting with physical care, giving medications, and observing effects and possible side effects. The nurse is challenged to avoid overstimulation when dealing with the client with mania. Using symptoms such as distractibility is often a way to avoid conflict. The nurse should recall that beneath the surface of this boastful, funny, often vulgar, and sexual facade is a person running away from depression. The comments are not personal. The nurse should set limits only on what is important.

Table 14–2	Goals, Interventions, Rationale, and Evaluation for Case Study	
Goal	**Intervention**	**Rationale**
Mr. Rally will take his medication as prescribed daily	Give medication and monitor blood level as ordered	Medication targets overactive behavior and, in turn, physical care
Mr. Rally will eat by himself in his room with supervision until overactivity and distractibility have decreased	Offer finger foods and high-calorie liquids	Meet nutritional requirements; can eat while moving about
	Remove to a nonstimulating area, such as his room	Decreased stimulation permits single focus
Mr. Rally will accept help with physical care and in selection of wearing apparel	Remind client to go to the toilet, to brush his teeth, to bathe	Meet physical care needs
	With his assistance, select comfortable and neat-appearing clothes for him	Offer choices, prevent embarrassment
Mr. Rally will contact only his assigned nurse for requests	Maintain a calm, matter-of-fact manner when he is making inappropriate remarks or gestures; do not take remarks personally; refer him to assigned nurse for requests	Non-defensive approach
	Use distraction when he is overactive; suggest an activity that can be completed in a short period of time	Utilize short attention span in a positive way
	As with all clients, maintain a suicide watch while he is in the manic phase	

Evaluation: One week after admission, the nurse records that Mr. Rally's rate of overactivity is beginning to diminish. He has eaten by himself in his room with supervision for the past 2 days. He is able to complete his personal care with limited assistance today and slept a total of 5 hours last night.

Critical Thinking Activities

1. Sit in a room. Become aware of all the actual sounds that surround you both in the room and outside of the room. React to each sound. Experience "distractibility."
2. Attend to the thoughts going on in your mind. Is each thought completed before you go on to the next thought? Experience "flight of ideas."

Review Questions

Multiple Choice—Choose the best answer to each question.

1. Which of the following is an explanation of reaction formation?
   a. Reaction is far beyond what the issue merits
   b. Acts as though there is no problem

c. Behaves the opposite of the underlying feeling

d. Separates the emotion from his/her behavior

2. How is bipolar type I defined?
   a. A major depression plus a manic/mixed episode
   b. A major depressive episode plus a hypomanic episode
   c. Chronic fluctuations between depressive symptoms and hypomanic symptoms
   d. Depressive reaction of psychotic proportions

3. Which medication is most closely linked with treatment of manic episodes?
   a. Benzodiazepines
   b. Anticonvulsants
   c. Vitamin B_6
   d. Lithium

4. What approach is suggested for the nurse dealing with the client during a manic episode?
   a. Calm, matter-of-fact
   b. Restrictive
   c. Confrontive
   d. Businesslike

5. Why does the client tend to overlook physical care needs during a manic episode?
   a. Feels that he or she does not deserve care
   b. Is suspicious of staff and other clients
   c. Out of touch with reality
   d. Too busy to eat, sleep, bathe, groom

References

American Psychiatric Association: *Diagnostic and Statistical Manual of Mental Disorders,* 4th ed. Washington, DC, American Psychiatric Association, 1994.

Bauer M: Bipolar disorders. In: Tasman A, Kay J, Lieberman J (eds): *Psychiatry,* vol 2. Philadelphia, WB Saunders Co, 1997.

Nolen-Hoeksema S: Understanding Depression: A Seminar for Health Professionals. Duluth, Minn, April, 1997.

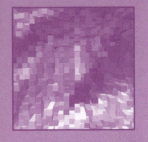

Anxiety and Somatoform Disorders

Outline

- **Anxiety Disorders**
  Levels of Anxiety
  Theories
  Categories and Symptoms
  Posttraumatic Stress Disorder
  Nursing Interventions
- **Case Study: Nursing Care Plan**

History and Data Collection
**Goals, Interventions, Rationale, and
  Evaluation**
- **Somatoform Disorders**
  Theories
  Categories and Symptoms
  Nursing Interventions

Key Terms

- agoraphobia
- anxiety
- body dysmorphic disorder
- compulsion
- conversion disorder
- generalized anxiety disorder
- hypochondriasis
- la belle indifference
- obsession

- pain disorder
- panic disorder
- posttraumatic stress disorder
- social phobia
- somatization
- somatization disorder
- somatoform disorder
- specific phobia

Objectives

Upon completing this chapter, the student will be able to:
1. Differentiate between anxiety and fear.
2. Discuss the levels of anxiety.
3. Describe the causes of anxiety and somatoform disorders.
4. Describe four categories of anxiety disorders.
5. Define five types of somatoform disorders.
6. Explain a nursing approach that is important in working with clients who have an anxiety or somatoform disorder.
7. List specific nursing interventions for clients with anxiety and somatoform disorders.

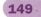

ANXIETY DISORDERS

Anxiety is a normal and often helpful emotion that alerts one to potential danger. It is distinguished from fear in that it is a vague, uneasy feeling, the source of which is nonspecific or unknown. The focus of anxiety is more internal than external. For example, a person might be anxious about "something bad happening." On the other hand, *fear* is usually directed toward an external object or situation, such as the fear of failing an exam.

Anxiety often occurs when a person is facing a new situation. It keys up the person's mind and body to increase focus and concentration. If an anxious person is aware of the anxiety and its cause, anxiety can be used to his or her advantage. Using the problem-solving process to move through the anxiety in a constructive way helps develop the person's character and personality. Review Figure 2–2 in Chapter 2 to see the paths that people take to cope with anxiety.

Levels of Anxiety

Anxiety affects a person physically, psychologically, and behaviorally. It can appear in many forms and levels of intensity. These levels of intensity can be described as follows (Robinson, 1996, p. 695; Murphy et al., 1996, p. 11):

- *Mild:* The person feels a vague uneasiness. At this level of anxiety, the person is aware, attentive, and able to solve problems. There is increased motivation to learn.
- *Moderate:* The person's tension and fear increase. He or she feels a sense of helplessness and irritability. Palms are sweaty, and pulse and respirations increase. Attention is focused on the present issue, but ability to think clearly is diminished. However, learning can still occur.
- *Severe:* The person perspires profusely, and breathing is shallow and rapid. Vital signs increase, and the person has urinary frequency, dry mouth, and numbness of extremities. The person is in distress and trembling. Sensory perception is greatly reduced, and learning cannot occur. The person is afraid of going crazy.
- *Panic:* The person's symptoms of severe anxiety escalate. He or she is emotionally overwhelmed and has feelings of dying. The person is unable to process information and may resort to primitive coping behaviors.

Some of the coping behaviors or defense mechanisms that are used to handle overwhelming anxiety include denial, displacement, repression, regression, reaction formation, and undoing. These are discussed in Chapter 2.

Theories

A number of theorists have attempted to explain the causes of anxiety disorders. Research indicates that anxiety is a combination of physical, psychosocial, and environmental factors. Some of the well-known theories are discussed here.

Biological Theory

Biological studies have focused on the brain stem, the limbic system, and the prefrontal cortex. *Neurotransmitters* are chemicals that allow electrical impulses to travel from nerve cell to nerve cell throughout the body. The electrical impulses can be affected by neurotransmitters and their receptors. The monoamine neurotransmitters, especially norepinephrine, may be responsible for increasing anxiety. Gamma-aminobutyric acid (GABA) is the most abundant transmitter in the brain; it is believed to have an inhibiting affect on anxiety. Antianxiety medication is used to alter neurotransmitter activity (see Chapter 22).

Genetic Theory

Based on what is known at this time, a general personality type that predisposes one to be overly anxious may be inherited (Bourne, 1995, p. 24). This type of personality is easily triggered by minor threats. Much depends on the person's particular environment and upbringing.

Psychoanalytic Theory

Freud believed that anxiety is the result of intrapsychic conflict between the ego and the id. When unconscious material threatens to enter consciousness, defense mechanisms help the person adapt. For example, a woman who is unable to express her negative feelings toward her husband may find fault with her co-workers. See Chapter 2 for a more detailed discussion of the relationship between the ego and the id, as well as defense mechanisms.

Interpersonal Theory

Harry Stack Sullivan attributed anxiety to interpersonal relationships that originate between child and caregiver. When early needs go unmet, the child does not receive the required unconditional love and nurturing. This initial anxiety becomes the model for coping with unpleasant events that occur later in life (Charron, 1998, p. 446). For example, a child who never received adequate love and caring during early years may find it difficult to have an intimate relationship in adult life.

Behavioral Theory

Behavioral theory claims that anxiety is a learned behavior that can be unlearned. For example, a parent who is afraid of heights and therefore will not fly may transmit this anxiety to a child. The child may carry this anxiety about flying into adult life. However, the anxiety can be reduced by persistently confronting the feared situation.

Categories and Symptoms

Some of the anxiety disorders included in the American Psychiatric Association's *Diagnostic and Statistical Manual of Mental Disorders, fourth edition* (DSM-IV) are panic disorder with or without agoraphobia, phobias, obsessive-compulsive disorder, posttraumatic stress disorder (PTSD), and generalized anxiety disorder (APA, 1994, pp. 393–436). These disorders are discussed here.

Panic Disorder

In **panic disorder**, brief episodes of intense fear are accompanied by multiple physical symptoms that occur repeatedly and unexpectedly in the absence of any external threat. The panic attacks that indicate panic disorder are believed to occur when the brain's normal mechanism for reacting to a threat— *the fight-or-flight response*—is triggered inappropriately (Bourne, 1995, p. 30). Panic attacks usually take a person completely by surprise while driving, working, or shopping.

Some or all of the following symptoms may occur during a panic attack (APA, 1994, p. 104):

- A sense of terror
- Chest pains
- Pounding heartbeat
- Difficulty breathing
- Dizziness or lightheadedness
- Sweating
- Fear of losing control or going crazy
- Fear of dying

In panic disorder, panic attacks recur, causing the person to develop an intense apprehension of having another attack. Those who are prone to panic attacks may also develop irrational fears called *phobias*. Phobias cause a person to avoid situations believed to trigger a panic attack, resulting in an increasingly limited life.

One phobia associated with panic disorder is **agoraphobia,** anxiety about being in places or situations from which escape might be difficult if panic-like symptoms occur. People with agoraphobia fear being in crowds, riding public transportation, standing in lines, or shopping in malls. They often restrict themselves to home or the immediate neighborhood.

Treatment involves cognitive-behavioral therapy and medications. In addition, self-help groups help people deal with their ongoing fears and offer support. Breathing and desensitizing exercises are also a part of therapy. For example, the person may learn not to add frightening thoughts on top of the fears, and to recognize that a panic attack, although uncomfortable, is not dangerous (see Chapter 27).

Reality Check

Marie is a 35-year-old woman who has confined herself to her home for the past year. She is afraid of leaving the house because of her inability to control her multiple physical symptoms. Marie has sought help from a therapist and is on medication, but she is still hesitant to travel or go shopping. One day, in a department store, she had a panic attack for no apparent reason and laid on the floor until the symptoms subsided.

Marie joined a support group and began to channel some of her internal feelings through painting. Her artwork is an expression of strong emotions that have now found a constructive outlet.

1. What was the phobia associated with Marie's panic attacks?
2. What defense mechanism(s) did Marie use?
3. What assumptions can you make about Marie's recovery?

Specific and Social Phobias

In addition to agoraphobia, the DSM-IV also includes specific and social phobias. **Specific phobia** is a marked and persistent fear that is excessive or unreasonable and involves the presence or anticipation of a specific object or situation: heights, open spaces, animals, electrical storms, closed spaces, etc. A **social phobia** is a marked and persistent fear of one or more social or performance situations in which a person is exposed to unfamiliar people. The person is afraid of humiliation or embarrassment. In both situations, exposure to the phobic stimulus or the feared social situation provokes an immediate anxiety response. The person is aware that the fear is excessive or unreasonable, but the feared situations are usually avoided or endured with intense anxiety (APA, 1994, pp. 410–411, 416–417).

"Real-life desensitization is the single most effective available treatment for phobias" (Bourne, 1995, p. 149). However, this approach is often uncomfortable and requires a strong commitment. Bourne (1995, p. 150) states three things that a person undergoing desensitization must be willing to do:

1. Take the risk to start facing situations the person may have been avoiding for many years.
2. Tolerate the initial discomfort that entering phobic situations, even in small increments, often involves.
3. Persist in practicing exposure on a consistent basis, despite probable setbacks over a long enough period to allow complete recovery (generally this takes from 6 months to 2 years).

Obsessive-Compulsive Disorder

Obsessions are recurrent and persistent thoughts, impulses, or images that are experienced as intrusive and cause marked anxiety. They are not simply excessive worries. The person attempts to ignore the thoughts, impulses, or images or substitute some other thought, realizing that these obsessional experiences are a product of the mind. **Compulsions** are repetitive behaviors that a person feels driven to perform in response to an obsession. These behaviors are aimed at preventing or reducing anxiety (APA, 1994, pp. 422–423). Some of the common compulsions or rituals people carry out include hand washing, checking, touching, and counting.

Obsessions and/or compulsions interfere with a person's normal routine. Activities that normally took a few minutes to perform now often take an hour or more. People who have obsessive-compulsive disorder (OCD) are usually perfectionists and need to be in control.

Many people experience some type of obsessive or compulsive behavior (e.g., "Did I turn off the stove or lock the door when I left home?"). If these ideas are not followed by a return visit home or a phone call, the person becomes anxious and has trouble concentrating on the task at hand.

Clinical observations indicate that antidepressants that are specific selective serotonin reuptake inhibitors (SSRIs), particularly clomi-pramine (Anafranil), are effective in weakening obsessive thoughts and compulsive actions. In addition to medication, behavioral therapy is help-ful. In this therapy, the client is exposed to progressive degrees of the stressor. In a controlled environment, he or she is encouraged to respond with a modified or delayed behavior (Robinson, 1996, p. 702). For a more complete discussion of this therapy, see Chapter 25.

The nurse can help the client interrupt obsessive thoughts and compulsive actions through relaxa-tion and cognitive techniques. If the ritual is excessive hand washing, the nurse needs to teach the client skin protection with special prepara-tions. Gradually limiting actions over a period of time can help decrease obsessive-compulsive behavior.

Posttraumatic Stress Disorder

People who are exposed to highly traumatic events, such as war, airplane or car crashes, natural disas-ters, or sexual abuse, are predisposed to developing **posttraumatic stress disorder** (PTSD). Some of the symptoms that occur after the traumatic event include the following (APA, 1994, p. 427–429):

- Difficulty falling or staying asleep, with flash-backs of the traumatic event or nightmares
- Irritability or outbursts of anger
- Difficulty concentrating
- Hypervigilence (being overly alert to danger)
- Exaggerated startle response
- A feeling of detachment from others

These symptoms can be grouped into two qualities that emerge in clients with PTSD: *deper-sonalization* (the experience of a sense of unreality, as if one is seeing oneself from a distance) and *entrapment* (the sense that escape routes are ex-tremely dangerous or costly). Both can result in feelings of personal vulnerability and emotional disconnection from others (Clark, 1997, p. 28).

One of the goals in PTSD treatment is to help the client gain a sense of control. Treatment involves a combination of cognitive-behavioral therapy and relaxation techniques. A technique called *positive dreaming* can help a person who has troubling nightmares. It involves asking the client to determine the end of the dream in advance. Before the client goes to sleep, he or she is encouraged to focus on dreaming the positive ending (Clark, 1997, p. 28).

One way to deal with numbing and dissociation is involvement in activities that reconnect the client to the outside world, such as doing sit-ups, taking a shower, or changing clothes (Clark, 1997, p. 28). Through these approaches, the nurse helps the client change behaviors, decreasing the dis-tressing symptoms.

Another valuable resource is a support group for PTSD survivors. In these groups, people have an opportunity to vent their feelings and share symptoms and memories in a supportive environ-ment.

Reality Check

Carl, a 48-year-old Vietnam veteran, is trou-bled with flashbacks of his wartime expe-riences. His closest buddy was killed while fighting next to him. Carl's flashbacks have affected his relationships with his wife and children. He is unable to hold his job and is on the verge of divorce. Carl has joined other veterans in a support group. Together they made a trip to Washington, D.C., and identified the names on the Vietnam Memo-rial of buddies killed in action.

1. What function might visiting the Vietnam Memorial serve for Carl and others from the support group?
2. When might relaxation techniques be most effective with Carl?

Generalized Anxiety Disorder

People with **generalized anxiety disorder** (GAD) are excessive worriers, anticipating that something terrible is going to happen: a natural disaster, illness, or harm to self or a loved one. These people are usually aware that their anxiety is extreme, and they try to conceal it, often making it worse. Some of the symptoms experienced by these people include the following:

- Restlessness or "edginess"
- A tendency to be easily fatigued
- Difficulty concentrating
- Muscle tension
- Irritability
- Sleep disturbance

GAD is diagnosed when excessive anxiety persists for at least 6 months with three or more of the above symptoms (APA, 1994, pp. 435–436). This constant state of worry can interfere with important areas of functioning. Medication is effective and is usually supplemented with relaxation techniques, stress management, and biofeedback. Another helpful approach is the use of cognitive-behavioral therapy, which teaches methods of challenging anxious thoughts (Living Without Anxiety, 1997, p. 4). The symptoms of anxiety are listed in Figure 15–1.

Nursing Interventions

Helping anxious clients deal constructively with their anxiety is the nurse's goal. Unless the nurse recognizes and evaluates his or her responses to anxiety, the nurse can unknowingly support the client's negative attempts to cope with anxiety. Because the client's problems may be similar to what the nurse is experiencing, there is danger of personalizing the problems. If this happens, the nurse loses objectivity and effectiveness in working with the client.

The most important quality for the nurse working with a client who is anxious is an attitude of acceptance. The nurse must remember that the client has the right to be as sick as he or she needs to be at this time. Whether the nurse approves of the client's behavior, the nurse must accept and realize that, at this time, this is the best the client can do.

The nurse relieves anxiety through concern and respect for the client, and through skill in working

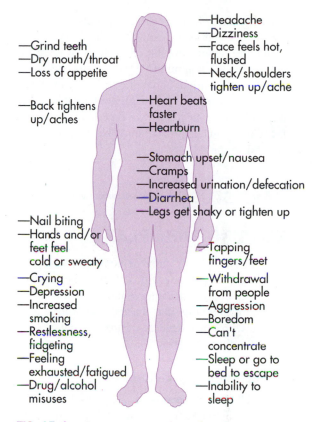

FIG. 15–1 Symptoms of anxiety. (Data from Anxiety Brochure, Bellin Psychiatric Hospital, Green Bay, Wis. Used with permission.)

with him or her. The nurse's willingness to spend time with the client is more effective than empty reassurance offered in phrases such as "Everything will be OK." It is important for nurses to evaluate what clients can and cannot do for themselves. In areas of care in which the client needs help, such as personal grooming, the nurse must use direct assistance.

In caring for a client with overwhelming anxiety, the focus of attention must be on the client, not on the symptoms. This means that every opportunity should be made to interact with the client when he or she is not talking about symptoms. When the client verbalizes many physical complaints, the nurse should listen and make a mental note for possible physical evaluation. The nurse should not comment about the client's symptoms or inquire about how the client feels. Rather, the nurse should communicate an understanding of how the client might be feeling inside by making a comment such as, "You seem anxious this morning, so I'll be with you for short periods throughout the day." This approach may be helpful in the general hospital.

CASE STUDY

NURSING CARE PLAN

The following case study demonstrates a nursing care plan for a client with anxiety. The example describes appropriate interventions for this client. Other interventions may be more appropriate for clients with other degrees of anxiety and/or other personal characteristics.

History and Data Collection

Mrs. Hattie Golden is a 42-year-old married woman who paces the floor and talks continuously about her difficulty breathing, the pounding of her heart, sweating, and smothering sensations. She says that she has a fear of dying and possibly going crazy. She talks about feeling insecure and inadequate; she is also indecisive.

Mrs. Golden was active in the local garden club and is known for her collection of African violets. Her medical exam revealed no reason for her symptoms.

The nurse uses the RN's nursing diagnoses and the data collected to detail nursing problems appropriate for intervention at the LPN/LVN level. Table 15–1 shows the result.

Goals, Interventions, Rationale, and Evaluation

Based on the nursing problem she has defined, the nurse proceeds to list appropriate goals and interventions, along with a rationale for each. With the RN's approval, she implements the interventions

and evaluates the result. The goals, interventions, and evaluation are shown in Table 15–2.

SOMATOFORM DISORDERS

The common characteristics of **somatoform disorders** are physical symptoms for which there are no known organic causes. The physical symptoms are not intentional, and they result in distress or impairment in functioning. These disorders are often encountered by the person's general medical physician (APA, 1994, p. 445). The physician frequently fails to realize that the person's "somatic complaints are metaphors for psychic suffering" (Muskin, 1997, p. 545). Such a person needs to be cared for by someone; he or she will go from doctor to doctor until some kind of help is received.

Somatization, then, is the expression of psychological stress through physical symptoms on an unconscious level. The purpose of the symptoms is to relieve anxiety. This is referred to as *primary gain*. Because the symptoms are very real to the person, medical advice is sought for relief. A continuation of the symptoms can lead to *secondary gains* by allowing the person to fulfill dependency needs, avoid responsibility, and receive special attention from others (Charron, 1998, p. 445). Often these gains can encourage the symptoms to continue.

Table 15–1	Nursing Diagnosis and Nursing Problem for Case Study
Nursing Diagnosis	**Nursing Problem**
Anxiety related to threat to self-concept as evidenced by dyspnea, palpitations, sweating, fear of dying	Mrs. Golden talks continuously about her difficulty breathing, heart pounding, sweating, and smothering sensations; symptoms are not due to any medical condition

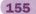

Table 15–2	Goals, Interventions, Rationale, and Evaluation for Case Study	
Goal	**Interventions**	**Rationale**
Mrs. Golden will take pre-scribed medication	Explain to Mrs. Golden about her medication—possible side effects, how long they might last, and what she can do to relieve them	Can give a sense of control over medication and side effects; this is her way of coping with anxiety at this time
	Listen to Mrs. Golden's complaints; do not tell her that they are not real	You are accepting her and at the same time diverting her attention away from herself
Mrs. Golden will observe nurse's care of African violets on unit for 1 week; Mrs. Golden will care for the African violets with nurse's assistance for the next week	Try to interest her in things outside of herself; provide simple activities, such as care of plants on unit, that are within her ability and at which she can succeed	

Evaluation: Mrs. Golden was receptive to taking medication. After 2 weeks, she was caring for the plants on the unit with the assistance of the nurse. As she became more involved in activities, her physical symptoms began to subside.

Theories

Some explanations exist for the cause of somato-form disorders. The influence of biological and genetic factors is being researched. There are indications that conversion disorder might have an organic basis related to arousal disturbances in the central nervous system (Charron, 1998, p. 482).

Many clinicians believe that somatoform disorders have psychodynamic origins. Freud thought that the psychological symptoms of illness and loss of physical functioning were related to repression of a conflict. He maintained that the physical symptom was symbolic of the conflict.

Behaviorists believe that symptoms are learned ways of communicating helplessness. Cognitive theorists believe that body sensations are misinterpreted by the person, who then becomes overly alarmed by them. This leads to hypochondriasis (discussed later in this chapter). These psychological theories emphasize the use of defense mechanisms as ways of dealing with anxiety. They include conversion, displacement, symbolism, pro-jection, somatization, and denial. These defense mechanisms are described in Chapter 2.

Categories and Symptoms

Some of the somatoform disorders included in the DSM-IV are somatization disorder, conversion disorder, pain disorder, hypochondriasis, and body dysmorphic disorder (APA, 1994, p. 445). These disorders are discussed here.

Somatization Disorder

The essential features of **somatization disorder** are multiple, recurrent somatic complaints beginning before age 30 and with no physical findings on medical examination. Some of the symptoms include the following (APA, 1994, pp. 449–450):

- Pain related to head, back, joints, and abdomen
- Nausea, bloating, and vomiting
- Sexual indifference
- Irregular menses

Although the person may present very colorful descriptions of the symptoms, the history of medical problems is limited. People with somatoform disorders are difficult to treat because they are not consciously aware of the causes for their difficulties.

Conversion Disorder

The predominant feature in **conversion disorder** is loss or alteration in voluntary motor or sensory function that suggests a neurological or other medical condition. Psychological factors are associated with this symptom because it is preceded by conflicts or other stressors. The symptom causes noticeable distress or impairment in daily functioning and cannot be explained by a medical condition (APA, 1994, p. 457).

Some of the most common neurological symptoms are paralysis, seizures, blindness, and coordination disturbances. These symptoms, although serious and sometimes dramatically present, are not intentionally produced. An identifying characteristic of conversion disorder is that the person does not seem concerned about the symptom. This calm attitude is referred to as **la belle indifference** (Thomas and Wimbush, 1996, p. 963).

The defense mechanisms involved in conversion disorder are repression and conversion. Chapter 2 discusses these mechanisms in further detail.

Reality Check

Thelma is a 35-year-old woman with six children. She was referred to the mental health center by the public health nurse. Thelma had been in a wheelchair for the past year. Her history revealed that before being in a wheelchair she was abused by her husband. Thelma and her husband lived across from a church and school that her children attended. The nuns at the school helped out with the children. Thelma was very calm about her condition and did not seem concerned that she was in a wheelchair. A complete medical examination revealed no organic basis for her condition.

1. What defense mechanisms did Thelma use?
2. What is the name for Thelma's lack of concern over her condition?
3. What might have been some of Thelma's secondary gains?
4. As Thelma's nurse, how might you have helped her develop more effective coping techniques?

Pain Disorder

In **pain disorder,** pain is the predominant focus of medical attention. The pain continues after extensive evaluation determines that there are no physical findings to account for the pain and its intensity. The pain causes significant difficulty in important areas of functioning. Psychological factors have a definite role in the initiation and severity of the pain. The pain is not intentional and is unrelated to other psychiatric disorders (APA, 1994, pp. 458, 459).

People with pain disorder spend considerable time going from doctor to doctor looking for relief. The use of excess amounts of pain medication and other treatments bring no relief. They deny that their pain has any relation to psychological factors (APA, 1994, p. 459).

Hypochondriasis

The person with **hypochondriasis** is preoccupied with fears of having a serious illness. This is based on the person's misinterpretation of bodily symptoms, usually heartbeat, breathing, or digestion. The preoccupation continues despite medical tests and reassurance that the symptoms are not physical in origin. These beliefs are not of delusional intensity and are not accounted for by the anxiety disorders. The duration of the beliefs causes disturbances in social, occupational, and other areas of functioning (APA, 1994, p. 463).

Body Dysmorphic Disorder

Body dysmorphic disorder is a preoccupation with an imagined defect in appearance where there are no obvious abnormalities. If there is a slight defect, the person's concern is noticeably excessive. This preoccupation, which usually focuses on a facial defect, interferes with the person's functioning. Such a person often seeks plastic surgery, which will not change the distorted thinking. This preoccupation is not associated with another mental disorder, such as dissatisfaction with the body in anorexia nervosa (APA, 1994, p. 466).

Nursing Interventions

The clue to successful nursing interventions is to determine which needs the client is fulfilling through somatization. This may be accomplished in the following ways:

- Establish a trusting relationship with the client
- Assess the secondary gains that the client might be receiving from the illness, such as receiving extra attention from others
- Avoid focusing attention on the complaints of the client after a thorough medical exam has been done
- Spend time with the client when the client is not complaining
- Observe and record frequency of complaints and when they occur (e.g., what is going on at the time the client has a complaint)
- If somatic complaints enter into the conversation, shift the focus to another topic or activity
- Do not try to convince the client that the symptoms are not real
- Focus on the client's strengths and use them to help fulfill the client's needs
- Involve the client in ways to reduce stress, such as relaxation, deep breathing, mild exercise, or visualization
- Help the client see the effect of his or her behavior on others
- Help the client express his or her feelings through assertive techniques
- Encourage the client to become as independent as possible in caring for self

SUMMARY

Anxiety is a vague, uneasy feeling of nonspecific or unknown origin. Whereas fear is directed toward an external object, the focus of anxiety is internal. The four levels of anxiety are mild, moderate, severe, and panic. Biological, genetic, interpersonal, and behavioral theories are several that attempt to explain the causes of anxiety disorders.

Five categories of anxiety disorders included in DSM-IV are panic disorder, phobias, obsessive-compulsive disorders, posttraumatic stress disorder, and generalized anxiety disorder. The categories of somatoform disorders discussed included somatization disorder, conversion disorder, pain disorder, hypochondriasis, and body dysmorphic disorder.

Nursing interventions for clients experiencing anxiety and somatoform disorders focus on the client and not on the symptoms that the client is expressing. Every opportunity needs to be made to interact with the client when he or she is not talking about his or her symptoms.

Critical Thinking Activities

1. Describe situations in your life when you have been anxious. What coping techniques did you use to deal with your anxiety?
2. What techniques have you used to help clients handle their anxiety?
3. What are your observations of instances in which the anxiety of staff influenced the behavior of clients on the unit?

Review Questions

Multiple Choice—Choose the best answer to each question.

1. Anxiety is
   a. an abnormal emotion.
   b. directed toward an external object.
   c. related to a specific source.
   d. a vague, uneasy feeling.

2. In severe anxiety, the client has
   a. a sense of helplessness and irritability.
   b. attentiveness with increased motivation to learn.
   c. profuse perspiration with rapid breathing.
   d. a sense of being emotionally overwhelmed.
3. An anxiety disorder that involves recurrent and persistent thoughts, impulses, or images followed by repetitive behaviors is known as
   a. generalized anxiety disorder.
   b. obsessive-compulsive disorder.
   c. panic disorder with agoraphobia.
   d. posttraumatic stress disorder.
4. A statement that a nurse might make when caring for a client with an anxiety or somatoform disorder is
   a. "Tell me more about your symptoms. I'll have the doctor see you."
   b. "Don't worry. Everything is going to be all right. I promise you."
   c. "Your complaints sound like something that I had awhile ago."
   d. "You seem anxious this morning, so I'll sit with you for awhile."
5. A person with a conversion disorder exhibits a
   a. preoccupation with fears of having a serious illness.
   b. calm attitude or la belle indifference about condition.
   c. group of multiple recurrent somatic complaints.
   d. preoccupation with an imagined defect in appearance.

References

American Psychiatric Association: Diagnostic and Statistical Manual of Mental Disorders, 4th ed. Washington, DC, American Psychiatric Association, 1994.

Bourne EJ: The Anxiety & Phobia Workbook, 2nd ed. Oakland, Calif, New Harbinger Publications, Inc, 1995.

Charron HS: Anxiety disorders and somatoform and dissociative disorders. In: Varcarolis EM (ed): Foundations of Psychiatric Mental Health Nursing, 3rd ed. Philadelphia, WB Saunders Co, 1998.

Clark CC: Posttraumatic Stress Disorder: How to Support Healing. Am J Nurs, 97(8):27–32, 1997.

Living Without Anxiety. The Johns Hopkins Medical Letter, 9(6):4–5, 1997.

Murphy MF, Moller MD, Billings JV: My Symptom Management Workbook: A Wellness Expedition. Richfield, Utah, Wellness Consultation and Education, 1996, p 11.

Muskin PR: Physical signs and symptoms. In: Tasman A, Kay J, Lieberman JA (eds): Psychiatry, vol I. Philadelphia, WB Saunders Co, 1997.

Robinson L: The journey threatened by stress and anxiety disorders. In: Carson VB, Arnold EN (eds): Mental Health Nursing: The Nurse-Patient Journey. Philadelphia, WB Saunders Co, 1996.

Thomas SA, Wimbush FB: The journey embedded in psychophysiological disorders. In: Carson VB, Arnold EN (eds): Mental Health Nursing: The Nurse-Patient Journey. Philadelphia, WB Saunders Co, 1996.

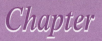

SIXTEEN

Dissociative Disorders and Sexual and Gender Identity Disorders

Outline

- **Dissociative Disorders**
    Diagnosis and Treatment
- **Sex and Sexuality**
- **Illness and Sexuality**
- **Sexual Disorders**
    Sexual Dysfunctions Related to
    Organic Causes

    Paraphilias
    Gender Identity Disorder
- **Case Study: Nursing Care Plan**
    History and Data Collection
    Goals, Interventions, Rationale, and
    Evaluation
- **Nursing Interventions**

Key Terms

- alternate personality
- coached memories
- depersonalization disorder
- dissociative amnesia
- dissociative fugue
- gender identity disorder

- paraphilia
- possession
- sex
- sexuality
- trance

Objectives

Upon completing this chapter, the student will be able to:

1. Explain the use of the coping mechanism of dissociation in dissociative disorders and sexual function disorders.
2. Discuss two major elements of a dissociative identity disorder.
3. Discuss three major factors in nursing intervention with the client experiencing a dissociative disorder.
4. Differentiate between the terms *sex* and *sexuality*.
5. Discuss how lack of factual information can cause the nurse to ignore client sexuality needs as part of a care plan.
6. Explain what is meant by *sexual dysfunction*.
7. Explain the role of the nurse with the client who is experiencing organic sexual dysfunction.
8. List three criminal paraphilias in the United States.
9. Name three characteristics of a gender identity disorder.

The dissociative and sexual and gender identity disorders are included in this chapter because the dissociative mechanism is used to cope with overwhelming stress (see Chapter 2). The dissociative mechanism is a common thread found in the dissociative disorders and sexual dysfunctions related to psychological factors. The client separates the painful event from consciousness.

DISSOCIATIVE DISORDERS

Dissociative disorders involve a sudden, temporary change in the functions of consciousness, identity, and behavior. The change is related to overwhelming stress that the person is unable to cope with in a healthy way. Whatever the stressor is, it is separated from consciousness. Dissociative amnesia, dissociative fugue, dissociative identity disorders, depersonalization disorders, and dissociative trance disorders are included in this category. Table 16–1 describes characteristics of each.

Of these disorders, the dissociative identity disorder (formerly known as *multiple personality disorder*) lends itself to the greatest controversy. Experts continue to disagree on whether it is a legitimate psychiatric disorder or a reflection of a social trend. The number of persons diagnosed with this disorder has increased considerably.

Some experts question whether there is a relationship between this increase and highly publicized stories such as *Three Faces of Eve, Sybil,* and *When Rabbit Howls.* All of these books are considered autobiographical and are related to sexual abuse.

A related concern is that nothing is usually done to validate a child's allegations of sexual abuse before the diagnosis of dissociative identity disorder. In some highly publicized cases, this has ruined the lives of people (often parents or stepparents) later discovered to be innocent of having sexually molested the client. Repressed memories in some cases turned out to be coached memories. **Coached memories** occur when the client is influenced during therapy by questions and statements made by the therapist. The client believes he or she has been molested, but no molestation took place.

Dissociative identity disorder may sound new, but it is not. The first description was offered in the 1800s. According to the American Psychiatric Association's *Diagnostic and Statistical Manual of Mental Disorders, fourth edition* (DSM-IV) (APA, 1997, pp. 447–449), the person with dissociative identity disorder has two or more distinct personalities or personality states. Each has its own relatively enduring pattern of perceiving, relating to,

Table 16–1	Characteristics of Dissociative Disorders
Disorder	**Characteristics**
Dissociative amnesia	Unable to recall important personal information (not related to organic causes); reversible by using hypnosis
Dissociative fugue	Leaves usual home/work area for hours to days, rarely months; assumes new identity; no memory of past
	When memory returns, has no recollection of fugue state
Depersonalization disorder	Feels detached from reality; views self/situation as though from the outside looking in; impairs social or occupational functioning
Trance-possession disorder	
Trance	Altered state of consciousness; selective or limited response to environmental stimuli
Possession	Believes he or she has been taken over by a spirit or other person; this is usually involved with the trance state

and thinking about the environment and the self. At least two of the personalities (or states) recurrently take full control of the person's behavior. The client usually presents with a complaint of blackouts (lapses in memory).

Curtin (1993, p. 29) defines the disorder as follows:

It originates in childhood when a child, repeatedly exposed to overwhelming abuse or trauma, mentally escapes or leaves the scene of abuse. The child may perceive the abuse as if he were watching it happen to him on a screen. This ability to dissociate or mentally escape is a defense mechanism used by a child who is unable to integrate or manage the trauma through healthier defense mechanisms. Dissociation is understood as a self-hypnotic state—different personalities are formed, each holding different memories and feelings and carrying out different functions. Because there is no conscious memory of the abuse, the child can continue to have a relationship with the abuser, on whom the child is often dependent.

The most common abuser is the stepfather. Clients with dissociative identity disorder often think they are "going crazy" because of the voices inside their heads. This symptom differs from hallucinations of schizophrenia, in which voices emanate from outside of self. The voices involved in dissociative disorder are the personalities conversing with each other. The conversations range from harmless comments to telling the person to hurt himself/herself or someone else. Because the personalities involved have different powers and strengths, they may vie for control and keep information secret from one another. Common separate personalities often include a protector, aggressor, persecutor, and helpmate. Initially, personalities are not aware of the existence of the others and are distressed by "signs" of others in their life.

Reality Check

Ruth Fredricks admitted herself to the psychiatric unit after discovering her "other life." During the past few months, she had been annoyed by calls from men who were suggestive in tone and seeking her "services" as advertised. Ruth hung up on the callers, initially considering these to be crank calls. However, she also discovered clothes—someone else's—in her closet. They were quite unlike her business suits—a prank, no doubt. There were also large sums of money missing from her bank account at different points. It was scary and not making sense. Finally, Ruth decided to ask the next male caller why he was calling her and what the source of his information was. The man referred to her small ad in the personal column, and said "Why are you asking, since we've had great times?" Ruth found the ad with her phone number. That's all she recalled until showing up at the hospital, begging for admission and saying "I think I'm going crazy." Shortly thereafter, she was demanding to leave.

1. What is your personal "gut" reaction to Ruth's story?
2. How do you visualize Ruth's appearance and behavior as the lady with the ad?
3. What caused the contradictory statements at the time of admission?

Diagnosis and Treatment

Diagnosis for people with dissociative identity disorder takes an average of 5 to 6 years. Many other diagnoses, including schizophrenia, are usually included within that time frame. People who have dissociative identity disorders do not respond to psychotherapeutic medication as might be expected with other diagnoses.

Treatment for dissociative identity disorders is long and difficult and is directed at integrating the personalities. Treatments of choice are psychotherapy and hypnosis. A screen technique is sometimes used during hypnosis to visualize disturbing behavior of other personalities as though they are appearing on a screen. The therapist must be highly skilled to be proactive with the separate personalities (Spiegel, 1997, p. 1159).

Nursing Interventions

Hospitalization may be precipitated by self-mutilative or violent behaviors of personalities involved. It is not always clear what incident or event causes a person to shift to an **alternate personality** (actor). Nurses need to be aware of this change and respond accordingly, often with decisiveness and speed. However, at no point is it wise to try to convince the client to assume his or her real (core) personality. In many cases, the client's life was brutal and disruptive during childhood. Authority figures were inconsistent and unreliable, creating a lack of trust. The client "may be very distrustful of staff and may try to manipulate nurses into behaviors that prove their unreliability. Thus, consistency in milieu is very important—particularly in conveying a caring, non-punitive, and predictable environment. Indeed, some clients will set up classic double-bind (no-win) situations so that nurses will look uncaring or insincere. For example, if nurses wake a patient for breakfast, they may be accused of being authoritarian; if they let the patient sleep, nurses may be accused of not caring whether or not the client gets enough to eat. In such a situation, a matter-of-fact, non-defensive manner has been observed to be effective" (Stafford, 1993, p. 19).

It is also helpful for the assigned nurse to request supervision. The nurse should take time to do advanced planning, check in as needed, and review the events of the day. In a sense, it is often as though one client has become a series of clients. If necessary, the nurse should seek help in recognizing when an alternate personality is emerging. The LPN/LVN must learn through supervision how to shift his or her approach to the client in a therapeutic way. The task is both challenging and interesting.

SEX AND SEXUALITY

Nursing is among the most intimate of professions. Nurses invade the client's personal space regularly as a part of nursing responsibility. They examine, probe, medicate, or wash a client's "private parts"

on an as-needed basis. However, nursing intimacy aside, both nurses and clients are often reluctant to speak openly of sex or sexuality issues. Nurses learn the mechanics of the male and female anatomy as a part of their education. Issues of sex and sexuality and implications for nursing care continue to be dealt with in general terms. The level at which the nurse identifies and responds to a client's needs may be limited to the nurse's own sex education and belief system.

Reality Check

1. Has your current source of information about sex and sexuality been adequate in relating to clients with sexual difficulties? Explain.
2. Where might you obtain more factual information if needed?

The terms *sex* and *sexuality* are often used interchangeably, but they have different meanings. **Sex** refers to the physical, erotic, and genital relationship. Sex is used to sell everything from clothes to cars. **Sexuality** means something much broader than sex. According to Zawid (1993, p. 8), sexuality is defined as the following:

It refers to the whole person, including his or her thoughts, experiences, learnings, ideas, values, fantasies, and emotions as they have to do with being male or female. Sexuality is also related to how we feel about ourselves and how we communicate those feelings to others by the way we act, walk, carry our bodies, talk, and dress. It also includes our interactions and relationships with people of the opposite sex and/or the same sex and how we respond to the messages we receive from them. Sexuality encompasses our lives, from birth to death.

ILLNESS AND SEXUALITY

A nurse's inability to separate the personal and professional self influences client care. Underlying personal values and prejudices may get in the way of providing compassionate care.

Reality Check

1. When you look at a client, do you see a whole person with needs in all areas, including sexuality? Or do you see a person too young, too old, too mentally or physically ill, too handicapped, and so on?
2. In assisting in developing a client care plan, do you include the sexuality needs?

Medical conditions can affect a client's sex and sexuality. The changes involved may be related to emotional or physical causes or both. Rarely do the changes affect the client alone. By providing skilled nursing intervention, the nurse affects lives beyond that of the client.

Sometimes the intervention is offering factual information such as an alternative position during sex that is less stressful physically. Sometimes it is providing reassurance that sexual feelings are normal, and that the person can make a *conscious choice not to act on them.* Sometimes the intervention involves providing or identifying structured sex education programs at the person's level of comprehension. When problems are beyond the scope of the nurse's knowledge, the intervention consists of providing information on sexual therapists and/or counselors. Sometimes the most important intervention is for the nurse to create a window of opportunity to talk about sexual changes and concerns.

When a loss in sexual functioning is involved, the client needs to grieve the loss before considering alternatives. The stages of grieving may be much the same as they are with death and dying. The manner in which the client ultimately copes may be related to previous coping style. Four factors influencing coping are the following:

- Chronic illness or state of being
- Involvement of fatigue
- Pain as part of the illness
- The depression that often accompanies losses

Each factor challenges nursing intervention.

SEXUAL DISORDERS

The DSM-IV (APA, 1994, p. 493) identifies three major categories of sexual disorders.

- *Sexual dysfunctions* related to organic causes, which include changes in the normal response cycle.
- *Paraphilias* that involve sexual dysfunctions and sexual identity difficulties. "A paraphilia is a disorder of *intention*, the final component of sexual identity to develop in children and adolescents. Intention, sometimes referred to as *atypical sexual expression,* refers to what a person wants to do with a sexual partner and what they want the partner to do with them during sexual behavior" (Levine and Rosenblatt, 1997, p. 1194).
- *Gender identity disorders* include a sense of discomfort and inappropriateness about one's anatomic sex and wish to be of another sex.

Sexual Dysfunctions Related to Organic Causes

Sexual dysfunctions related to organic causes may involve psychological (emotional), organic (physical), or a combination of these. The major categories are related to sexual desire, arousal, orgasm, and sexual pain.

Cancer

Physiological reactions to cancer include depression and high anxiety. Disfiguring tumors may result in loss of self-esteem. Treatment for many kinds of cancer may cause pain, loss of attractiveness, stigma, myths, and loss of sexual desire. In addition, many forms of treatment for cancer cause complications.

Sexual complications for both men and women include loss of desire, loss of sex organs (surgical castration), infertility, changes in hormonal balance, and damage to nerves and/or blood supply of adjacent organs. For men, complications that interfere with sexuality may also include problems with the following:

- Erection
- Ejaculation

- Retrograde ejaculation
- Impotence

In women, complications that interfere with sexuality may include the following:

- Loss of breasts
- Stenosis and/or atrophy of vagina
- Menstrual irregularities

Cardiovascular Disorders

Sexual activity in clients with cardiovascular disorders is usually subject to physical limitations. Reasons include side effects of medication, poor circulation, decreased physical stamina, and fear of having a heart attack during sex. Additional restrictions may affect clients, depending on the specific disorder. For example, people who have had a myocardial infarction (MI) may experience the following:

- Lack of information on when and how to resume sex
- Discomfort in asking questions about sex
- Fear of discussing the possibility of "coital coronary" (couples with a long-term relationship)
- Possibility of "motel coronary" with extramarital partner or during sex in unfamiliar surroundings

Clients with cardiovascular disorders may also be subject to confusion because of changing roles. The partner may become overprotective, or the client may experience depression related to multiple losses.

Diabetes

Diabetes also has an effect on a person's sex and sexuality. It affects blood supply and nerves and lowers sexual desire in both men and women. In men, it may also cause the following:

- Difficulty achieving and maintaining an erection
- Retrograde ejaculation
- Change in fertility
- Increase in abnormal sperm production

In women, diabetes may:

- Affect the excitement phase of the response cycle

- Cause more vaginal dryness
- Require an increased amount of stimulation to reach orgasm
- Cause problems with conception

Diabetes may also increase the difficulty of regulating insulin while a woman is pregnant. The status of the fetus and newborn and mother need careful monitoring.

Genitourinary Disorders

Diseases related to genitalia often require multiple intrusive procedures. These may result in body-image issues and embarrassment. Many clients have difficulty asking sex-related questions. Specific problems depend on the type of genitourinary (GU) disorder.

Kidney disorders affect all stages of sexual response. Common problems include the following:

- Life-threatening changes
- Body-image changes
- Dependency issues
- Mood changes (depression, mood swings)
- Chronic fatigue
- Infertility
- Side effects from medication
- Excess weight gain and fluid retention

In addition, some clients with kidney disease are dependent on dialysis for life. Their lives therefore become disease-focused.

Other GU disorders that may affect a person's sexuality include bladder and prostate disorders. Bladder problems, such as bladder cancer and cystitis, may cause pain, increased urinary frequency, and urinary burning. Prostate cancer and prostatitis may result in loss of desire and uncomfortable, painful contractions during orgasm. Benign prostatic hypertrophy may cause difficulty voiding, dribbling, and increased urinary frequency, urgency, and nocturia. All of these may affect sexual desire. In addition, treatment side effects may include retrograde ejaculation, infertility, and erectile dysfunction.

Respiratory Disorders

Respiratory disorders that can affect a person's sexuality include chronic obstructive pulmonary disease (COPD), asthma, chronic bronchitis, and emphysema. These problems commonly occur in the 40- to 70-year age group, in which normal age-related sexual changes are also taking place. These normal changes may be confused with illness-related changes, some of which are treatable. For example, impotence related to Leriche's syndrome (clogging of iliac arteries to the pelvis) can be treated with surgery.

Medications for respiratory illness also have an effect on sexuality. Some medications improve sexual functioning by relieving shortness of breath and congestion. Others impair functioning by causing infertility, menstrual irregularities, mood swings, erectile dysfunction, and nightmares.

Negative emotional responses to respiratory illness can affect a person's sexuality. These include the following:

- Depression and anxiety
- Sleep deprivation or sleep apnea
- Feelings of anger or hopelessness
- Financial issues
- Personal identity issues
- Body-image issues because of physical changes
- Barrel chest
- Distended neck veins
- Bluish coloring (cyanosis) of skin
- Increased cough and mucous production

Nursing Interventions

Clients who experience sexual dysfunction caused by illness have probably had a previous successful sexual relationship. Unfortunately, the client may not tell about the relationship and the nurse may not want to know. Providing an opportunity to explore worries and realities will open the door to education and/or counseling if needed. Their motivation is based on their previous level of sexual functioning.

Regardless of the type of organic illness that affects the client sexually, some common interventions apply:

- Clients need education regarding the sexual response cycle and how their illness affects functioning.

- Involve both the client and partner in discussions. Both are affected, and two sets of ears are better than one.
- Listen carefully and respond first to the client's priority concern(s). The issue worrying the client and getting in the way of learning may be something else. For example, there may be financial or child-care issues with which the client needs assistance.
- Explore myths and belief systems about the illness. Special ties to religion or culture may limit exploration of alternative sexual expression.

Table 16–2 gives suggestions for dealing with the specific diseases discussed in this section.

Paraphilias

Paraphilias include socially destructive behaviors such as pedophilia (sex with children), voyeurism (peeping Tom), exhibitionism (flashing), sadistic rape (forced sex), and more. Some of these behaviors are sexual crimes; some are not.

Characteristics of Paraphiles

According to DSM-IV (APA, 1994, pp. 526–532), three characteristics common to all persons who have a paraphilia are the following:

1. *A long history of preoccupation with unusual, highly erotic fantasy.* The fantasies are preoccupied with aggression. The source of arousal may be fantasized in daydreaming during masturbation, looking at explicit sexual films or magazines, and so on. The object of arousal can be human or nonhuman. If human, there is no sense of love, caring, respect, or human attachment. The theme of the fantasy often shifts and changes over time. The shift of greatest concern is from fantasy to sexual behavior; for example, shifting from fantasizing rape to raping.
2. *An internal drive to play out the fantasy.* Initially it may be preoccupation with a behavior. As it intensifies, there is the pressure to act out the fantasy in a sexual behavior. Usually this behavior is masturbation. Sometimes it involves locating a person to shock; for

Table 16–2	Suggestions for Dealing With Specific Diseases

Cancer	The nurse may discuss the following suggestions with the client as appropriate: • Fertility issue options such as advance egg or sperm banking • Ways to enhance sexual interest • Communicating intimacy needs to partner • Sexual positions to reduce discomfort and/or pain • Information on dealing with body-image issues (e.g., American Cancer Society [ACS] program "Look Good Feel Better") • Grieving for losses; many hospitals have ongoing grief counseling available • Reducing depression and anxiety by using counseling, guided imagery, or medication if needed • Involvement with other clients recovering from cancer (e.g., ACS "I Can Cope" program) • Sexual counseling as needed Resources include ACS publications: • *Sexuality and Cancer for the Man Who Has Cancer and His Partner* • *Sexuality and Cancer for the Woman Who Has Cancer and Her Partner*
Cardiovascular Disorders	Medical health dictates safety and timing of sexual activity; the nurse can provide a sense of hope by providing the following factual information: • It is common to masturbate while in the hospital (heart rate does not get as high as with intercourse) • Discuss when sexual activity can be resumed; the usual criteria include the ability to walk up two flights of stairs without undue stress and pain • Need to start slowly with hugging, kissing, massaging • Discuss use of less stressful positions such as missionary position—any position that is comfortable is appropriate; direct client to listen to the body—what does not create dyspnea? • Discuss sexual side effects of medication, if any • Explain the negative effect of smoking on sex (constricts blood vessels) • Explain the negative effect of alcohol on sex (respiratory depression) • Avoid heavy meals before sex • Discuss importance of cardiac rehabilitation program • Stress the need for open, honest communication with partner, doctor, nurse • Encourage sexual counseling as needed
Diabetes	The following suggestions are appropriate for both men and women: • Healthy diet and moderate exercise to maintain proper glucose level, blood pressure, and weight • Discuss effect of smoking (vasoconstrictor) and alcohol (respiratory depressant)

Table 16–2	Suggestions for Dealing With Specific Diseases *Continued*
Diabetes *Continued*	• Discuss need for more sexual stimulation • Encourage sexual counseling as needed • Fertility issues may involve artificial insemination *Males:* • Impotence may have treatable causes such as out-of-control blood sugar level, drug side effects, Leriche's syndrome, or depression; observe for signs and symptoms *Females:* • Use of water-based lubricants for vaginal dryness • Prone to yeast infections; teach use of cotton underpants, eating properly, dry bathing suits, increased fluids, avoiding stress
Genitourinary Disorders	***Kidney*** • Grieve losses • Affects mental state; may include role reversal • Resources include the Trio and Kidney Organization ***Bladder*** Ways to avoid cystitis include: • Use water-soluble vaginal lubrication • Urinate before intercourse • Avoid diaphragm use, which *increases* the possibility of cystitis • Wear cotton underpants • Drink 2–3 quarts of fluid per day, including cranberry juice • Urinate every 2 hours • Use unscented toilet tissue; wipe front to back • Avoid bubble baths ***Prostate*** • Provide factual information on illness • Invite questions about myths and facts and sexual functioning
Respiratory Disorders	Encourage client to participate in rehabilitation program to increase respiratory reserve. Factors to increase sexual functioning include: • Some medication may help sexual functioning (e.g., bronchodilators relieve shortness of breath) • Plan for sex during the time of day when client feels most energetic; room temperature (68°) and humidity (40%) may be helpful • Increase oxygen saturation by exhaling through pursed lips several minutes before sex • Avoid heavy meal before sex • Side-lying position or male seated and straddled may be less tiring • Encourage sexual counseling as needed

example, "flashing" an erection to a woman. The amount of time spent masturbating becomes time consuming—perhaps 10 to 15 times per day. This is disrupting to activities of daily living: work, school, home responsibilities, and so on. The preoccupation often includes viewing and collecting pornographic materials. The person may use uncommon sexual services such as prostitutes, phone sex, and Internet sex to meet needs.

3. *A severe sexual dysfunction when a partner is involved.* The wives of men who are paraphiles report lack of interest in sex on the part of the paraphile and inability to perform. Some partners, however, are willing to play out a role with the person experiencing a paraphilia (e.g., dressing like a little girl).

Table 16–3 reviews some criminal and noncriminal paraphilias as defined in the United States. The source of intense sexual arousal, fantasies, urges, or behaviors is listed under the heading *Definition.*

Treatment

Sexual disorders are often not recognized, diagnosed, or treated unless they interfere with relationships, harm the person or others, or violate the law. For the client with paraphilia, the sexual urges and fantasies may be so entrenched that the client is resistive to psychotherapeutic intervention. If the behavior is violent and destructive, the legal system will become involved. The person will be removed from society as punishment. Families and communities become involved by refusing to condone "secrets." External controls are provided for future acting out by letting others know what is going on.

Gender Identity Disorder

According to DSM-IV, the client with a **gender identity disorder** strongly and persistently identifies as a member of the other sex. This may involve childhood, adolescence, or adulthood. Gender identity disorder is not connected with a physical sexual disorder.

Characteristics

In children, four or more of the following characteristics are present.

- A stated desire or insistence that he or she is of the other sex
- Cross dressing: in boys, dressing in female attire, and in girls, wearing the usual male attire
- Make-believe play and fantasy involves being the other sex
- Participation in stereotypical games and pastimes of the other sex
- Preference for playmates of the other sex

Adolescents and adults manifest the disorder by stating that they wish to be of the other sex, passing frequently as the other sex, desiring to live and be treated as the other sex, and believing that he or she has the feelings and reactions of the other sex.

Both males and females with gender identity disorder are uncomfortable with their sex and gender role. Boys indicate that their penises and testes are disgusting, will disappear, or that it would be better not to have a penis. They have an aversion for rough and tumble play and reject stereotypical male toys, games, or activities. Girls with this disorder reject urinating in a sitting position and insist that they will grow a penis. They do not want to grow breasts or menstruate and have an aversion to the usual female clothing.

Adolescents and adults are preoccupied with getting rid of their primary and secondary sexual characteristics. They believe they were born the wrong sex. Their feelings and concerns create significant stress and difficulties in social, occupational, or other important functioning areas.

Treatment

No one really knows how to cure an adult's gender disorder. Many clients insist on getting rid of primary and secondary sexual characteristics through hormones, surgery, and other procedures. These treatments alter the current sexual characteristics to simulate the other sex. Psychotherapy is useful if a trusting client-therapist relationship exists to deal with underlying feelings in a con-

Table 16–3 Paraphilias

Paraphilia	Definition	Special Features	Sex Crime (Felony)	Noncriminal
Pedophilia	Men who erotically and romantically prefer children or young adolescents	At least 16 years old and at least 5 years older than child or children (usually age 13 or younger)	X	
Voyeurism	Watch unsuspecting person who is naked, disrobing, or engaged in sex	Some men who watch women break into buildings; may result in rape or nonsexual violence	X	
Exhibitionism	Usually teenagers or men who expose penis to another person to shock or elicit sexual interest (fantasy)	May or may not masturbate during or after episode	X	
Sadism	Intense, sexually arousing fantasies, urges, or behaviors involving psychological or physical suffering, including humiliation of the victim	Paraphilic sadism is present in only a small number of rapes; diagnosis includes rapists' erotic scripts, which involve a partner's fear, pain, humiliation, and suffering	X (if rape)	
Frotteurism	Touching and rubbing against a nonconsenting person	Unaware of the fear they cause; often involves socially isolated men	X	
Masochism	Pain inflicted to person; ranges from being spanked to the point of becoming sexually excited to near-fatal means	Most common form of female paraphilia; sometimes sadists and masochists pair up to meet each others' needs		X
Transvestite fetishism	Involves cross-dressing; limited to articles of female clothing	Heterosexual male		X
Fetishism	Use of nonliving objects for sexual gratification	Arousal related to holding or wearing article; person is considered a paraphile if he or she uses one object for decades		X

structive way. Group therapy helps the client find support in discovering other people with similar problems.

CASE STUDY

NURSING CARE PLAN

The following case study demonstrates a nursing care plan for a client with sexual dysfunction secondary to a myocardial infarction. The example describes appropriate interventions for this client. Other interventions may be more appropriate for clients with other types of sexual dysfunction.

History and Data Collection

Mrs. Charles, age 56, has had a myocardial infarction. She works full time as a science teacher and is active in several volunteer organizations. Her husband of 5 years seems bewildered by what has happened. Mrs. Charles is doing well physically, but is resistant to having sexual intercourse with her husband. She shows her resistance by becoming distraught and weeping.

The nurse uses the RN's nursing diagnoses and the data collected to detail nursing problems appropriate for intervention at the LPN/LVN level. Table 16–4 shows the result.

Table 16–4	Nursing Diagnosis and Nursing Problem for Case Study
Nursing Diagnosis	**Nursing Problem**
Sexual dysfunction related to misconceptions about resuming sexual activity after myocardial infarction	Client is fearful that she will have a heart attack during intercourse

Goals, Interventions, Rationale, and Evaluation

Based on the nursing problem she has defined, the nurse proceeds to list appropriate goals and interventions, along with a rationale for each. With the RN's approval, she implements the interventions and evaluates the result. The goals, interventions, and evaluation are shown in Table 16–5. ▲

NURSING INTERVENTIONS

It is important for nurses and students who feel unsure or uninformed to seek additional information and education in the area of sexual disorders. The client needs and is entitled to compassionate care. He or she needs to be able to verbalize and explore the conflicting feelings and emotions without fear of judgment. Physical treatments, when involved, cause discomfort, and skilled nursing care is expected. Clients also need to learn about available community support groups.

SUMMARY

Dissociative disorders rely on the coping mechanism of dissociation to separate painful events from consciousness. In this way, the person sets aside the psychological pain associated with the overwhelming traumatic events. Use of this mechanism can result in dissociative amnesia unrelated to organic injury, dissociative fugue, depersonalization disorder, dissociative trance disorder, or dissociative identity disorder (formerly multiple personality disorder).

Treatment involves psychotherapy and hypnotherapy. Nursing intervention calls for great skill to maintain a consistent therapeutic milieu.

Nurses need to become familiar with more than the anatomical information. Otherwise, myths and prejudices may keep them from collecting data and dealing respectfully with the client.

Clients may develop sexual dysfunction as a part of a physical illness. Understanding the human sexual response and at what stage the response is

Table 16–5	Goals, Interventions, Rationale, and Evaluation for Case Study	
Goal	**Intervention**	**Rationale**
Mrs. Charles will learn the facts of when and how she can resume sexual activity	Explore beliefs and myths Mrs. Charles holds about heart attacks and future sexual activity	Find out which beliefs are fact and which are fiction
	Make a plan with Mrs. Charles on topics she needs to learn about; request that her husband be included	Provide a sense of control for what will be discussed Encourage a sense of partnering, a "second set of ears" Answer his questions and concerns at the same time

Evaluation: By day 2, Mrs. Charles was able to state the guidelines for resuming sexual activity with her husband.

affected gives clues to intervention. Clients need factual information and education on how to cope with sexual changes caused by illness. Their partner needs to be educated as well.

Paraphilic behavior as defined in the United States is often carried on in private or with a partner who plays out a role. Criminal sexual behaviors include pedophilia, voyeurism, exhibitionism, sadism (with rape), and frotteurism (when sexual arousal or orgasm is achieved by rubbing up against another person who is unaware of the activity, usually without specific genital contact). Noncriminal paraphilia includes masochism, transvestite fetishism, and fetishism. Clients may be resistive to treatment and/or change. The law becomes involved when harm occurs to self or others.

Gender identity disorders in childhood, adolescence, or adulthood find the client strongly and persistently uncomfortable in being their sex. They feel that they are trapped in the wrong body. Many seek medical means to make physical changes to that of the opposite sex.

Critical Thinking Activities

1. View the videos *Three Faces of Eve* or *Sybil*. Check with your school or local library for availability. Both are also available in some video stores. Discuss how movies such as these may influence the frequency with which dissociative identity disorders are diagnosed.

2. Review the sexual problems listed in Table 16–2 for a physical condition of interest to you. Develop a statement of how you might approach a client to encourage him or her to talk about sexual problems related to the illness.

Review Questions

Multiple Choice—Choose the best answer to each question.

1. How does the coping mechanism of dissociation work in dissociative disorders and sexual function disorders?
   a. Separates the painful event from consciousness
   b. Changes unacceptable thoughts and feelings into a socially acceptable outlet
   c. Offers believable reasons that are untrue for not fulfilling a responsibility
   d. Responds to others as though his or her thoughts and feelings belong to them

2. Why was dissociative identity disorder previously confused with personality disorders?
   a. It was assumed to be a maladaptive way of responding to stress
   b. The seriousness of the disorder was not recognized
   c. The previous name, *multiple personality disorder,* made the diagnosis sound like a personality disorder
   d. The psychotic state of the client made it difficult to diagnose
3. What is a major challenge for the nurse working with the client who has a dissociative identity disorder?
   a. Maintaining consistency in approach, regardless of the alternate personality
   b. Making a therapeutic shift in approach when an alternate personality emerges
   c. Providing continuous rationale regarding emerging alternate personalities
   d. Recalling the abuse to which a client was subjected, leading to dissociation
4. Why are client concerns of sex and sexuality often ignored by nurses?
   a. Instructors do not include sex and sexuality in nursing courses
   b. Concern that client will not do as he or she is told to do by the nurse
   c. Lack of factual information, leading to personal discomfort in the nurse
   d. Respect for privacy in this area of human response

5. What is pedophilia?
   a. Men who erotically and romantically prefer children or young adolescents
   b. Usually teens or men who expose their penis to other persons to shock or elicit interest
   c. Touching and rubbing against a nonconsenting person
   d. Use of nonliving objects for sexual gratification

References

American Psychiatric Association: Diagnostic and Statistical Manual of Mental Disorders, 4th ed. Chicago, 1994.

Curtin SL: Recognizing multiple personality disorder. J Psych Nurs 31(2):29–33, 1993.

Levine SB, Rosenblatt EA: Sexual disorders. In: Tasman A, Kay J, Lieberman JA (eds): Psychiatry, vol II. Philadelphia, WB Saunders Co, 1997.

Spiegel D: Dissociative disorders. In: Tasman A, Kay J, Lieberman JA (eds): Psychiatry, vol II. Philadelphia, WB Saunders Co, 1997.

Stafford LL: Dissociation & multiple personality disorder. J Psych Nurs 31(1):15–20, 1993.

Zawid C: Medical issues and sexuality. In: Sexual Health: A Nurse's Guide. Western Schools Press, South Eaton, Mass, 1993.

Eating Disorders

Outline

- **Types of Eating Disorders**
  Anorexia Nervosa
  Bulimia Nervosa
  Compulsive Overeating
- **Causes of Eating Disorders**
  Biological Factors
  Social Factors
  Psychological and Psychodynamic
  Factors
- **Therapies**
  Psychoeducation
  Nutritional Management

Pharmacotherapy
Behavior Modification
Psychodynamic Psychotherapy
Family Therapy
Group Therapy
- **Nursing Interventions**
- **Case Study: Nursing Care Plan**
  History and Data Collection
  Goals, Interventions, Rationale, and
  Evaluation
- **Resources for Prevention and Support**

Key Terms

- anorexia nervosa
- binge eating
- body image
- bulimia nervosa
- compulsive overeating

- eating disorder
- obesity
- purging
- transitional objects

Objectives

Upon completing this chapter, the student will be able to:
1. Describe three distinct eating disorders.
2. Discuss the possible causes for eating disorders.
3. Explain why obesity may be considered an eating disorder.
4. Discuss four therapies that are significant in working with people with an eating disorder.
5. Define the nurse's role in working with a client with an eating disorder.
6. State the resources that are available to people with eating disorders.

Fairburn and Walsh (1995, p. 135) define an **eating disorder** as a "persistent disturbance of eating or eating-related behavior that results in the altered consumption or absorption of food and that significantly impairs physical health or psychosocial functioning."

A common theme found in various eating disorders is a distorted body image. **Body image** is the reflection of how a person feels, thinks, and perceives his or her personal appearance. It is an important part of self-concept, which relates to self-esteem. "Of all psychological factors that are believed to cause eating disorders, body image dissatisfaction is the most relevant and immediate antecedent" (Rosen, 1995, p. 369).

TYPES OF EATING DISORDERS

Our society is obsessed with being thin and having a perfect body. This obsession has contributed to the development of eating disorders. The American Psychiatric Association's *Diagnostic and Statistical Manual of Mental Disorders, fourth edition* (DSM-IV) (APA, 1994, p. 538) classifies two conditions, anorexia nervosa and bulimia nervosa, as eating disorders. Disorders that do not meet specific criteria for these two listed conditions are included under "eating disorders not otherwise specified," or what could be called *atypical eating disorders.*

One example of an atypical eating disorder is frequent binge eating that is not followed by self-induced vomiting as in bulimia nervosa. This becomes **compulsive overeating**. Although people who engage in this behavior are often obese, obesity in itself is not considered an eating disorder. **Obesity** is an excess of body fat, usually 20% over acceptable standards. According to DSM-IV, obesity is not listed as an eating disorder because it has not been definitely established that it is associated with mental health or behavioral problems. However, many physical and psychological concerns are associated with the distress of being overweight.

Anorexia Nervosa

DSM-IV (APA, 1994, pp. 544–545) includes the following criteria for a diagnosis of **anorexia nervosa:**

- A refusal to maintain body weight at or above a minimally normal weight for age and height (weight loss leading to maintenance of body weight less than 85% of that expected)
- Intense fear of gaining weight or becoming fat, even though underweight
- Disturbance in the way in which one's body weight or shape is experienced, such as denial of the seriousness of the current low body weight or undue influence of body weight or shape on self-evaluation
- In females, amenorrhea (the absence of at least three consecutive menstrual cycles when they are otherwise expected to occur)

These criteria "point to three sets of related features: (1) an intense preoccupation with weight and shape; (2) behaviors that are directed at the relentless pursuit of thinness; and (3) the physical consequences of these behaviors, such as emaciation, disturbance of endocrine function, and other nutritional abnormalities" (Beumont, 1995, p. 151).

Some of the physical, behavioral, and emotional symptoms that occur in anorexia nervosa include the following:

- *Physical:* extreme weight loss, resulting in the body's inability to maintain heat; insomnia; constipation; skin rash or dry skin; loss of hair or nail quality; dental problems; and cessation of the menstrual period
- *Behavioral:* unusual eating habits, such as severely restricted food intake or food rituals; distorted body image; frequent weighing; high interest in exercise and high achievement
- *Emotional:* denial, low sense of self-worth, low self-control, perfectionism, masked anger, "good" and "bad" food lists

Table 17–1 describes the effect of anorexia nervosa on various physical systems.

Table 17–1	Medical Problems Related to Anorexia Nervosa
Heart	Starvation causes the heart muscles to shrink; the heart slows down or beats irregularly
Amenorrhea	Menstruation ceases frequently in anorectic patients
Kidneys	Dehydration can occur with ano- rectic behavior; kidney stones and kidney failure are a result of a lack of fluids in the body
Lanugo	Lanugo is a fine body hair that can develop on the bodies of anorectics
Muscle atrophy	Muscle and tissue can deteriorate with a substantial loss of weight
Digestive problems	Bowel irritation and constipation can be problems related to restrictive eating
Osteoporosis	Anorectics can develop osteopo- rosis later in life

Data from Bellin Psychiatric Center, Green Bay, Wis.

Bulimia Nervosa

DSM-IV (APA, 1994, pp. 549, 550) lists the fol- lowing criteria for a diagnosis of **bulimia nervosa:**

- Recurrent episodes of binge eating and a sense of lack of control over how much one is eating
- Recurrent, inappropriate compensatory behavior to prevent weight gain, such as self-induced vomiting, or misuse of laxatives or diuretics
- Binge eating and inappropriate compensatory behavior both occur, on average, at least twice a week for 3 months
- Self-evaluation is unduly influenced by body shape and weight

Some of the physical, emotional, and behavioral symptoms that may occur in bulimia nervosa include the following:

- *Physical:* People with bulimia nervosa are usu- ally within normal weight range, but excessive vomiting may lead to dehydration and electro- lyte imbalance, as well as irritation and tearing of the throat, esophagus, and stomach. Vomiting may also cause stomach acids to erode tooth enamel. Laxative dependence, emetic toxicity, and swollen glands can also occur (Bellin Psychiatric Center, Green Bay, Wis).
- *Emotional:* Eating binges are often followed by self-criticism and depressed mood—what some call "postbinge anguish" (Kaplan, Sadock, and Grabb, 1994, p. 696).
- *Behavioral:* Binges are secret, with a feeling of loss of control or inability to stop eating and an obsession with body image and appearance.

Contrary to common belief, bulimia nervosa does not occur exclusively during episodes of an- orexia nervosa. Bulimia nervosa is more common than anorexia nervosa. Isolated episodes of binge eating and purging have been reported in as high as 40% of college women (Kaplan, Sadock, and Grabb, 1994, p. 695). This disorder can also occur in men and older women. **Binge eating** is eating in a distinct period of time an amount of food that is definitely more than most people would eat under the same conditions (APA, 1994, pp. 545–546). **Purging** is usually self-induced vomiting or the misuse of laxatives, diuretics, or enemas.

Reality Check

You notice that Mary Ellen, a co-worker, sneaks leftover food off of clients' trays. She tries to be very secretive about it. As Mary Ellen's behavior continues, she con- sumes larger quantities of food. After eating, Mary Ellen disappears from the unit for a short period. This behavior seems to occur whenever Mary Ellen is unable to com- plete her assignments.

1. How is Mary Ellen coping with stress?
2. What might you, as a co-worker, do to help Mary Ellen?
3. What resources might be helpful for Mary Ellen?

Compulsive Overeating

Obesity has several causes. They include overeating, heredity, lack of sufficient exercise, and complicated neurochemicals that control appetite and eating behaviors. Faulty eating behaviors can begin in childhood. **Compulsive overeating** is a disorder in which people learn to use food as a means of coping with stress.

As a person becomes overweight, his or her body image is affected. The person may feel less attractive, rejected, and lonely, and uses food to ease the pain. A vicious cycle is created, and the person finds comfort in food. The symptoms of compulsive overeating include the following:

- Overweight (usually)
- Body dissatisfaction
- Gorging on large quantities of food without purging
- Unsuccessful dieting
- Eating alone or hiding eating

Reality Check

Catherine, a 45-year-old housewife, spends her day watching TV soap operas. She continually eats snacks, including cookies, candy, and chips, and she drinks sodas. She has gained 30 lb in the last 3 months. Her children have all moved out, and she is alone all day while her husband works. She has been told that she has diabetes.

1. What might explain Catherine's behavior?
2. How might Catherine be helped in changing her behavior?
3. What could you do to educate Catherine about diabetes?

Compulsive overeating can have serious physical effects. It can cause joint problems, high blood pressure, high cholesterol levels, and heart disease. It puts a strain on the heart muscle, forcing it to work harder. People who are overweight also have an increased risk of diabetes (Bellin Psychiatric Center, Green Bay, Wis.).

CAUSES OF EATING DISORDERS

An eating disorder becomes a way of coping with anxiety (see Fig. 2–2). Biological, social, and psychological factors are implicated as possible causes of eating disorders.

Biological Factors

Some of the findings from research indicate that there are neurochemical changes in people with anorexia nervosa and bulimia nervosa. However, it is difficult to know if the chemical changes precede or follow other changes that occur in these disorders, such as amenorrhea, constipation, and insomnia. In anorexia nervosa, many of the biochemical changes resulting from starvation are also present in depression, such as hypercortisolemia and non-suppression by dexamethasone. In bulimia nervosa, cycles of binge eating and purging have been associated with differing levels of various neurotransmitters, such as serotonin and norepinephrine. People with bulimia nervosa can often be helped with antidepressants (Kaplan, Sadock, and Grabb, 1994, pp. 690, 695).

Social Factors

Eating disorders are one response to a society that emphasizes thinness and exercise. There are indications that people with anorexia nervosa have close but strained relationships with their parents. Anorexia nervosa can be a way of gaining control over the pressure exerted by society and parents to achieve in life. People with bulimia nervosa also are high achievers, and they respond to society's pressure to be thin. Their family relationships are less close and tend to be conflicting. In both conditions, many of the people are depressed and have a history of familial depression (Kaplan, Sadock, and Grabb, 1994, pp. 690, 695).

Psychological and Psychodynamic Factors

The underlying psychodynamic pathology is varied. Each person needs to be "understood as a person." He or she wants others to understand why the illness occurred—the pressures, the person's vulnerability, and the factors that prevent recovery (Beumont, 1995, p. 152).

Anorexia nervosa appears to result from societal demands on adolescents for more independence. Those with the disorder substitute their focus on eating and weight gain for other adolescent social activities. People with anorexia nervosa often lack a sense of autonomy and self-identity. "Self-starvation may be an effort to gain validation as a unique and special person" (Kaplan, Sadock, and Grabb, 1994, p. 690).

Like those with anorexia nervosa, people with bulimia nervosa have difficulty meeting the demands of adolescence, although they are more outgoing and angry. Many people with bulimia nervosa have a history of problems with separation from a caretaker. This may be evidenced by the lack of transitional objects during their childhood years (Kaplan, Sadock, and Grabb, 1994, p. 695). **Transitional objects** (such as relatives, friends, favorite toys, a blanket) provide support to the child during the changes that he or she goes through.

THERAPIES

Therapies for eating disorders include psychoeducation and psychotherapy, as well as nutritional management and medical interventions (pharmacotherapy). This section discusses the various therapeutic approaches.

Psychoeducation

This approach provides information to the person about the disorder and ways of overcoming it. The purpose is to promote attitudinal and behavioral change. Therapists must have a background in the scientific material that they plan to present. This approach imparts to the client an attitude of respect; the educational process becomes a collaborative effort to help him or her recover. Educational information includes the following: (Olmsted, Kaplan, 1995, pp. 299-301):

- The complex nature of eating disorders: people need to understand that what made them suscep-

tible to developing an eating disorder may be different from what is maintaining the problem
- Medical complications that result from vomiting, diuretic use, and laxatives
- Basic nutritional information, including the food pyramid
- Body-image issues and sociocultural factors; discussion of society pressures on women to be thin through advertisements and in the media; the goal is to help the person focus on his or her strengths rather than on appearance
- Prevention of relapse: it is important for people to know that the process of recovery takes time and to differentiate between "slips" and relapse

Nutritional Management

Nutritional counseling should focus on achieving and maintaining the following (Beumont, Touyz, 1995, p. 307):

- Normal nutrition (adults) or normal growth (adolescents)
- Normal eating behavior
- A normal attitude about food
- Normal responses to hunger satiety cues

Before any nutritional education can be effective, the person's trust needs to be gained. This may be established not only by giving accurate information but also by being a good listener.

Pharmacotherapy

Use of medication for anorexia nervosa does not usually occur until acute medical problems have been addressed and the person has gained weight. If the person is depressed, the selective serotonin reuptake inhibitors (SSRIs) may be preferred to other antidepressant medications.

Investigations show that the use of medication, mainly antidepressants, in the treatment of bulimia nervosa is more effective than in anorexia nervosa. Some think that this difference is due to an increase of mood disturbance associated with bulimia. However, it is recommended that psychotherapy be tried before medication with people who are not seriously depressed (Walsh, 1995, p. 36).

Behavior Modification

The techniques of behavior modification are an effective form of treatment for people with eating disorders. The key to successful implementation of such a program is to help the person develop a sense of control. The person contracts with the therapist and participates in setting goals as well as rewards for achievement of the goals, such as weight gained or not vomiting (Decker, Freeman, 1996, p. 919).

Psychodynamic Psychotherapy

Psychodynamic psychotherapy is used in eating disorders to help the client to do the following (Herzog, 1995, p. 330):

- Regain a sense of feeling and caring about self and others
- Express his or her feelings related to the disorder, such as inadequacy, power, or dependency
- Develop more constructive coping strategies
- Achieve physical and emotional health

This therapy is usually used on a long-term basis with the person who has anorexia nervosa. The relationship between client and the therapist is the primary treatment tool.

Family Therapy

Family therapy helps family members make positive changes in their lives. The focus is on the family as a whole and off the person with the eating disorder. These families usually have poor communication patterns, with vague boundaries and roles. Through a family systems approach, the treatment team helps the family make connections between changes in family patterns and resulting changes in the person's eating behaviors. The therapist treats the family in an understanding and nonjudgmental way. Positive feedback is important, as well as making the person with the disorder responsible for his or her own behavior (Conant, 1994, p. 723).

Group Therapy

Group therapy can be helpful for people with eating disorders. Sharing problems with others can help reduce the stigma, shame, and isolation that these people feel. Other advantages of group therapy are that members can learn from one another, and that it is a more cost-effective approach. The group leader functions as a facilitator, encouraging members to use skills learned in group sessions with family and friends. Assuming personal responsibility and reaching out to others in mutual support are difficult goals to achieve, but they are necessary (Conant, 1994, p. 723).

NURSING INTERVENTIONS

Many people with eating disorders are treated on an outpatient basis unless their condition is life threatening. The nurse working with a client who has an eating disorder needs to collect data on the client's weight, eating behavior, activity (exercise), family relations, physical signs and symptoms, and perception of self. Some of the important interventions in working with a client with an eating disorder include the following:

- Establishing a trusting relationship by being honest and accepting and keeping promises
- Helping the client re-examine negative perceptions of self and recognize and focus on strengths
- Helping the client identify the real feelings and fears that contributed to inappropriate eating behavior
- Exploring with the client how food is used to provide comfort and relieve anxiety
- Offering positive reinforcement for independently made decisions affecting the client's life
- Helping the client own angry feelings and learn to deal with them in acceptable and appropriate ways
- Promoting feelings of control within the environment by encouraging participation and independent decision making
- Helping the client identify specific concerns within the family and ways of possibly relieving those concerns
- Explaining to the client the details of specific programs ordered by the physician, such as behavior modification

CASE STUDY

NURSING CARE PLAN

The following case study demonstrates a nursing care plan for a client with anorexia nervosa. The example describes appropriate interventions for this client. Other interventions may be more appropriate for clients with other types of eating disorders.

History and Data Collection

Sally, a 14-year-old freshman, was admitted to the psychiatric unit because of severe weight loss. She had lost 20 lb in the last 2 months. Her mother told the nurse that her daughter thinks she is too fat and has been skipping meals. She also found her exercising in her bedroom at night after everyone had gone to bed. Sally has a sister who is ill and receives a lot of medical care.

Every time the parents come to visit Sally, the first questions that they ask the nurse are "Did Sally eat yesterday?" and "How much weight did she gain?"

Sally spends her time drawing pictures. One of her drawings was printed in the school newspaper.

The nurse uses the RN's nursing diagnoses and the data collected to detail nursing problems appropriate for intervention at the LPN/LVN level. Table 17–2 shows the result.

Table 17–2	Nursing Diagnosis and Nursing Problem for Case Study
Nursing Diagnosis	**Nursing Problem**
Alteration in nutrition (less than body requirements) related to not eating and physical exertion as evidenced by weight loss	Sally has lost a significant amount of weight because of improper eating habits and excessive exercise

Goals, Interventions, Rationale, and Evaluation

Based on the nursing problem she has defined, the nurse proceeds to list appropriate goals and interventions, along with a rationale for each. With the RN's approval, she implements the interventions and evaluates the result. The goals, interventions, and evaluation are shown in Table 17–3. ▲

RESOURCES FOR PREVENTION AND SUPPORT

The organizations listed provide a range of services to help people prevent and treat eating disorders. Information about their services is either free or available at a minimal charge for the cost of printing and mailing.

- Eating Disorders Awareness, Inc. (EDA)
  2661 Bel-Red Road
  Bellevue, WA 98009
  (206) 867-0700

  This is an international program founded in 1987 and dedicated to the prevention of eating disorders. The organization promotes healthy attitudes toward eating and weight.

- National Association of Anorexia Nervosa and Associated Disorders (ANAD)
  PO Box 7
  Highland Park, IL 60035
  (708) 831-3438

  ANAD was founded in 1976 and was the first national nonprofit educational and self-help organization in America dedicated to alleviating eating disorders. Their free services include counseling, information, and referrals; self-help groups for victims and parents; and a newsletter.

- Bulimia Anorexia Self-Help, Inc. (BASH)
  PO Box 39903
  St. Louis, MO 68139
  1-800-227-4785

  This organization began in 1981 as a small support group. Eight years later, it began to

Table 17–3	Goals, Interventions, Rationale, and Evaluation for Case Study	
Goal	**Intervention**	**Rationale**
Sally will gain 1-2 lb of body weight per week	Establish a trusting relationship with Sally Collect data on Sally's nutritional status	The nurse-patient relationship is based on trust Need to have a nutritional baseline
Sally will develop effective coping techniques to replace her inappropriate eating behavior by discharge	Focus on Sally's strengths; help her identify the feelings and fears that contributed to her eating pattern; explore with her how food can be used for comfort and relief of anxiety; using Sally's artistic talents, encourage participation in activities	Self-awareness is important in changing behavior patterns; positive reinforcement helps increase self-esteem when it is task-specific; support strengths
Involve Sally's family in family therapy	Give positive reinforcement; support the recommendation for Sally's family to participate in family therapy	Family therapy opens communication among all the members and supports them in making changes in their lives

Evaluation: With much encouragement, Sally began to eat. By the end of one week, she had gained ½ lb. Family therapy helped her parents realize that with all the attention focused on the sister who was ill, they were neglecting Sally. Sally began to use her artistic ability to channel her feelings.

provide information on problems related to overweight and dieting. The 24-hour crisis line number is 1-800-762-3334.

- Overeaters Anonymous (OA)
  PO Box 92870
  Los Angeles, CA 90009
  (213) 542-8368

This is a self-help group for people who compulsively overeat. The program is modeled after the 12-step program of Alcoholics Anonymous. With the support of members, compulsive overeaters are helped to change their eating habits.

- National Food Addiction Hotline
  1-800-USA-0088

The hotline is associated with the Florida Institute of Technology, School of Psychology, 50 West University Boulevard, Melbourne, FL 32901-6988 (Moe, 1991, pp. 133–137).

SUMMARY

Millions of Americans suffer from eating disorders in a society that is obsessed with thinness and body appearance. Types of eating disorders discussed in this chapter are anorexia nervosa, bulimia nervosa, and compulsive overeating.

Some of the causes for eating disorders include biological factors, social factors, and psychodynamic factors. The symptoms of the eating disorders revolve around an obsession with body image and appearance and a low sense of self-control and self-worth. In anorexia nervosa, the person has extreme weight loss; in bulimia nervosa, there is binge eating and purging. The obese person who is a compulsive overeater finds comfort and stress relief in food.

Many medical problems are related to eating disorders. These problems can involve the heart, kidneys, muscles, digestive organs, and electrolyte balance.

Therapies that are helpful with eating disorders are psychoeducation, nutritional management, pharmacotherapy, behavior management, psycho-dynamic psychotherapy, family therapy, and group therapy. Nursing interventions need to focus on establishing a trusting relationship with the client, and re-examining with the client the negative perceptions of self. The nurse helps the client explore more effective means of coping with feelings by focusing on the client's strengths and using positive reinforcement. Some resources for prevention and support groups are listed.

Critical Thinking Activities

1. How much is your thinking influenced by a person's weight and body shape?
2. How might the advertisements and TV programs that focus on body weight and appearance affect young people's body image?
3. What is your reaction to the weight-reducing plans and diet pills that are being marketed today?

Review Questions

Multiple Choice—Choose the best answer to each question.

1. A common theme found in eating disorders is
   a. autonomy and self-identity.
   b. participation in socialization.
   c. distortion of body image.
   d. personal responsibility.
2. A feature of anorexia nervosa is
   a. gorging on large quantities of food.
   b. an intense preoccupation with weight and shape.
   c. recurrent binge eating and purging.
   d. an excess of body weight.
3. Which of the following is an important nursing intervention in working with a client with an eating disorder?
   a. Using a confrontational approach with the client

   b. Using scare tactics about the ill effects of eating disorders
   c. Complimenting the client on how thin he or she looks
   d. Promoting feelings of control within the environment
4. A medical problem related to compulsive eating is
   a. lanugo.
   b. electrolyte imbalance.
   c. high blood pressure.
   d. amenorrhea.
5. The goal of behavior modification in the treatment of a person with an eating disorder is to
   a. help the person develop a sense of control.
   b. restore the person's ability to feel and care.
   c. improve communication patterns within the family.
   d. improve the mood of the person.

References

American Psychiatric Association: Diagnostic and Statistical Manual of Mental Disorders, 4th ed. Washington, DC, American Psychiatric Association, 1994.

Beumont PJV: The clinical presentation of anorexia and bulimia nervosa. In: Brownell KC, Fairburn CG (eds): Eating Disorders and Obesity: A Comprehensive Handbook. New York, The Guilford Press, 1995.

Beumont PJV, Touyz SW: The nutritional management of anorexia and bulimia nervosa. In: Brownell KC, Fairburn CG (eds): Eating Disorders and Obesity: A Comprehensive Handbook. New York, The Guilford Press, 1995.

Conant MJ: People who defend against anxiety through eating disorders. In: Varcarolis EM (ed): Foundations of Psychiatric Mental Health Nursing, 2nd ed. Philadelphia, WB Saunders Co, 1994.

Decker WA, Freeman M: The journey challenged by eating disorders. In: Carson VB, Arnold EN (eds): Mental Health Nursing: The Nurse-Patient Journey. Philadelphia, WB Saunders Co, 1996.

Fairburn CG, Walsh BT: Atypical eating disorders. In: Brownell KD, Fairburn CG (eds): Eating Disorders and Obesity: A Comprehensive Handbook. New York, The Guilford Press, 1995.

Herzog DB: Psychodynamic psychotherapy for anorexia nervosa. In: Brownell KD, Fairburn CG (eds): Eating

Disorders and Obesity: A Comprehensive Handbook. New York, The Guilford Press, 1995.

Kaplan HI, Sadock BJ, Grabb JA: Synopsis of Psychiatry, 7th ed. Baltimore, Williams & Wilkins Publishing, 1994.

Moe B: Coping With Eating Disorders. New York, The Rosen Publishing Group, Inc, 1991.

Olmsted MP, Kaplan AS: Psychoeducation in the treatment of eating disorders. In: Brownell KD, Fairburn CG (eds): Eating Disorders and Obesity: A Comprehensive Handbook. New York, The Guilford Press, 1995.

Rosen JC: Assessment and treatment of body image disturbance. In: Brownell KD, Fairburn CG (eds): Eating Disorders and Obesity: A Comprehensive Handbook. New York, The Guilford Press, 1995.

Walsh BT: Pharmacotherapy of eating disorders. In: Brownell KD, Fairburn CG (eds): Eating Disorders and Obesity: A Comprehensive Handbook. New York, The Guilford Press, 1995.

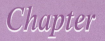
Personality Disorders

Outline

- **Classification of Personality Disorders**
  Antisocial Personality Disorder
  Borderline Personality Disorder
- **Case Study: Nursing Care Plan**

History and Data Collection
Goals, Interventions, Rationale, and
  Evaluation

Key Terms

- **destructive manipulation**
- **object constancy**

- **personality disorder**
- **splitting**

Objectives

Upon completing this chapter, the student will be able to:

1. Define *personality disorder*.
2. Describe the characteristics of personality disorders based on clusters A, B, and C.
3. Describe the predisposing factors of an antisocial personality disorder.
4. List symptoms associated with antisocial personality disorder.
5. Describe specific nursing interventions for the client with an antisocial personality disorder.
6. Discuss the predisposing factors of a borderline personality disorder.
7. Identify symptoms of a borderline personality disorder.
8. List three characteristics that are present in a person with borderline personality disorder.
9. List the nursing intervention that may be used to meet the challenges presented by a client with borderline personality disorder.

According to the American Psychiatric Association's *Diagnostic and Statistic Manual of Mental Disorders, fourth edition* (DSM-IV), a **personality disorder** is one in which a person's behavior and inner experience are markedly different from the expectations of his or her culture. In addition, the disorder has the following characteristics (APA, 1994, p. 629):

- Is pervasive and inflexible
- Has an onset in adolescence or early adulthood
- Is stable over time
- Leads to distress and impairment

CLASSIFICATION OF PERSONALITY DISORDERS

The DSM-IV has grouped the personality disorders into clusters based on descriptive similarities (APA, 1994, pp. 629, 630). Table 18–1 describes the clusters of personality disorders and their characteristics.

This chapter will focus on the antisocial personality disorder and the borderline personality disorder from Cluster B. These two disorders present many challenges for the nurse in both the inpatient and outpatient settings.

Table 18–1 Clusters of Personality Disorders and Characteristics

Cluster/Behavior	Main Characteristics
Cluster A	
Paranoid personality disorder	Overall suspicion and distrust, without cause, that others are exploiting, harming, or deceiving him or her
Schizoid personality disorder	Detachment from social relationships; restricted range of expression of emotions in interpersonal settings; the person is a loner
Schizotypal personality disorder	Pattern of social and interpersonal deficits, marked by odd beliefs or magical thinking, that influences relationships
Cluster B	
Antisocial personality disorder	Diffuse pattern of disregard for and violation of the rights of others that begins in childhood or early adolescence
Borderline personality disorder	Diffuse pattern of unstable internal relationships, poor self-image, unstable mood, and marked impulsivity, beginning in early adulthood
Histrionic personality disorder	Excessive emotionality and attention seeking, beginning in early adulthood; people with this disorder are uncomfortable unless they are the center of attention
Narcissistic personality disorder	Diffuse pattern of grandiosity, need for admiration, and lack of empathy toward others
Cluster C	
Avoidant personality disorder	Pattern of social inhibition, feelings of inadequacy, and hypersensitivity to negative evaluation, beginning in early adulthood
Dependent personality disorder	Excessive need to be taken care of by others; this leads to submissive and clinging behavior with fear of separation; develops by early adulthood
Obsessive-compulsive personality disorder	Preoccupation with orderliness and perfectionism; the person is reluctant to delegate tasks and displays rigidity and stubbornness; pattern of behavior begins in early adulthood

Antisocial Personality Disorder

Antisocial personality disorder has been known as *psychopathic, sociopathic,* or *dyssocial personality disorder.*

Predisposing Factors

There is evidence that multiple factors are present in the cause of antisocial personality disorder. These factors include the following (Gunderson, Phillips, 1995, p. 1442):

- Genetics
- Frequent exposure to substance abuse and criminal behavior
- A childhood with erratic, neglectful, harsh, or physically-abusive parenting
- Attention deficit/hyperactivity or conduct disorder in childhood
- Sociological factors such as poverty, urban environment, large families, divorce, and poorly structured early schools

Symptoms

People with an antisocial personality disorder appear to operate on the pleasure principle: "I want what I want when I want it." Their behavior varies, but is most commonly associated with areas in which strong values are held, such as aggressiveness and sexual impulses.

The antisocial pattern begins early in life. The adult is remembered as the child who "never did mind, regardless of tears and promises." In adolescence, patterns of truancy, casual sexual relationships, drug and alcohol abuse, fights, stealing, and vandalism are common. From early on, the person usually has had repeated bouts with the law, despite promises not to repeat the offenses. He or she feels no remorse for hurtful actions, and may explain a brutal act with a statement such as " I just wanted to see what it felt like to cut the dog in half." This person engages in a variety of criminal activities that frequently include rape.

The personality of the client with antisocial behavior is usually superficially charming, and the client is quick to play one staff member against another. This **destructive manipulation** is a way of getting something from another person for one's own purpose without considering the needs of that person. Occasionally, the client can persuade a new nurse to believe that the nurse is the only one who has ever understood or listened to the client. According to the client, all he or she needs is a chance, some money, a place to stay, and some help finding a job. For example, the nurse may comply, only to find out too late that a characteristic of this disorder is pathological lying.

The person may be seen in a mental health setting for a variety of reasons. He or she may be experiencing a superimposed psychosis, may have abused alcohol or drugs, or may have been sent by the courts for evaluation or as an opportunity to work on his or her underlying problems. The chances of making a healthy adjustment are guarded because the person with an antisocial personality disorder continues to engage in antisocial behavior. Studies indicate that some of these people finally begin to "burn out" around age 40 and consequently settle into more socially acceptable behavior.

Nursing Interventions

Nursing interventions for people with antisocial personality disorder include the following:

- A thorough *orientation* to rules, regulations, and expectations.
- A firm, yet respectful, *attitude.* The nurse should remember that the client's behavior represents his or her defense against anxiety. The client deals with anxiety by immediately discharging it onto the environment in many destructive ways.
- Involving the client in a discussion about what is to be accomplished during hospitalization.
- Developing a structured plan for each day's activities. The nurse should review the plan with the client, being sure it is understood. It is important that the client have a copy of the plan.
- Making *no* exceptions to the plan once it is instituted.
- Having the client limit all requests to his or her assigned caregiver on each shift. The nurse should make sure that all staff are aware of the plan.

- Recording compliance with the plan on each shift. The client is entitled to honest feedback on how he or she is progressing.
- Interrupting behavior in which the client begins to use negative techniques, and pointing out what the client is doing.
- Knowing where the client is at all times. He or she may seek out clients with like problems or defenseless clients (e.g., withdrawn clients) to exploit them.

If the client has superimposed problems, such as psychosis or substance abuse, specific additional interventions will have to be incorporated into his or her care.

Borderline Personality Disorder

Borderline personality disorder is the personality disorder most commonly seen in clinical settings. It occurs in 2% to 3% of the general population (Gunderson, Phillips, 1995, pp. 1439, 1440).

Predisposing Factors

Borderline personality disorder includes a variety "of probably nonspecific predisposing neurobiological, early developmental, and socializing factors" (Gunderson, Phillips, 1995, pp. 1439, 1440). Studies have suggested that people with borderline personality disorder have histories of early parental loss or traumatic separations. In the search for maternal substitutes, these people use transitional objects from childhood for an extended time, which can continue into adulthood. Also, the relationship with the mother is hostile and full of conflict. This is not balanced by a positive relationship with the father. Both parents usually have significant psychological problems. The mother is often erratic and depressed; the father is absent or disturbed. The family history often includes alcoholism and physical or sexual abuse.

Symptoms

Criteria used to diagnose a borderline personality disorder include the following (APA, 1994, p. 654):

- Frantic efforts to avoid real or imagined abandonment

- A pattern of unstable and intense interpersonal relationships characterized by an alternation between extremes of idealization and devaluation
- Identity disturbance: markedly and persistently unstable self-image and sense of self
- Impulsivity in at least two areas that are potentially self damaging (e.g., spending, sex, substance abuse)
- Recurrent suicidal behavior, gestures or threats, or self-mutilating behavior
- Affective instability caused by a marked reactivity of mood
- Chronic feelings of emptiness
- Inappropriate or intense anger or difficulty controlling anger
- Transient, stress-related paranoid ideation or severe dissociative symptoms

Three significant characteristics present in clients with a borderline personality disorder are the following:

1. *Lack of object constancy:* **Object constancy** is the ability to remember or think of an important person or object as "real" when that person or object is not present. This capacity begins developing during the toddler stage and is not complete until school age. An example of this is when parents leave a young child with a baby-sitter; the child sometimes feels the parents are not returning. In the client with borderline personality disorder, object constancy is limited or does not exist. This explains the person's frantic efforts to avoid abandonment.
2. *Splitting:* **Splitting,** for people with borderline personality disorder, is "like living in a world of one or ten, and two through nine do not exist" (Dresser, 1996). It becomes difficult to relate to others because things are right or wrong, black or white. These people live in extremes, which can be very frustrating and exhausting.
3. *Self-mutilation:* This behavior results from the client's need to feel alive. When he or she sees blood, it is a sign of living rather than death. Staff often accuse the client of seeking attention, depriving the client of the opportunity to learn ways of reconnecting to the self (Dresser,

1996). It is generally not the client's intent to commit suicide. Suicide occurs when the client miscalculates his or her actions.

Statements from clients with borderline personality disorder reflect estrangement, inadequacy, and despair. Examples include the following (Miller, 1994, p. 1217):

- "I had a lot of friends, but I never felt part of the group."
- "I can't explain it, but . . . you feel you're useless, you're worthless."
- "I wouldn't wish this on someone else. If someone said that you could get rid of it by giving it to someone else, I don't think I would do it, knowing what I have been through."

Nursing Interventions

Clients with borderline personality disorder can cause dissension and disruption among staff. Open communication among all caregivers, with specific guidelines, can have positive benefits for clients and their nurses (Piccinino, 1990, p. 27). Interventions include the following (Dresser, 1996):

- Being consistent and honest
- Admitting mistakes
- Learning the client's language
- Asking about both thoughts and feelings (they are often different)
- Constantly clarifying what both the nurse and the client heard and what it meant
- Limiting acting out; the nurse should set limits when he or she is not angry
- Keeping consequences clear, consistent, and upfront; a written contract can help in teaching new coping behaviors
- Teaching the client to recognize, label, and share feelings verbally
- Teaching the client realistic goal setting and self-acknowledgment
- Teaching use of humor
- Helping the client recognize personal "warning signs"
- Assisting in creating "bridges" for effective coping during crisis

Treatment

Treatment for antisocial and borderline personality disorders focuses on interpersonal relationships such as limit setting and controlling manipulation. Psychotropic medications must be administered with caution to clients with personality disorders. These clients generally do not like taking medicine. They are fearful of taking something over which they have no control. Despite the problems, antipsychotics may be useful for brief periods to control agitation. A client with borderline personality disorder may be helped at times with antidepressants (Profiri, 1998, p. 526).

Reality Check

Tina, a 35-year-old single parent, was admitted to the mental health center for cutting her wrist. This is her fifth admission for self-mutilation. The same nurse who cared for Tina during her other hospitalizations was assigned to work with her. The nurse explained to Tina the rules of the unit, and asked Tina to repeat what she heard. Tina said that the nurse was the only one who understood her, and that she would do all that she could to follow the rules. Later on in the day Tina approached her nurse, stating that she hated her and had done nothing to help her.

1. What type of behavior is Tina showing?
2. What response might the nurse make regarding Tina's accusations?
3. What interventions might help Tina develop better coping skills?

CASE STUDY

NURSING CARE PLAN

The following case study demonstrates a nursing care plan for a client with an antisocial personality disorder. The example describes appropriate interventions for this client. Other interventions may be more appropriate for clients with other symptoms or a different personality disorder.

History and Data Collection

Fred Marker, age 19, is admitted to the mental health center. He had been on the children's unit for 6 weeks at the age of 13. Fred has a history of numerous problems, such as truancy from school, lying, running away from home, using drugs and alcohol, and frequent fights. Because of drug use and stealing, he appeared in juvenile court at age 15, but the case was dismissed for lack of evidence. This is the first time Mr. Marker has been in adult court for selling drugs. The judge listened to Mr. Marker's plea for a chance to "straighten out" and sent him to the mental health center for 2 weeks of observation.

Mr. Marker is a tall, good-looking, charming young man who quickly involved himself in unit activities. Later in the week, three clients reported missing money. Although the money was located in Mr. Marker's room, he denied taking it, adding "Somebody planted it there. Another bum rap!" Later in the day, he sought out a new staff nurse. He talked to her about needing someone to understand him and give him a chance. He told her she was the first one who had ever listened to him.

The nurse uses the RN's nursing diagnoses and the data collected to detail nursing problems appropriate for intervention at the LPN/LVN level. Table 18–2 shows the result.

Table 18–2	Nursing Diagnosis and Nursing Problem for Case Study
Nursing Diagnosis	**Nursing Problem**
Impaired social interaction related to communication barriers as evidenced by exploitation of others for the fulfillment of own desires	Mr. Marker has taken money from other clients' rooms; uses his personal charm to influence staff

Goals, Interventions, Rationale, and Evaluation

Based on the nursing problem she has defined, the nurse proceeds to list appropriate goals and interventions, along with a rationale for each. With the RN's approval, she implements the interventions and evaluates the result. The goals, interventions, and evaluation are shown in Table 18–3.

▲

SUMMARY

Personality disorders present a persistent pattern of behavior that is markedly different from the expectations of the person's culture. The two personality disorders discussed are antisocial personality disorder and borderline personality disorder. These disorders present many challenges for the nurse in the inpatient and outpatient settings.

The person with an antisocial personality disorder displays a complete disregard for others. The cause of this disorder includes multiple factors. People with antisocial personality disorder seem to operate on the pleasure principle: "I want what I want when I want it." They use destructive manipulation to fulfill their desires. Their way of dealing with anxiety is to discharge it onto the environment immediately.

The person with antisocial personality disorder requires specific limits and a structured plan for each day's activities with no exceptions. It is best to have one assigned caregiver for the client, with clear communication among *all* staff regarding the plan of care. The staff person needs to be firm, respectful, and not influenced by the charming ways of the client.

The person with borderline personality disorder presents a pattern of instability regarding interpersonal relationships, self-image and affects, and noticeable impulsivity. Studies suggest that people with borderline personality disorder have histories of early parental loss or traumatic separations. Three significant characteristics present in people with borderline personality disorder are lack of object constancy, splitting, and self-mutilation. Clients with borderline personality disorder can

Table 18–3	Goals, Interventions, Rationale, and Evaluation for Case Study	
Goal	**Intervention**	**Rationale**
Mr. Marker will behave in a socially acceptable manner while on the unit for a 2-week observation	Provide Mr. Marker with a thorough orientation to unit rules, regulations, and expectations; give him a copy of the unit orientation booklet for reference	Identify expectations
	Instruct Mr. Marker to limit all of his requests on each shift to the staff person assigned to him; make no exceptions to the rules	Define limits
	Know where Mr. Marker is at all times, because he is under court observation; do not allow passes or independent activities during the 2-week observation period; police department has requested that they be notified should he leave	Standard procedure per court
	Deal with all attempts at destructive manipulation by interrupting the cycle and explaining to Mr. Marker what he is doing	Decrease destructive manipulation
	Note and carefully record Mr. Marker's behavior on each shift	Required for court observation
	Instruct all staff to read and follow Mr. Marker's care plan	Provide continuity, consistency, and safety checks against destructive manipulation

Evaluation: During the second week of observation, Mr. Marker did not take money and did not try to talk staff into special favors.

cause dissension and disruption among staff. Open communication is essential. The nurse needs to be consistent, honest, and limit acting out. A written contract can keep consequences clear and up-front. Such a tool is helpful in teaching new coping behaviors.

Critical Thinking Activities

1. What nursing interventions would be appropriate in a care plan for a client who plays one staff member against another?
2. What types of interventions could be used to help a client with borderline personality disorder deal with the feelings of abandonment?

Review Questions

Multiple Choice—Choose the best answer to each question.

1. Which of the following is an example of a Cluster B personality disorder?
   a. Schizotypal personality disorder
   b. Avoidant personality disorder
   c. Dependent personality disorder
   d. Antisocial personality disorder
2. Which of the following is a symptom of an antisocial personality disorder?
   a. Splitting
   b. Destructive manipulation

c. Self-mutilation

d. Lack of object constancy

3. A specific nursing intervention for a client with an antisocial personality disorder is

a. rotating the staff who care for the client.

b. allowing the client to plan the day's activities.

c. interrupting negative techniques used by the client.

d. believing that the client is trying to do what is right.

4. The self-mutilation in a client with a borderline personality disorder results from

a. a need to feel alive.

b. a need for attention.

c. a need to die.

d. a need to control staff.

5. A nursing intervention that may be used for a client with a borderline personality disorder is to:

a. confront the client about manipulative behavior.

b. avoid the client when he or she is acting out.

c. keep consequences clear, consistent, and up-front.

d. allow the client to have the benefit of the doubt.

References

American Psychiatric Association: Diagnostic and Statistical Manual of Mental Disorders, 4th ed. Washington, DC, American Psychiatric Association, 1994.

Dresser JG: Workshop on Life in Black and White: Living With Borderline Personality Disorder, May 1996.

Gunderson JG, Phillips KA: Personality disorders. In Kaplan HI, Sadock BJ (eds): Comprehensive Textbook of Psychiatry, 6th ed, vol 2. Baltimore, Williams & Wilkins, 1995.

Miller SG: Borderline personality disorder from the patient's perspective. Hospital and Community Psychiatry, 22(9):1215–1219, 1994.

Piccinino S: The nursing care challenge: borderline patients. J Psychosoc Nurs 28(4):22–27, 1990.

Profiri F: Personality disorders. In: Varcarolis EM (ed): Foundation of Psychiatric Mental Health Nursing, 3rd ed. Philadelphia, WB Saunders Co, 1998.

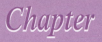
Mental Health Problems in Non-Psychiatric Settings

Outline

- **Loss and Grief**
  - The Grief Process
  - Nursing Interventions
- **Intensive Care Unit Psychosis**
  - Reasons for Psychosis
  - Nursing Interventions
- **Suicide**

- Myths and Realities
- Data Collection
- Nursing Interventions
- **Domestic Violence**
  - Signs of Abuse
  - Nursing Interventions
- **AIDS: Dealing With Emotional Aspects**

Key Terms

- bereavement
- body mapping
- domestic abuse
- grief
- grief process

- ICU psychosis
- lethality
- mourning
- psychological autopsy
- suicide

Objectives

Upon completing this chapter, the student will be able to:

1. List types of losses a person may experience in a lifetime.
2. Give three reactions that a person might have to a loss.
3. Describe the grief process.
4. List two obstacles to grieving.
5. Describe how the nurse can support the client and family during the grief process.
6. Explain what is meant by *ICU psychosis*.
7. Give examples of two perceptual distortions experienced during ICU psychosis.
8. List three nursing interventions that may alleviate the fear experienced by the client during ICU psychosis.
9. Discuss three myths regarding suicide.
10. Give an example of questions a nurse might ask a client regarding his or her suicidal thoughts, feelings, and plans.

Objectives—cont'd

11. Describe nursing support for the client who is suicidal.
12. Explain what is meant by *domestic violence*.
13. Describe victims of domestic violence.
14. Discuss why people have difficulty leaving a violent relationship.
15. List two helpful nursing interventions.
16. Discuss two emotional issues that may be faced by the client with AIDS.

It is difficult to separate body, mind, and spirit. The client with a physical illness is affected emotionally and spiritually. The client with an emotional illness is affected physically and spiritually. It is therefore important to view the client in a holistic sense. This is why so much time in a psychiatric facility is spent on activities of daily living such as eating, personal hygiene, sleeping, elimination, etc. The client with emotional problems may have a co-existing physical illness or injury. Sometimes spiritual needs are overlooked, especially for the client with emotional problems. Psychiatric problems, especially anxiety and depression, can be symptoms of physical illnesses.

Emotional reactions, from mild to severe, are a part of every physical illness. Treatment of physical illness is a priority because of concerns related to increasing severity of illness. *Total care* implies dealing with the emotional effect of illness as soon as physical needs are stabilized. Sometimes nursing intervention is as basic as active listening while completing physical care tasks.

LOSS AND GRIEF

Grief is a normal and healthy response to a loss. Throughout the life cycle, from birth to death, people encounter numerous losses. Some of these losses may include the following:

- The death of a family member, friend, or pet
- Moving away from friends and loved ones
- Loss of a job or failure to receive a promotion
- Financial losses
- Loss of health, a body part, or self-worth
- Loss of a sense of identity because of a disability
- Losses related to the stigma and prejudice associated with mental illness

A loss can be viewed positively, as an opportunity for growth, or negatively, as a bad omen. Responses to a loss are very individual. These responses, both psychological and physiological, are the essence of **grief**. Some people, after a loss, may withdraw into a world of their own; others may be very expressive and verbalize their anger, guilt, loneliness, and despair. It is important to recognize the range of feelings and deal with them to gain resolution.

Grief has been compared to an open wound. If the wound does not heal from the inside out, it will ulcerate and cause the scab to reopen. A person must heal from the inside out. The grieving process helps the person work through the many feelings associated with the loss or anticipated loss. Grief work is hard but necessary. The alternative is that, like the wound, the emotions held in will begin to cause other difficulties, such as physical illnesses. Prolonged grief that becomes incapacitating can result in depression, and the person needs to seek counseling.

Grief can be good. A person often gets in touch with a side of himself or herself that previously was unknown. Although there are similarities in the grief process, each person is unique. This is important for the nurse to remember in caring for a client experiencing a loss. Table 19–1 lists some of the common reactions to grief.

The Grief Process

The **grief process** involves learning to cope with a specific loss. Within the grief process, both bereavement and mourning occur. **Bereavement** is suffering the death of a loved one. **Mourning** includes the processes by which grief is resolved. There is no time line for grieving. Everyone

Table 19–1	Common Reactions of Grief			
Physical Reactions	**Emotional Reactions**	**Behavioral Reactions**	**Intellectual Reactions**
Weakness and fatigue	Numbness	Searching for what was lost	Difficulty concentrating
Rapid heartbeat	Confusion		Forgetfulness
Increased blood pressure	Sadness	Detached from surroundings	Inattention
Muscular tension	Guilt		Loss of productivity
Sleep disturbance	Despair	Withdrawn from friends and activities	Memory loss
Decreased resistance to illness	Hopelessness		Oriented to past rather than present or future
	Helplessness	Crying	
Weight and appetite change	Feeling of being lost	Seeking solitude	Preoccupation
	Anger	Unable to initiate/complete activities	Rumination
Neglect of self	Bitterness		Thoughts of death or suicide
Headaches	Agitation	Use of alcohol and/or drugs	
Sexual disinterest	Difficulty in relationships		Worrying
	Irritability	Nightmares	Disoriented to time and place
	Loss of self-esteem		

Data from Kathleen Baumann, Counseling Services, 1992. Used with permission.

grieves in a different way. Much depends on what the loss is and the circumstances surrounding it. The grief process is difficult and demanding. Because of this, many people try to avoid or postpone it.

Some obstacles to grieving include the struggle with the pain of loss and the time and energy involved in the healing process. However, if the person does not deal with the grief, the associated feelings are repressed and can cause problems later in life. Becoming involved in a grief support group encourages the person to participate actively in the grief process.

The grief process has been compared to the seasons of nature. Nature appears dormant in autumn and winter, but underneath changes are taking place and new growth is beginning. There will be a spring again. In the grief process, it may not seem like much is changing. However, as the person deals with the feelings and accepts the reality of the loss, changes occur with the hope of a new life (Baumann, 1997, p. 1).

In her book *On Death and Dying*, Dr. Elizabeth Kubler-Ross describes five stages involved in the grief process. They include denial, anger, bargaining, depression, and acceptance. Other authors list as many as 10 stages. The simplest model of the grief process includes three phases. The initial phase is one of shock and denial. The denial is an important coping mechanism that allows the body to adjust to the reality of the situation. After this period, there is a working phase in which the person deals with many feelings of anger and/or blame, guilt, loneliness, despair, depression, and other emotions. This is the hardest and longest part of the grief process. In the final phase, the person accepts or becomes resigned to the loss. This last step is not always achieved.

Nursing Interventions

To help the client and family deal with anticipatory loss or actual loss, the nurse needs to examine his or her feelings about loss, especially death. The focus in health care has been to save lives. The Hospice Foundation of America has helped to refocus these goals so that the emphasis is on the client enjoying as much of the life that he or she has left, as well as ensuring that his or her life is handled with the utmost dignity. Specific things that the nurse can do to make the client and family more comfortable include the following:

- Being available to the client and family
- Giving the client and family members permission to grieve
- Listening attentively; giving feedback on what the nurse has heard, such as "It sounds like you are feeling (frightened, worried, etc.)"
- Helping the client and family identify and express their feelings, allowing crying and talking
- Not giving advice; avoiding statements such as "I know just how you feel" or "time will heal"; the nurse should let the client and family tell how they feel
- Not making judgments; "the nurse should remember the three Bs: Be sensitive, Be available, Be QUIET" (Gambill, 1996)
- Supporting the client and family in the grief process by encouraging them to use their positive coping skills
- Remembering that a great deal of patience is needed in the grief process; offering support to clients and families is exhausting and demanding for all involved

Reality Check

Paul, a 45-year-old teacher, has pancreatic cancer. He has been readmitted to the hospital for further tests. The results of the tests are discouraging; the doctor has told Paul and his family that he has a month to live. Hospice care has been recommended. This is a terrible shock to Paul and his loved ones. He was hoping for more positive news.

1. What can the nurse do to support Paul and his family?
2. What is a resource that would be helpful to Paul's family?

INTENSIVE CARE UNIT PSYCHOSIS

Most clients who are admitted to the intensive care unit (ICU) experience some level of confusion. When this confusion extends to psychotic symp-

toms, the client is said to have an **ICU psychosis.** These symptoms may be difficult to detect at first, primarily because the nurse has no history with the client. Characteristics of ICU psychosis include the following:

- Impaired intellectual function
- Difficulty in judging reality
- An altered emotional state

These characteristics are caused by the high-stress situation perceived by the client (Fossett, Nadler-Moodie, 1996, p. 126).

Perceptual symptoms involving visual and auditory hallucinations, illusions, and delusions are common. Behaviors are a response to the perceptual changes. Table 19–2 describes examples of perceptual and behavioral symptoms.

Reasons for Psychosis

An ICU admission is often unplanned and involves a person who is already experiencing sleep deprivation. Suddenly the person has no control of his or her life. Confusion is increased by many unsettling experiences, including the following:

Table 19–2	Perceptual and Behavioral Symptoms

Perceptual Symptoms	Example
Hallucinations (visual or auditory)	Sees or hears family members or spirits
Illusions	Misidentifies medical staff as co-workers, etc.
Delusions	Has delusions of persecution, often related to painful or uncomfortable procedures

Behavioral Symptoms	Example
Tries to escape perceived danger	Tries to get out of bed to escape danger; pulls out intravenous tubing, catheters, etc.

- Lack of privacy
- Being close enough to other clients to hear and smell them
- Hearing new, unfamiliar sounds
- Having lights on day and night
- A variety of nurses and doctors who pick and probe
- A mix of medications, often including sedation

Life for the client becomes a blur of reality and unreality. An added dimension may include alcohol and/or other drug intake not mentioned by the client during admission. The nurse must continuously collect data, report it, and reassure the client.

Nursing Interventions

Nursing intervention begins with skill and an attitude of respectfulness. The client's often bizarre behavior is powered by *fear*, lack of control, and total dependency. As part of basic intervention, the nurse should do the following:

- Introduce himself or herself the same way at every encounter until the confusion clears
- Explain (in nonmedical terms) what he or she is going to do and continue to explain during each step of the procedure
- Make changes that do not jeopardize care. For example, what is the client's view from the bed? Sometimes moving equipment a bit provides a better view. Turning off suction when it is not being used reduces the noise level.
- Deal with perceptual distortions by reflecting understanding of what the client is going through and the fear that is being experienced. If the nurse knows specifically that the perception is related to the illness (i.e., injury, medication, sedation) and will subside as the client continues to heal, the nurse should say so. The message the nurse should impart is "We are here to protect you and assist you."
- Be aware that, because of the client's current state, he or she will exaggerate any implication of criticism.
- Intercoms often feed into a client's hallucinations and delusions. The nurse should add a matter-of-fact explanation of what it is and how it works as often as needed.

- Dim the lights whenever appropriate. However, the nurse should be aware of any shadows that are created. These may be frightening to the client and require additional explanation.
- Be as quiet as possible. The night shift must remember that the client is trying to sleep.

Fortunately, symptoms related to ICU psychosis usually subside within 24 hours. The client probably will not remember what happened. It serves no purpose to recount potentially embarrassing behaviors.

SUICIDE

Most people think about a person who is suicidal as being housed safely in a psychiatric unit with trained staff. This is not so. The client may be in the ICU, in the general medical/surgical unit, or out in the community. What all of these people share in common, regardless of age or where they are located, is a sense of hopelessness. They see no alternative other than death. The highest rate of suicide is among people with schizophrenia, manic episodes, and depression with high anxiety. However, it is incorrect to assume that all people who consider suicide are mentally ill. Adolescents have been known to commit "copy cat" suicides. When a teen commits suicide, others in the area may follow suit.

In the United States, 30,000 to 40,000 people commit suicide each year. Women make more attempts; men succeed more often. Men tend to use more immediately lethal means, such as guns. The actual number of yearly suicides is probably higher than the official figure. Some people hide their suicide by making it seem accidental. Other suicides remain unreported.

Suicide takes place in all cultures, in all religions, in all social classes, and at all education levels. Common reasons include cumulative losses, recent catastrophic loss, severe ongoing pain as part of a chronic or terminal illness, and alcohol or other drug abuse/dependency. An interesting but unexplained phenomenon is an increase in suicide in well-educated, successful men over age 40. There is speculation that it is related to cultural expectation. Furthermore, certain cultures use suicide as a way of dealing with overwhelming problems they encounter living in a new society.

Myths and Realities

Suicide, the deliberate ending of one's life, continues to be surrounded with myths. Table 19–3 lists common suicide myths and explains the corresponding realities.

Reality Check

What myths about suicide have you heard?

Data Collection

Possible clues of impending suicide include the following:

• Previous suicide attempts
• Threats of committing suicide
• Preparation for leaving, such as putting affairs in order, giving away prized possessions, contact-

ing family and friends not seen for awhile, and saying good-bye in a special way
• Acquiring the means to commit suicide
• A sudden lift in spirits that can mean the person is relieved because they think their problems will be over soon—"the calm before the storm"

Nurses occasionally fear that they will put suicidal ideas into their client's head by bringing up the subject. This belief is false. If a nurse thinks a client is suicidal, he or she should ask in order to determine potential and **lethality** (being able to cause death). Questions for determining suicide potential could include the following (Fossett, Nadler-Moodie, 1996, p. 43):

• Are you thinking of killing yourself? Have you thought of taking your life?
• Have you been considering ways to harm yourself?
• Do you feel like hurting yourself?

Table 19–3 Myths and Realities About Suicide

Myth	Reality
1. People who talk about suicide do not commit suicide.	Approximately four fifths of those who talk about suicide end up killing themselves.
2. Suicide happens without prior warning.	Suicide may seem sudden, as a "cry for help"; often these clues are identified after the fact.
3. People who are suicidal are determined to kill themselves.	The desire to live is part of the human condition. People who think of suicide are struggling with ambivalent desires to live or die. The basic wish to live provides a key for intervention. Many people who have attempted suicide and recovered say it seemed like the only way to relieve their overwhelming emotional pain.
4. Improvement after a suicide attempt means the suicidal risk is gone.	Not so. For example, the most dangerous time for the person with depression and high anxiety is during the convalescent period. The antidepressant begins to take effect; the person is capable of making a plan and has energy to carry it out.
5. People who commit suicide are mentally ill.	Some are. However, many times the actual suicidal act is an impulsive one resulting from unhappiness or anger, especially among the younger population.
6. It is not a suicide unless there is a note.	Only a small percentage of those who actually commit suicide leave notes. Many of the deaths listed as accidents, such as one-car incidents, are actually suicides.

- Do you mean you are feeling suicidal?
- Have you been thinking of hurting yourself?

If the client admits to being suicidal, the nurse should proceed with questions to determine lethality:

- Do you have a plan?
- What is your plan?
- Do you have the (gun, pills—whatever the client indicated) to carry out the plan?
- When are you planning to kill yourself? (Is there an immediate risk, such as jumping out of a window or down an open stairwell in the hospital?)

Other issues such as previous attempts, a family history of suicide that is often interpreted as "permission," religion, social support system, serious illness, and losses are all part of data collection. Generally, guns are the most lethal means of suicide and drug overdose (depending on the type and amount of drug taken) the least.

Nursing Interventions

The person who is considering suicide needs active emotional support. The nurse must not, however, get trapped into promising that he or she will keep the client from committing suicide. This may be interpreted as a challenge, and the nurse can be proved wrong by a person determined to die. Some guidelines for interacting with the suicidal client include the following:

- Listening carefully and trying to understand the feelings behind the words. The nurse should look at the body language. If the client is hearing voices, what are the voices telling him or her to do?
- Evaluating the seriousness of the person's thoughts and feelings. If the person has a plan and means to carry it out, the problem is more acute.
- Evaluating the intensity of the emotions. For example, high anxiety, agitation, and restlessness in a person who is depressed are causes for alarm.
- Seriously accepting every complaint and feeling the person expresses. It is important to not undervalue what the person is saying.
- Asking the person directly about suicidal thoughts. Talking about it frankly can help prevent the person from carrying out his or her plan. The person usually welcomes the opportunity to talk because he or she tends to feel all alone, unnoticed, and uncared for.
- Following up on a person's comment that the crisis is over and he or she no longer feels suicidal. Such a statement may be a deliberate attempt to mislead.
- Giving strong, definite guidelines. These are essential for a distressed person. The nurse can provide emotional strength by communicating that he or she knows what the client is doing and that everything possible is being done for the client.
- Evaluating the client's resources (internal and external), previous coping mechanism, and social support system.
- Acting specifically. The nurse should give the person an assignment, such as a no-decision suicide contract (Drye, Goulding, and Goulding, 1973, p. 172). Under the contract, the person agrees not to do anything to himself or herself accidentally or purposely for a specified time period. It is important to stress the accidental aspect of the agreement. Although this method is not foolproof, people tend not to break their word if they agree to something in writing and sign their name.
- Asking for assistance and advice when needed. Student nurses should rely heavily on the instructor and staff assigned to the client for guidelines regarding their approach (and role).
- Making the environment as safe and unchallenging as possible. If necessary, the nurse should maintain constant supervision during the suicide crisis period. The nurse must assume nothing. For example, Ms. A. was permitted plastic dinnerware only. All items used were to be accounted for at the end of each meal. Someone did not notice that the spoon was missing. Her bed was next to the wall. At night she gradually worked the handle of the spoon against the block

wall. A staff person was, as always, posted with her for the night. The staff person generally sat in a chair in the doorway reading a magazine. One morning, the staff person heard Ms. A. gasp and ran for the bed. Ms. A. had pressed the now-sharp point between her ribs. She narrowly missed puncturing her lung.

- Reassuring the person that the feelings of despair and pain are temporary and will pass (intense feelings usually pass within 24 to 48 hours). The nurse might encourage a change of pace, such as exercise or relaxation techniques. The nurse should not make statements such as "Everything will be all right" or "Don't worry." These statements are useless. The nurse cannot guarantee a positive outcome regarding the client's problems. Statements such as these indicate a lack of sensitivity to the client's problems.
- Mentioning that as long as life exists, there is a chance for help. The client is choosing a permanent solution to a temporary problem. Understanding the client's cultural and religious values and beliefs can be helpful. Does the client, for example, believe that if he or she does not solve problems in this lifetime, the problems repeat in the next? Is the value, according to the client's belief, to "get it right this time"? Some clients contemplate suicide to get even with someone. A reminder that they will no longer be alive to enjoy the other's misery may be a timely reminder that a far better form of getting even is to live and live well!
- Talking about people the client cares about who will become victims if the person follows through by killing himself or herself.
- Avoiding challenges or taunts. The nurse's anger can easily get in the way of effective intervention. For example, statements by nurses such as "You haven't the guts to do it" or "It was stupid to take the radio in the bathtub with you. Don't you know it has to be plugged in to kill you?" can be not only unhelpful, but actively harmful. The last comment provoked a successful suicide the day the client went home. This time he "did it right" and was found dead in his bathtub with the radio plugged in.

- Avoiding arguments regarding the client's motives; these arguments are also useless. Comments such as "You're just talking that way because you've had too much to drink" or "How can you think of suicide; you have so much to live for!" fall on deaf ears.

If the client succeeds in taking his or her life, the nurse can gain support from participating in a psychological autopsy. During a **psychological autopsy,** feelings are shared, insights are gained, and peers provide support. The nurse and other members of the staff share feelings they may have of grief, anger, guilt relief, etc., in a straightforward way. It is also a time to look at what could have been done differently, any signals that were missed, and what was done correctly.

DOMESTIC VIOLENCE

Domestic abuse involves ongoing emotional and psychological abuse with periodic physical abuse. It was originally thought to be limited to women, but there is increasing evidence that men are being victimized as well. One reason that less evidence has emerged of violence against males is that friends (and professionals) tend not to take their complaints seriously. Another factor may be the "macho mystique," which creates embarrassment and shame for the male victim. Domestic violence involves all social, cultural, and religious groups. People may be single, married, or in same-sex relationships. Nurses will meet these clients in all areas of nursing, including the following:

- *Psychiatric unit:* Clients may be admitted because of attempted suicide, depression, panic attacks, or alcohol and/or other drug abuse
- *Emergency room:* Clients may receive treatment for fractures, head and face injuries, internal injuries, etc.; if the partner accompanies the injured person, he or she often speaks for the person and explains the injuries as accidental
- *Obstetric visit:* Visits are often missed because abuse of pregnant women increases during pregnancy; if visits continue, the male significant other speaks for the pregnant woman

- *Pediatric unit or clinic:* Often both parents show up; the abused parent and child may be especially passive, whereas the abusing parent does the talking and explaining; the child may seem to be trying to fade into the background
- *Any general hospital unit:* The abusing partner may seem especially solicitous and concerned
- *Home visits:* Sometimes visits are forbidden by the abusing partner; attempts to isolate are common; clients with chronic disease tend not to comply with suggested treatment

Common denominators exist to some degree for all people who experience domestic abuse: fear of reprisal, embarrassment, shame, self-blame, social isolation, and inability to identify alternatives.

Reality Check

Judy, age 36, is a student nurse who left her husband a year ago. She described it this way.

I was flattered by his attentiveness during our courtship. He never let me out of sight and let everyone know I was his! My dad tried to warn me it was possessiveness, but . . .

The abuse started shortly after our honeymoon and increased in intensity when our child, Jill, was born. He found us a place in the country about 2 miles in from the main road. Jack had a great job and was well liked—a hard worker. Each morning, he left with our car, the telephone, and my shoes. None of the neighbors knew us, and the closest one was a mile away.

Everything had to be just so when he arrived home at 6 PM: his beer, his bath, his food, the house, and the baby had better not cry. I never could predict what would set him off, and he would always blame me. ''If you hadn't,

I wouldn't have gotten mad and had to hit you. See what you made me do.''

Usually by morning he would apologize and tell me he loved me ''faults and all, no one loves you like I do.'' I kept trying to believe that today would be different if I could just do everything right. When my family came, which was rare, I was ashamed to admit what was happening to me. I made up excuses for any bruises at the time. After all, my father had tried to warn me. Besides, I was afraid. Jack had warned me he would kill me if I told anyone.

1. Identify the feelings that kept Judy from seeking help.
2. How would you handle suspicions of domestic abuse if it involved a friend?

Signs of Abuse

Today, most nurses learn about identifying and responding to domestic violence. They learn that both males and females are involved. Blaming the victim is counterproductive. They learn about available resources and how to connect clients with these resources. Nurses also learn facts about domestic violence, such as the following:

- People stay in abusive relationships because of fear of reprisal, not because they get perverse pleasure from the abuse
- Victims do not deliberately provoke abusers because they have a need to suffer
- Victims do not adjust to the pain and discomfort after awhile
- Injuries such as burns, cuts, bruises at various stages of healing, bites, or dislocations may be signs
- Physical complaints such as dizziness, chest pains, stomach pains, rapid heartbeat, premature labor, miscarriage, and sexual problems are possible clues (Nelson, 1996, p. 2)

Nursing Interventions

A major part of nursing intervention involves setting aside personal prejudices and myths and replacing them with facts. Intervention guidelines include the following:

- *Providing privacy:* Sometimes this means being creative in separating the client from his or her partner.
- *Asking direct questions:* "Did someone hit you?" or "Is anyone hurting you?" may not initially bring forth the truth, but these are the proper questions. Rapport with the client often takes several separate encounters before a sense of trust is developed. Pressuring the client for an answer does not accomplish the desired response.
- *Body mapping:* **Body mapping** is a way of using a body diagram to record where the client's cuts, bruises, burns, fractures, and other injuries are located.
- *Recording the story:* Record the story as told by the client, noting date, time, place, who was involved, and what happened.
- *Assessing potential danger:* Location of guns and other weapons is important to assess immediate danger to the client.
- *Assessing potential support system:* Sources for money, housing, safety, transportation, and family are important as part of assessing the client's support system.
- *Making an escape plan:* With client's permission, provide information on local resources and referral for a quick, safe getaway.
- *Counseling:* Once the client is out safely, dealing with painful emotional issues can be considered.

Reality Check

Many states have laws about nurses reporting abuse. Does your state have such a law? What is stated as the nurse's responsibility?

ACQUIRED IMMUNODEFICIENCY SYNDROME: DEALING WITH EMOTIONAL ASPECTS

"AIDS, a fatal, relatively new disease, has predominantly affected groups that are socially stigmatized: homosexual men, injectable drug users, and racial minorities. It also occurs in a social climate that does not approve of homosexuality, sexual promiscuity, or drug use. This, coupled with discrimination, prejudice, and the fear of contagion, causes significant psychological response to HIV."

L. Delorenzo (1996, p. 29)

Discrimination and ignorance are averted through learning facts and integrating the knowledge into nursing care. Most nursing programs now include information on cultures, lifestyles, and human sex and sexuality. Fear of contagion is replaced by learning universal precautions and applying this knowledge. Box 19–1 discusses the difference between the personal values and professional responsibilities of nurses.

Myths about casual contact and acquired immunodeficiency syndrome (AIDS) are dispelled by learning how contagion takes place and facts about the course of the illness. An appreciation is gained for the psychological effect of the diagnosis: the person's life is changed forever. The face of AIDS continues to change. "The number of AIDS cases among women is rising more quickly than among men, and sex with infected men has overtaken drug use as the leading cause of infection among women," federal researchers say.

Clients with AIDS are admitted to all nursing areas, including home care. In each area, nurses need to deal with emotion-laden issues, some of which are listed below by clinical area.

- *Family practice clinic:* The client may have just learned that he or she has AIDS. The nurse may be the one to listen to immediate reaction and concerns about the future; the nurse may also be

BOX 19–1	Personal Values vs. Professional Responsibilities

Florence Nightingale reflected on nursing as a calling and provided nursing care for people in all circumstances. Modern theorists speak of nursing as an art and science and develop statements of social policy. Part of the art of nursing is the service that is provided. The client, in essence, buys a service and is entitled to the most skilled care a nurse can deliver. This is what a nurse promises as part of the nursing oath. It is also what a nurse is hired to do. It is curious, then, to hear some nurses mix up their personal values with their professional responsibilities. For example, at a statewide nursing conference, three nurses were conversing during a presentation on AIDS. "It is God's wrath being visited on these evil men," stated the male nurse. A female nurse chimed in, "They deserve to die for their sinful ways." The other female nurse continued "and I for one will not soil my hands to comfort even one." Wrong profession, perhaps? As a nursing student, would you have said anything to the three nurses if you overheard their conversation? If so, what?

the one to provide factual information on resources.

- *Obstetric/prenatal clinic:* The client has AIDS, is newly pregnant, and is trying to decide whether to continue the pregnancy. The nurse needs to present information in a clear, concise way so that the client bases her decision on facts about prognosis and alternatives.
- *Pediatric/neonatal unit:* The infant of the mother with AIDS has been admitted.
- *Oncology unit:* The client has developed Kaposi's sarcoma. The nurse listens, provides physical care, and offers factual information about the illness and community resources.
- *Medical unit:* The client has been admitted with severe respiratory distress diagnosed as *Pneumoniae carinii*. The nurse listens and provides skillful care, reassurance, and information as needed.

- *Psychiatric unit:* The client is severely depressed. He was diagnosed with AIDS 6 weeks ago. The nurse seeks out the client for one-to-one, low-key contact and, later, for opportunities to talk about feelings regarding the illness.
- *Nursing home:* The client has developed AIDS-related dementia. The nurse provides physical care, orientation as needed, and supportive care.
- *Home care:* Their "child" with end-stage AIDS has come home to die. The nurse provides physical care and an opportunity for the client and family to deal with impending death and associated feelings.

Although many clients can live longer and better because of newly developed medications, nurses are still the compassionate key. They collect data, identify client needs, and provide nursing intervention to meet these needs. Confidentiality remains a major issue in the case of clients with AIDS, which continues to evoke attitudes leading to discrimination and prejudice. Because these attitudes are fueled by ignorance, it is up to the nurse to learn the facts, apply the knowledge, and educate others.

SUMMARY

Throughout the life cycle, a person experiences numerous losses. Grief is a normal and healthy response to loss. Grief is good. It often gets a person in touch with a part of the personality that was unknown before the loss. Grief work is hard, but necessary. It is important to work through the many feelings that result from loss or anticipated loss.

Everyone grieves differently and goes through several distinct phases. There is no specific time line for grief. Nurses need to support clients and families in times of loss by being available and listening attentively. By listening and reflecting, they can help clients use positive coping skills in dealing with their grief.

ICU psychosis is experienced by almost every client during the initial 24-hour period in the ICU. The client's often bizarre behavior is powered by fear, lack of control, and total dependency.

Many people have suicidal feelings at some time during their life but do not act on them. Suicide takes place in all cultures, in all religions, in all social classes, and at all education levels. The nurse must understand the myths and realities associated with suicide, as well as appropriate responses and questions to assess the intent of the client.

Domestic violence involves women and men of all social, cultural, educational, and religious groups. They may be single, married, or in same-sex relationships.

Nursing attitudes influence the quality of care received by clients with AIDS. Because AIDS continues to evoke attitudes leading to discrimination and prejudice, confidentiality is imperative. It is also up to the nurse to learn the facts, apply the knowledge, and educate others.

Critical Thinking Activities

1. What are losses that you have had in your lifetime?
2. What is your way of coping with a loss?
3. What additional loss does a person with mental illness face?

Review Questions

Multiple Choice—Choose the best answer to each question.

1. Which of the following is a desirable nursing intervention for a client experiencing grief?
   a. Give advice on how to cope
   b. Encourage the client to "be strong and not cry"
   c. Be sensitive; be available; be quiet
   d. Avoid contact with the client until he or she is under control
2. What is meant by *ICU psychosis?*
   a. Confusion that may extend to the client being out of touch with reality
   b. A syndrome precipitated by the nurse's response to the client

   c. The client's response to serious diagnostic information
   d. A chronic psychiatric illness resulting in hallucinations and delusions
3. Which intervention is appropriate when dealing with a client who is suicidal?
   a. Challenge the client that you do not think he or she is capable of committing suicide
   b. Ask "Have you had thoughts of taking your life?"
   c. Leave the client alone to show you trust him or her
   d. Promise the client you will keep him or her from committing suicide
4. Which of the following is a common characteristic of domestic abuse?
   a. It is limited to females and children
   b. The victim sets off the abuser in some way
   c. It is limited to poor, undereducated people
   d. The victim believes that he or she is to blame
5. Which of the following is an emotional issue faced by the client with AIDS?
   a. Contagion of others by droplet infection
   b. Attitudes of discrimination and prejudice
   c. Passing on illness through casual contact
   d. Knowing that illness is limited to men

References

Baumann K: Though Leaves Fall, There's A Hint of Green. Tomorrow Fall, 2(3):1, 1997.

Delorenzo L: HIV/AIDS: A 1-Hour Overview. South Eaton, Mass, Western Schools Press, 1996.

Fossett B, Nadler-Moodie M: Nursing management of the suicidal patient. In: Psychiatric Aspects of General Patient Care, 3rd ed. South Eaton, Mass, Western Schools Press, 1996.

Gambill A: Do & Don't Suggestions for Bereaved and Their Caregivers. Colorado Springs, Colo, Bereavement Publishing, Inc, 1996.

Nelson M: Domestic Violence: A Nursing Concern, 3rd ed. South Eaton, Mass, Western Schools Press, 1996.

Drye R, Goulding RL, Goulding M: No-suicide decisions: patient monitoring of suicidal risk. Am J Psychiatry 130(2): 171–174, 1973.

Older Adults and Mental Health

Outline

- Myths of Aging
- Stresses in Later Life
- Mental Health Problems in Older Adults
- Concerns of Older Adults
    Elder Abuse
    Fraudulent Solicitations
    Compulsive Gambling
- Barriers to Mental Health Care for Older Adults
- Nursing Interventions
- Promotion of Mental Health in Older Adults

Key Terms

- ageism
- Coalition on Mental Health and Aging
- elder abuse
- golden gamblers
- KISS
- scams

Objectives

Upon completing this chapter, the student will be able to:

1. Compare the myths with the facts that exist about aging.
2. Describe the changes that may cause stress in the life of the older adult.
3. Discuss the mental health problems that the older adult may experience.
4. List the different types of elder abuse.
5. Describe two scams or rip-offs that may involve older adults.
6. Explain the barriers to mental health care for older adults.
7. Describe how the nurse can foster independence and meaning in the life of the older adult.
8. List ways of promoting mental health in the older adult.

Many terms are used to describe persons in the last period of the life cycle: *aged, elderly, seniors,* and *older adult.* No matter which term is used, the older person often resents it because of the derogatory meanings it conveys. Our society maintains a bias against the process of growing old. It is not limited to the young and how they view older people, but also includes how older persons view themselves (Holzapfel, 1998, p. 955). This bias or prejudice is referred to as **ageism.**

The ability to reach old age is now expected for people in the United States. "One in every eight people in the country is 65 years of age or older, and that proportion will increase to one in five by 2030. Very old people (over age 85) . . . by 2050 will comprise 5 percent or more of people in the United States" (La Rue, 1995, p. 2527).

MYTHS OF AGING

Negative attitudes about growing old are perpetuated by existing myths. Table 20-1 lists some of these myths, along with the facts of aging. More

positive attitudes toward aging need to be developed, especially by nurses who provide much of the direct care to older adults.

STRESSES IN LATER LIFE

Mental health in the older adult depends on how he or she perceives and adapts to the changes that occur in life. These can include physical, mental, social, emotional, and economic changes. Any new event may cause stress in the person. "The mental and emotional health of people of all ages is related to how well they cope with or adapt to the stresses and changes in their lives" (Solomon, 1996, p. 46). Some of the occurrences in later life that can cause stress include the following:

- *Physical changes:* Chronic conditions such as cardiovascular disease, diabetes, cancer, stroke, impaired vision, and chronic obstructive pulmonary disease (COPD) are prevalent among older adults. The persistence of these conditions can lead to emotional problems.

Table 20–1	Myths and Facts of Aging

Myths	Facts
Older adults are not able to learn new tasks, or the old refrain "You can't teach an old dog new tricks."	After retirement, older adults often develop new skills and hobbies. Creativity can occur at any age.
As people grow older, they become more set in their ways.	The ability to adapt to changes in life is related to a person's personality and flexibility throughout life.
There is inevitable mental deterioration as one grows older.	The personality of a person does not change unless altered by pathological conditions. Learning is possible at any age.
Sexual interest declines with aging.	Sexual interest and activity continue to be important to the older adult.
Older adults are comfortable financially and have nothing to worry about.	Although a small number of older adults may be very well-off and some moderately comfortable, a large segment remain poor.
Many older adults are lonely and socially isolated.	Loneliness comes from losses. Many older adults have support systems to deal with their losses.

Data from Holzapfel SK: The elderly. In: Varcarolis EM (ed): Foundations of Psychiatric Mental Health Nursing, 3rd ed. Philadelphia, WB Saunders Co, 1998.

- *Mental changes:* The inability to remember specific information causes great concern in older adults. They may fear they are losing their minds. The more stress created by this fear, the less the older adult is able to remember. It simply takes longer for an older adult to recall information. Because of the public attention that is focused on Alzheimer's disease, many think that they have dementia.
- *Social and emotional changes:* The older adult is faced with many losses, including loss of family and friends, function, freedom, and a future. The degree of stress caused by these losses is related to the importance that each loss holds for the person. It is important to help the older adult grieve his or her loss.
- *Economic changes:* Retirement can cause stress if the older adult retires *from* life, instead of *to* life. If the person has a strong work ethic, retirement can cause a feeling of uselessness with a loss of identity. Also, retirement usually results in a change of economic status. Income and health care often become major concerns.

MENTAL HEALTH PROBLEMS IN OLDER ADULTS

The stresses that the older adult experiences can cause mental health problems. Some of these problems include the following:

- *Depression:* Depression is the most widespread and incapacitating mental disorder among older adults. Depression is *not* a normal part of growing older. Many older adults who have clinical depression are misdiagnosed with other illnesses. Also, the older person often does not seek help because he or she thinks the symptoms are an inevitable part of aging, or because of the stigma associated with mental illness (Gomez and Gomez, 1993, p. 32).
- *Alcohol abuse:* Alcohol abuse is a serious problem for about 2% to 5% of older adults (Coalition on Mental Health and Aging, 1994). There are usually two types of problem drinkers among

older people. The first type is the person who has consumed alcohol all of his or her life. The effects of drinking begin to show when physical changes occur because of the aging process. The second type is the older person who begins to drink in excess as a way of coping with stress. Stresses may include the loss of a loved one, retirement, or declining health.
- *Polydrug use and misuse of prescription medications:* Older adults in America use more prescriptions and consume more over-the-counter drugs than any other age group (Coalition on Mental Health and Aging, 1994). Many drugs have a long half life: that is, they remain in the body for a long time. Drugs are eliminated by the liver and kidneys. In the older person, liver metabolism decreases. Therefore medication can accumulate in the system.
- *Anxiety disorders:* Anxiety disorders are prevalent in 10% to 20% of people age 65 and over (Coalition on Mental Health and Aging, 1994). They can result in poor nutrition and sleep deprivation. See Chapter 15, "Anxiety and Somatoform Disorders," for more information about anxiety disorders.
- *Suicide:* "Suicide rates among the elderly are the highest of any age group, perhaps as high as double the rate seen in the general population. White men over age 85 are at the greatest risk . . ." (Devons, 1996, p. 67). The losses that an older adult experiences—retirement, health status, death of loved ones—may occur at a time when the person is vulnerable and unable to cope. This can result in feelings of isolation and loneliness. Many suicides can be prevented by identifying older adults who may be at risk for suicide and encouraging them to seek treatment (Devons, 1996, p. 72).

CONCERNS OF OLDER ADULTS

Older adults have many medical and nonmedical concerns that can affect their mental health either directly or indirectly. Among these are elder abuse, fraudulent solicitations, and compulsive gambling.

Elder Abuse

"Up to two million older adults are abused each year—and the numbers seem to be growing" (Lynch, 1997, p. 27). The four main types of **elder abuse** are physical abuse, material/financial abuse, psychological abuse, and neglect by self or caregiver.

- *Physical abuse* is the infliction of physical pain or injury. It includes hitting, bruising, pushing, shoving, lacerating, slapping, sexually molesting, restraining, etc. Without intervention, abuse tends to escalate.
- *Material/financial abuse* is the illegal or unethical exploiting of funds, property, or other assets of an older person for personal gain. Many times the older person does not realize what is happening when family members offer to handle the person's business.
- *Psychological abuse* is the infliction of emotional pain or distress on the older person by derogatory name-calling, insulting, ignoring, humiliating, isolating, or threatening the person. This type of abuse can be hard to detect unless actually observed. The nurse needs to be aware of changes in the older client's behavior, such as being withdrawn, fearful, or depressed.
- *Neglect by self or caregiver* is probably the most common of reported cases of elder abuse. The older adult is considered to be at risk because of lack of attention to self and environment. Case workers often find older adults living alone in deplorable conditions. Neglect can also occur when the caregiver is unable to provide the necessary services, such as a spouse trying to care for a disabled partner, or a caregiver ignoring an older client's needs.

Abuse-reporting laws vary from state to state, but all include protection from liability for people who report elder abuse (Lynch, 1997, pp. 30, 32). In local areas, the Adult Protective Services (APS) provides service and information about resources for elder abuse.

Reality Check

Alma Vander, a 78-year-old woman, is active in senior groups, participating in their educational and exercise programs. She lives alone in her own home and has one child, a married daughter. After an educational program at the hospital, Alma confided in the nurse that her daughter wanted her to sign over her house to the daughter. In fact, the daughter threatened Alma, and said that she would not speak to her unless Alma gave her the house. Alma was very distressed to think that her only child would do this. As a result of this stress, Alma was having physical problems. When it was suggested that Alma consult an attorney, she said that she and her daughter had the same attorney.

1. How would you classify what Alma's daughter is doing to her?
2. What sources are available to help Alma?
3. How might this type of abuse be prevented?

Fraudulent Solicitations

Older adults grew up in a time when many families did not feel the need to lock their doors at night. This feeling of safety no longer exists. Some unscrupulous operators specifically target senior citizens as their prey. Studies have shown that seniors are the most vulnerable population and the least likely to report rip-offs or scams (Bureau of Consumer Protection, 1997, p. 10).

Older adults are often tricked by **scams** presented as legitimate contests or offers, such as the following:

- *Prize offers* use attention-getting gimmicks such as fancy certificates, official entry numbers, or envelopes that look like telegrams. No matter how they are packaged, these offers will cost money. Con artists lure consumers into calling a a special telephone number for more information. After making the call, consumers find they must pay claim fees, shipping costs, or purchase merchandise to be eligible for the offer.

- *Bank examiner* schemes use con artists to get older adults to withdraw large amounts of cash from their bank accounts. They pretend to need help from the older adult to conduct an investigation of the bank. To do the investigation, the older adult needs to withdraw money and give it to the scam artist, who promises to return the money after the investigation. Of course, this never happens.
- *Social security scams* are mailed in official-looking envelopes marked "Urgent!, Important! Social Security and Medicare Information Enclosed!" There is often an official-looking government postage-paid stamp in one corner and a return address that appears to be that of a government agency. Several nonprofit organizations use these official-looking envelopes to send direct-mail solicitations to older Americans for funds to support lobbying efforts to "save" the social security system. Many older adults are scared into thinking that their financial security depends on their support of these lobbying efforts (Bureau of Consumer Protection, 1997, p. 33).
- *Other scams* include switching long-distance telephone service, work-at-home schemes, hearing aids, insurance, medical quackery, recreational property, and home improvements and repairs. These scams may lead directly to mental health problems in older adults.

Some groups and individuals have banded together to foster cooperation between law enforcement agencies and senior citizens to reduce criminal victimization. If there is any doubt about a product, service, or offer made to an older adult, the nurse should encourage that person to contact the local office of the Consumer Protection Agency.

Reality Check

Millie is an 83-year-old woman who lives alone in an upstairs apartment. She has traveled extensively, never married, and continues to drive her own car. Much of her time is spent in answering sweepstakes mail. She is convinced that soon a van will be pulling up with a prize, such as 1 million dollars, or a trip to a far-off land. Despite the fact that she has never won, Millie continues to send for expensive merchandise in order to enter contests. She lives on a limited income and hopes that the prize money will help her financially.

1. What might be some of the reasons Millie engages in this activity?
2. Discuss some problem-solving approaches that might be used to change Millie's focus.

Compulsive Gambling

The phrase **golden gamblers** refers to older adults who take bus trips to the casinos. When gambling becomes a preoccupation, an avoidance of dealing with unresolved grief issues, a substitute for loneliness, or a chasing of losses, then it becomes a serious problem for the older adult. Gambling can lead to desperation and suicide. Throughout the country, support groups are available for problem and compulsive gamblers.

BARRIERS TO MENTAL HEALTH CARE FOR OLDER ADULTS

Gaining access to mental health services can be very difficult for older adults. Some of the primary impediments to services include the following (Coalition on Mental Health and Aging, 1994):

- The stigma associated with emotional disorders and mental illness, which makes older people reluctant to seek services.

- Ageism toward the older adult. The general public and professionals believe that depression, forgetfulness, and other disorders are a normal part of aging. They assume that older people cannot benefit from mental health treatment.
- Lack of mental health care in some nursing homes for those residents who have mental health and cognitive disorders.
- Medicare's limited outpatient mental health benefits, which require high deductibles and copayments.
- Private health insurance, which provides minimal benefits for mental health treatment.
- Lagging federal support for community mental health services.
- Lack of professional staff trained to provide mental health care to older people. This includes physicians, mental health professionals, and people trained in aging.
- Limited interaction between the mental health and aging service systems.

NURSING INTERVENTIONS

Good mental health in older adults depends partly on the person's attitudes and mental health throughout his or her life. People who have developed the following skills are likely to have better mental health as they grow older (Eliopoulos, 1996, p. 652):

- Meaningful roles and interests
- Methods to manage stress effectively
- Good communication skills
- Problem-solving capabilities

Nurses play an important role in the care of the older adult and have contact with this population in many different settings. Box 20–1 can serve as a guideline in working with the older client.

In communicating with the older adult, the nurse needs to remember the acronym **KISS**—"Keep It Short and Simple." To help older adults stay mentally fit, nurses should encourage them to do things that depend on memory, such as taking

---

BOX 20–1	Bauer's A, B, Cs of Relationships With the Older Adult

*A*llow the older adult to make choices and decisions.
*B*elieve in the older adult. He or she is our legacy.
*C*apabilities of the older adult need to be recognized and fostered.
*D*evelop dependable relationships so that the older adult can count on you.
*E*xercise improves the quality of life.
*F*oster rewarding experiences.
*G*oals need to be small, realistic, and attainable. Keep your eyes on the goal; if not, you see obstacles.
*H*umor can help develop trust, thus improving self-confidence and understanding.
*I*nvolve the older adult in his or her daily life.
*J*ustice and security are the right of all older adults.
*K*ind words communicate warmth and empathy.
*L*isten to the older adult and share his or her memories.
*M*oving to music is a motivator.
*N*eeding to feel worthwhile is an essential factor of self-esteem.
*O*pen up areas for exploration.
*P*rovide an abundance of patience and a nonjudgmental attitude.
*Q*uestion what effect your behavior and comments might have on the older adult.
*R*eminisce with the older adult over days gone by.
*S*timulate the senses—hearing, sight, smell, taste, and touch.
*T*ake time; let the older adult set the pace.
*U*nrealistic expectations can lead to frustration and anger.
*V*alue what the older adult has to offer.
*W*isdom of age needs to be sought and utilized.
*X*L (extra large) dose of respect and dignity.
*Y*ield to the rightful requests of the older adult.
*Z*oom into the needs of the older adult.

B. B. Bauer

---

classes, playing cards, doing crossword puzzles. In other words, older adults should heed the warning to *"Use it or lose it!"* One does not *grow* old—one becomes old by not growing.

PROMOTION OF MENTAL HEALTH IN OLDER ADULTS

Life-long learning has become a part of our culture. To provide learning opportunities for older adults, educational programs have been developed at university campuses for people in retirement. Classes in history, art, music, government, language, geography, and other subjects provide intellectual stimulation as well as camaraderie and socialization.

The Older Americans Act (OAA) distributes federal funds to states to provide services for people age 60 and above. These services include long-term care and information, senior centers, nutrition programs, and volunteer opportunities. In 1991 the **Coalition on Mental Health and Aging** was organized to address the mental health service needs of older people by doing the following:

- Advocating for appropriate mental health treatment and care for older adults
- Decreasing the stigma associated with mental and emotional problems
- Improving access to mental health services by older adults
- Drawing attention to the importance of emotional well-being, prevention, and self-help programs for older adults
- Educating professionals, the general public, decision makers, and older people on the mental health issues of our older population
- Encouraging older adults to use the services of mental health professionals, volunteer programs, and self-help programs

SUMMARY

Reaching old age is now expected of people in the United States. Negative attitudes about growing old are perpetuated by existing myths. These attitudes are held by the young as well as the old.

Changes in later life that cause stress include chronic physical conditions, cognitive changes, many losses, and changes in economic status because of retirement. Some of the mental health problems in older adults are depression, alcohol abuse, polydrug use and misuse of prescription medications, anxiety disorders, and suicide. Areas of concern with older adults include elder abuse, fraudulent solicitations, and compulsive gambling.

One of the barriers to mental health care for the older adult is gaining access to mental health services. Insurance provides minimal benefits for mental health treatment.

Nurses are significant in the care of the older adult. By following "Bauer's A, B, C's of Relationships with the Older Adult," the nurse can help the client utilize the strength he or she has to deal with changes that occur (Bauer, 1997). The nurse can help promote mental health in the older adult by raising awareness of the resources available in the community.

Critical Thinking Activities

1. Draw yourself as you think you will appear at the age of 80.
2. Where do you think you will be when you are 80 years old?
3. List the *strengths* that you think you will have at age 80.
4. List the *weaknesses* that you think you will have at age 80.

Review Questions

Multiple Choice—Choose the best answer to each question.

1. Which of the following statements is a myth about aging?
   a. Learning is possible at any age
   b. A large segment of older adults remain poor
   c. Sexual interest declines with age
   d. Support systems help older adults deal with losses
2. A mental health problem that an older adult may experience is
   a. hearing loss.
   b. depression.
   c. impairment of vision.
   d. arthritis.

3. A barrier to mental health care for older adults is
   a. stigma associated with emotional disorders and mental illness.
   b. an attitude that the older person can benefit from mental health treatment.
   c. sufficient mental health care for the older adult in the nursing home.
   d. adequate insurance benefits for mental health treatment of older adults.

4. The nurse can foster independence and meaning in the life of the older adult by
   a. helping the older adult with the activities of daily living.
   b. setting unrealistic expectations to challenge the older adult.
   c. encouraging the older adult to do things as quickly as possible.
   d. listening to the older adult and sharing his or her memories.

5. One form of physical abuse of the elderly involves
   a. exploiting funds and property.
   b. inflicting emotional pain or distress.
   c. hitting, pushing, or shoving.
   d. neglecting attention to self and environment.

References

Bauer BB: Bauer's A, B, C's of Relationships With the Older Adult. Unpublished, Green Bay, Wis, 1997.

Bureau of Consumer Protection: Preventing Senior Citizen Ripoffs. Madison, Wis, Dept of Agriculture, Trade and Consumer Protection, 1997.

Coalition on Mental Health and Aging: Key Issues in Aging and Mental Health, Washington, DC, American Association of Retired People, 1994.

Devons C: Suicide in the elderly: How to identify and treat patients at risk. Geriatrics 51(3):67–72, 1996.

Eliopoulos C: The elderly traveler. In: Carson VB, Arnold ED (eds): Mental Health Nursing: The Nurse-Patient Journey. Philadelphia, WB Saunders Co, 1996.

Gomez GE, Gomez EA: Depression in the elderly. J Psychosoc Nurs 31(5):28–33, 1993.

Holzapfel SK: The elderly. In: Varcarolis EM (ed): Foundations of Psychiatric Mental Health Nursing, 3rd ed. Philadelphia, WB Saunders Co, 1998.

La Rue A: Geriatric psychiatry. In: Kaplan HI, Sadock BJ (eds): Comprehensive Textbook of Psychiatry, 6th ed, vol 2. Baltimore, Williams & Wilkins, 1995.

Lynch SH: Elder abuse: What to look for, how to intervene. Am J Nurs 97(1):27–32, 1997.

Solomon R: Coping with stress: A physician's guide to mental health in aging. Geriatrics 51(7):46, 1996.

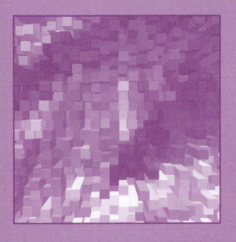

Interventions

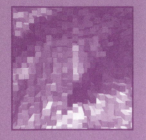

Stress, Crisis, and Crisis Intervention

Outline

- **Stress**
    - **Stages of Stress**
    - **Coping With Stress**
- **Crisis**
    - **Types of Crisis**
    - **Recognizing a Person in Crisis**
- **Crisis Intervention**
- **Case Study: Nursing Care Plan**
    - **History and Data Collection**
    - **Goals, Interventions, Rationale, and Evaluation**

Key Terms

- burnout
- coping
- crisis
- crisis intervention
- distress
- empathy
- generic approach
- individual approach
- maturational crisis
- situational crisis
- stress
- stressor
- sympathy

Objectives

Upon completing this chapter, the student will be able to:

1. Explain the difference between stress and distress.
2. Identify four effective ways of coping with stress.
3. Describe a physical, emotional, and behavioral symptom of burnout.
4. Differentiate between a situational crisis and a maturational crisis.
5. List six common emotional, cognitive, and behavioral signs and symptoms of a person in crisis.
6. Define *crisis intervention*.
7. Describe the three balancing factors in Aguilera's model for problem solving with a person in crisis.
8. Discuss three areas of focus for nursing intervention with a client in crisis.

To live is to grow, and growing involves change. With change comes stress. Change is a natural mechanism to prevent stagnation and decay. Many times the first response to change is resistance. Often the person responds by saying, "We've always done it this way, why change?" or "If it isn't broken, why fix it?"

Some of the stress associated with change can be decreased by allowing ourselves to grieve the loss associated with change. Any change—adverse or pleasant—involves loss (Vander Zyl, 1996, p. 16). By recognizing and grieving the loss, the person makes energy available to adapt to change. How one handles the change determines the quality of one's life.

STRESS

Stress is the body's reaction to the demands made on a person. Animals and humans have protective responses to deal with stressful situations. The adrenal glands secrete a hormone called *adrenaline,* which increases the heart rate and makes a person more alert. These changes help the body prepare for fight or flight from real or perceived danger. If they are short-lived, all of these responses are good because they can motivate a person during competition and emergencies.

Stages of Stress

The initial adrenaline reaction is referred to as the *alarm stage* in Dr. Hans Selye's description of general adaptation syndrome (GAS). If the stress remains, the body moves to the next stage, which is one of resistance. The final stage is one of exhaustion. When the body is constantly wound up and cannot relax, a whole array of undesirable results can occur. A wide range of physical disorders can occur when body chemistry is upset. It is the uncomfortable stress or **distress** that causes problems.

Humans have a creative imagination; it suggests unreal dangers and gives rise to unnecessary fears. Stress is not an event, but the result of a person's *perception* of an event. One often focuses on what happened in the past or what will occur in the future. This causes distress. The person's focus needs to be on how to make stress work for—not against—him or her. Selye sees stress as the "spice of life" (Selye, 1974, p. 85).

Coping With Stress

One person may see a stressful event as incapacitating, whereas another may view the same event as a challenge. "Simply defined, a *challenge* is anything that calls for special effort or dedication" (Frisch, Kelley, 1996, p. 5). For example, a person is asked to give the keynote address at a large conference. This could be seen as very stressful or as a challenge depending on the experience and personality of the presenter. The way a person handles the threatening or challenging situation is referred to as **coping**.

Holmes and Rahe (1967) developed a method of comparing the effects of certain life events with the occurrence of an illness. Their Social Readjustment Rating Scale (SRRS) lists 43 situations that can occur during a lifetime. As a result of their research, the events were rank-ordered and assigned a mean value (Table 21–1). A common theme to all of the listed life events was "the occurrence of each usually evoked or was associated with some adaptive or coping behavior on the part of the individual" (Holmes and Rahe, 1967, p. 217). Their findings indicated that the higher the score on the SRRS during a 1-year period, the greater the probability of developing a serious illness within the next 2 years. As the score decreased, so did the risk.

Ineffective Coping Methods

The defense mechanisms described in Chapter 2 are often used to deal with stressful situations. However, these unconscious mechanisms, when overused, can interfere with healthy living by distorting one's thinking, feeling, and acting. People who are mentally ill have used ineffective ways of dealing with life's problems.

Caring for a client who is mentally ill can produce stress and possibly burnout for the nurse. This can result in job dissatisfaction and lack of concern for others. **Burnout** is a process marked

Table 21–1   Holmes and Rahe's Social Readjustment Rating Scale

Rank	Life Event	Mean Value	Score
1	Death of spouse	100	_____
2	Divorce	73	_____
3	Marital separation	65	_____
4	Jail term	63	_____
5	Death of close family member	63	_____
6	Personal injury or illness	53	_____
7	Marriage	50	_____
8	Fired at work	47	_____
9	Marital reconciliation	45	_____
10	Retirement	45	_____
11	Change in health of family member	44	44
12	Pregnancy	40	_____
13	Sex difficulties	39	_____
14	Gain of new family member	39	_____
15	Business readjustment	39	_____
16	Change in financial state	38	38
17	Death of close friend	37	_____
18	Change to different line of work	36	_____
19	Change in number of arguments with spouse	35	_____
20	Mortgage over $10,000	31	31
21	Foreclosure of mortgage or loan	30	_____
22	Change in responsibilities at work	29	29
23	Son or daughter leaving home	29	_____
24	Trouble with in-laws	29	_____
25	Outstanding personal achievement	28	_____
26	Spouse begin or stop work	26	_____
27	Begin or end school	26	26
28	Change in living conditions	25	_____
29	Revision of personal habits	24	_____
30	Trouble with boss	23	_____
31	Change in work hours or conditions	20	20
32	Change in residence	20	_____
33	Change in schools	20	_____
34	Change in recreation	19	_____
35	Change in church activities	19	_____
36	Change in social activities	18	_____
37	Mortgage or loan less than $10,000	17	_____
38	Change in sleeping habits	16	_____
39	Change in number of family get-togethers	15	_____
40	Change in eating habits	15	_____
41	Vacation	13	13
42	Christmas	12	12
43	Minor violations of the law	11	
		Total:	186

From Holmes TH, Rahe RH: The social readjustment rating scale (SRRS). J Psychosom Res 11:217,1967. (Used with permission.)

by physical, emotional, and behavioral symptoms. Some of the symptoms include the following (Greenstone and Leviton, 1993, p. 40):

Physical

- Constantly tired
- Trouble sleeping
- Frequent illness
- Gastrointestinal disturbances and headaches
- Loss of appetite

Emotional

- Absence of positive feelings toward clients
- Negative self-concept, feelings of failure
- A sense of helplessness and losing control
- Resistance to change

Behavioral

- Resistance to going to work, increased absenteeism
- Anger, resentment, and discouragement evidenced by statements such as "It doesn't make any difference what I do, nothing changes"
- Isolation
- Avoidance of conversation with clients
- Trouble listening and concentrating

Staff often start out very enthusiastic in the mental health setting. However, those who have the most contact with clients usually have the least power to change the system. A lack of positive feedback from supervisors and clients results in staff becoming very frustrated. They become apathetic and, unfortunately, many remain in the situation because of the fringe benefits.

Effective Coping Methods

There are many ways to deal effectively with stress. Nurses should understand these coping methods, both for their personal use and to share with clients. Box 21–1 lists several effective coping methods.

CRISIS

A **crisis** is an acute, time-limited reaction to an overwhelming emotional experience that can result in a state of disequilibrium or imbalance. It comes from the Greek word meaning "decision," but the Chinese definition is that of "danger" and "opportunity" (Arnold, 1996, p. 334). Being in crisis is not pathological. Crisis is a struggle for equilibrium when problems seem insolvable (Varcarolis, 1998, p. 366). A crisis can be a turning point in one's life.

Types of Crisis

There are two main types of crises: situational and maturational. A **situational crisis** develops from an external event such as an accident, loss of job, death, illness, retirement, or financial troubles. The life events listed in Table 21-1 can become situational crises, depending on a person's emotional status, ability to cope, and the support received. **Maturational crisis** includes the many issues that arise in progressing from one stage of development to the next. Erikson's theory of personality development in Chapter 2 lists undesirable behaviors for each stage of development. These behaviors may lead to crises if development outcomes are not achieved.

Recognizing a Person in Crisis

Greenstone and Leviton (1993, pp. 5–6) describe the profile of a person in crisis:

Bewilderment:"I never felt this way before."
Danger:"I am so nervous and scared."
Confusion:"I can't think clearly."
Impasse:"I feel stuck."
Desperation:"I've got to do something."
Apathy:"Nothing can help me."
Helplessness:"I can't take care of myself."
Urgency:"I need help now!!!!!!!!"
Discomfort:"I feel miserable, restless, and unsettled."

Table 21-2 lists common signs and symptoms of psychological reactions to crisis.

CRISIS INTERVENTION

Crisis intervention is the act of interrupting a person's downward spiral as skillfully and quickly as possible, returning the person to a pre-crisis

BOX 21–1	Effective Methods for Coping With Stress

- Identify the **stressor** (the cause of the stress). Tune into the body signal system, especially migrating aches and pains, such as headaches, backaches, constant fatigue, irritability, and sleeping problems.
- Differentiate between feelings of empathy and sympathy. **Empathy** is respectful, detached concern. The nurse understands what the client is experiencing but does not experience the emotion with him or her. **Sympathy**, on the other hand, leaves the nurse vulnerable to identifying with the client and sharing the client's emotions. The nurse is no longer in control of the situation and has limited long-range value to the client. Thus a long-term sympathetic response is very stressful. What started out as a caring relationship becomes—through overinvolvement—detrimental to both client and nurse.
- Take a long walk, a swim, or a bike ride. Exercise is the most natural way to change from stress to relaxation. It can calm anxiety, reduce depression, relax tense muscles, and improve self-esteem.
- Maintain a sense of humor. It is an equalizer among staff and, in many instances, between client and nurse. According to Robinson (1991, p. 50), humor in the work setting accomplishes three functions. It communicates important messages, promotes social relationships, and diminishes the discomfort of delicate situations.
- Focus on the positive aspects of what is occurring at the moment.
- Call emotions being experienced by their real names, such as *anger* instead of *guilt*. Sometimes under the guilt is a feeling of anger.
- Remember that there is always more than one way to solve a problem. Use the imagination to brainstorm all possible solutions.
- Identify positive outlets that have worked before in dealing with emotional discomfort.
- Differentiate between what can be changed and what cannot be changed, and allocate energies accordingly.
- Beware of chronic complainers and the temptation to do their work just to quiet them down.
- Associate with positive people. The nurse, by taking care of himself or herself in a positive way, can serve as a desirable role model for both co-workers and client.

level of functioning (Greenstone and Leviton, 1993, p. 1). There are two approaches to crisis intervention: generic and individual. The **generic approach** is based on certain recognized patterns of behavior that are present in most crises, such as bereavement, disaster, or chronic illness. According to Aguilera (1998, pp. 18–19), this approach "focuses on the characteristic course of the *particular kind of crisis* rather than on the psychodynamics of each individual in crisis. Specific intervention measures are designed to be effective for all members of a given group rather than for the unique differences of one individual. Recognition of these behavioral patterns is an important aspect of preventive mental health."

The **individual approach** is used in select cases when the generic approach is not effective. This approach focuses on the unique needs of the person and the events that caused the crisis. Whichever approach is used, the goal of crisis intervention is resolution of the immediate crisis. The focus is on the present and on restoration to pre-crisis level of functioning. The therapist is an active participant and uses a direct and supportive approach. Thus crisis intervention is short term, usually lasting one to eight sessions. This intervention differs from psychoanalysis and brief psychotherapy, which have a different focus and length of treatment.

A model for problem solving with a person in crisis is presented by Aguilera (1998, p. 32). The focus is on three *balancing factors:* perception of the event, situational support, and coping mechanisms. Figure 21–1 shows Aguilera's model. The upper portion of the model diagrams the initial reaction of a person to a stressful situation. In column A of Figure 21–1, all balancing factors are present; therefore, a crisis is avoided. In column B, one or more of the balancing factors are missing;

thus the problem may be unresolved, resulting in a crisis (Aguilera, 1998, p. 32). The three balancing factors are further detailed below:

- *Perception of the event* is the way a person takes in and uses information from the environment. A person's perception determines his or her way of coping with life stresses. For example, a woman did not see the need to grieve the death of her spouse. After returning to work, she became physically ill but refused to see a physician. A distorted perception of the effects of her loss on herself caused a state of disequilibrium.
- *Situational supports* are significant others who help a person cope with the stresses of life. With reference to the previous example, if the widow

had significant others in her environment to nurture and support her, she may have been able to avoid such a crisis.
- *Coping activities* are ways that people use to handle stressful situations. Defense mechanisms, as discussed in Chapter 2, are techniques for dealing with discomfort. Many develop early in childhood when a person is placed in stressful situations that he or she cannot handle. Many defense mechanisms operate at an unconscious level. Depending on the degree to which they are used, defense mechanisms can have a healthy or unhealthy effect on a person. In the earlier example, the widow used denial by refusing to see a doctor about her physical symptoms. If this coping technique were to continue, her health might be in danger.

Table 21-2	Common Signs and Symptoms of Psychological Reactions to Crisis	
Emotional	**Cognitive**	**Behavioral**
Anticipatory anxiety	Confusion	Withdrawal
Generalized anxiety	Poor attention span	Sleep disturbance
Shock	Poor concentration	Angry outbursts
Denial	Flashbacks	Change in activity
Insecurity	Loss of trust	Change in eating habits
Fatigue	Difficulties in decision making	Increased fatigue
Uncertainty	Nightmares	Excessive use of sick leave
Fear		Alcohol or drug abuse
Helplessness		Irritability
Depression		Difficulty functioning at normal ability level
Panic		Antisocial acts
Feeling out of control		Frequent visits to physician for nonspecific complaints
Grief		Loss of desire to attend religious services
Outrage		Regression
Numbness		Crying
Frustration		Change in communications
Inadequacy		Preoccupation with the crisis to the exclusion of other areas of life
		Diminished job performance
Feeling overwhelmed		Unresponsiveness
Anger		Hysterical reactions

Data from Greenstone JL, Leviton SC: Elements of Crisis Intervention. Pacific Grove, Calif, Brooks/Cole Publishing Co, 1993, pp 6–7.

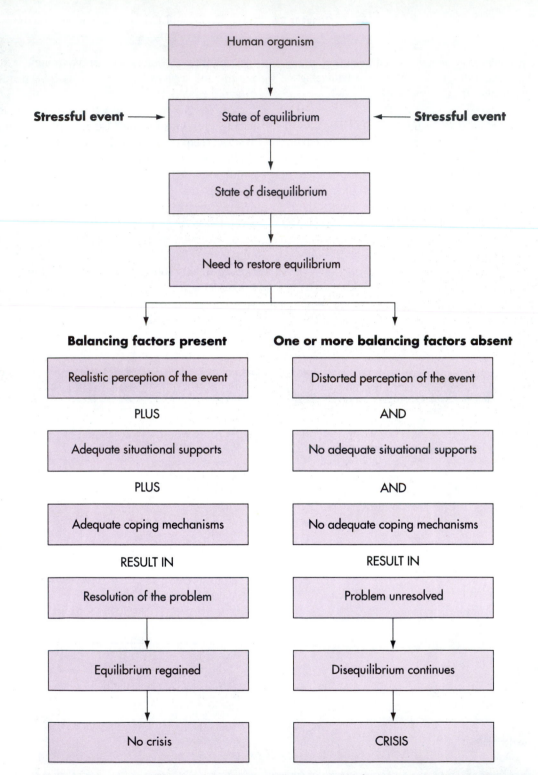

FIG. 21–1   Aguilera's model as a problem-solving approach to crisis intervention. (From Aguilera DC: Crisis Intervention: Theory and Methodology, 8th ed. St. Louis, Mosby, 1998, p 33. Used with permission.)

Reality Check

Joe and Marie, both professional people, have been married 25 years. They are heavily in debt because of Joe's excessive use of credit cards. Marie has allowed the situation to continue for many years, claiming she has no control over her husband. Joe manages their money and feels that, as the primary wage earner, he has the right to control their finances. Joe and Marie have now lost their credit rating and do not qualify for a loan.

1. What type of crisis are Joe and Marie facing?
2. Using Aguilera's model, what balancing factors are absent in Joe and Marie's life?
3. What problem-solving factors may be used in Joe and Marie's life to restore equilibrium?

Aguilera's model provides a helpful framework for nurses attempting to understand the factors involved in crisis and crisis intervention. Some people are more prone to crises than others. In fact, certain people, because of their lifestyle, become accustomed to living in crisis. Nursing interventions for persons need to focus on the following (Frisch and Kelley, 1996, pp. 11, 14):

- Increasing the client's sense of self-worth. This can be done by reframing the crisis so that the client perceives the situation as a challenge rather than a threat.
- Promoting the perception of control. Many clients do not feel that they have control. This sense of control can be fostered by encouraging the use of client's strengths. The nurse should use positive reinforcement when the client shows control.
- Promoting some resolution to the crisis so that the client will be as healthy as can be.

CASE STUDY

NURSING CARE PLAN

The following case study demonstrates a **nursing care plan** for a client in crisis. The example describes appropriate interventions for this client.

History and Data Collection

Steve Cole, a 40-year-old mechanic, just lost his job because of downsizing. This job is the only work he has ever done. Steve spent all his free time working on cars. Since his layoff, he has begun drinking and has threatened to shoot himself. His wife and children, afraid that they might be injured, have left. They called the police, and Steve was admitted to the mental health center.

The nurse who is collecting data (assessing) notes that balancing factors are absent in Steve's case; he has no situational support and no adequate coping mechanisms. She uses the RN's nursing diagnoses and the data collected to detail nursing problems appropriate for intervention at the LPN/LVN level. Table 21–3 shows the result.

Goals, Interventions, Rationale, and Evaluation

Based on the nursing problem she has defined, the nurse proceeds to list appropriate goals and interventions, along with a rationale for each. With the RN's approval, she implements the interventions

Table 21–3	Nursing Diagnosis and Nursing Problem for Case Study
Nursing Diagnosis	**Nursing Problem**
Risk for violence: self-directed related to recent job loss as evidence by threatening to harm self	Steve started drinking and threatened to kill himself after losing his job; wife and children left because of fear

Table 21–4	Goals, Interventions, Rationale, and Evaluation for Case Study	
Goal	**Interventions**	**Rationale**
Steve will not harm himself while in the hospital	Give medication as ordered; create a safe environment by removing harmful objects	Client's safety is a priority
	Initiate a verbal contract with Steve that he will not accidentally or purposely harm himself for a specific period of time; when that time has expired, set another period of time and continue the process	The client assumes responsibility with a contract; trust is developed between the client and nurse
Steve will discuss his feelings of hopelessness on losing his job	Encourage Steve to explore his negative feelings; help him work on positive ways of handling stress, using his mechanical skills	Finding constructive ways of dealing with stress will avoid the use of destructive behavior; support groups help keep a person from feeling isolated and alone
	Identify community resources that will support Steve during unemployment; encourage family counseling	

Evaluation: Steve Cole did not harm himself while in the hospital. Medication, the verbal contract, and using strengths to cope with the stress of unemployment helped Steve regain his equilibrium.

and evaluates the result. The goals, interventions, and evaluation are shown in Table 21–4.

▲

SUMMARY

Growing involves change, and with change comes stress. Stress is the body's reaction to the demands made on it. It can be a very positive force in accomplishing tasks and reaching goals. Prolonged stress can result in an array of physical and emotional problems.

Working in the mental health field can produce various stresses that can lead to burnout. Burnout results in physical and emotional exhaustion. This can lead to job dissatisfaction and decreased performance.

Some effective coping methods include exercising, having a sense of humor, and maintaining a focus on the positive aspects of the moment. There is always more than one way to solve a problem.

A crisis is an acute, time-limited reaction to an overwhelming emotional experience that can result in a state of disequilibrium or imbalance. There are two types of crises: situational and maturational. A situational crisis develops from an external event, whereas a maturational crisis relates to issues that arise in development. Signs that indicate a person is in crisis can include bewilderment, desperation, helplessness and apathy.

The goal of crisis intervention is resolution of the immediate crisis and return to a pre-crisis level of functioning. Aguilera's model for problem solving with a person in crisis focuses on three balancing factors: perception of the event, situational support, and coping mechanisms. Nursing interventions need to focus on increasing the client's self-worth and perception of control with some resolution to the crisis.

Critical Thinking Activities

1. Recall a stressful event that you have had in your life, such as a death in the family, an accident, starting school, an illness, or having children. Use Aguilera's model to answer the following questions.

   - What was your perception of the event?
   - What type of situational support did you have?
   - What coping mechanism(s) did you use?
   - Was a crisis avoided?

2. How might you interact with a staff member who lacks a concern for clients and co-workers?

Review Questions

Multiple Choice—Choose the best answer to each question.

1. A behavioral symptom of burnout is
   a. trouble sleeping.
   b. absence of positive feelings.
   c. isolation.
   d. frequent illness.
2. An effective method for coping with stress is
   a. associating with chronic complainers.
   b. exercise such as a long walk or bike ride.
   c. focusing only on the negative.
   d. trying to change what cannot be changed.
3. Which of the following is an example of a maturational crisis?
   a. Problems with interpersonal relationships
   b. Personal injury or illness

c. Death of a close family member
d. Change in work conditions
4. Crisis intervention involves
   a. brief psychotherapy treatment.
   b. a nondirective approach.
   c. a focus on the past.
   d. resolution of immediate crisis.
5. A common cognitive sign of a psychological reaction to crisis might be:
   a. feeling overwhelmed.
   b. change in eating habits.
   c. difficulties in decision making.
   d. generalized anxiety.

References

Aguilera DC: Crisis Intervention: Theory and Methodology, 8th ed. St. Louis, Mosby, 1998.

Arnold EN: Crisis intervention. In: Carson VB, Arnold EN (eds): Mental Health Nursing: The Nurse-Patient Journey. Philadelphia, WB Saunders Co, 1996.

Frisch NC, Kelley J: Healing Life's Crises: A Guide For Nurses. Albany, NY, Delmar Publishers, 1996.

Greenstone JL, Leviton SC: Elements of Crisis Intervention. Pacific Grove, Calif, Brooks/Cole Publishing Co, 1993.

Holmes TH, Rahe RH: The Social Readjustment Rating Scale (SRRS). J Psychosom Res 11:213–218, 1967.

Robinson V: Humor and the Health Professions: The Therapeutic Use of Humor in Health Care, 2nd ed. Thorofare, NJ, Slack, Inc, 1991.

Selye H: Stress Without Distress, Philadelphia, JB Lippincott Co, 1974, p 85.

Vander Zyl S: Taking Care of You: Stress Management for Nurses. Madison, Wis, Madison Newspapers, Inc, 1996.

Varcarolis E: Crisis and crisis intervention. In: Foundations of Psychiatric Mental Health Nursing, 3rd ed. Philadelphia, WB Saunders Co, 1998.

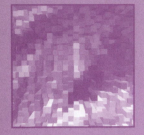

Chapter

TWENTY-TWO

Psychopharmacology

Outline

- **Antipsychotic Medications**
  Common Antipsychotic Medications
  Uses for Antipsychotic Medications
  Side Effects
  Future Implications
- **Anticholinergic Medications**
- **Anxiolytic (Antianxiety) Medications**
  Traditional Anxiolytics
- **Antidepressant Medications**
  Tricyclic Antidepressants
  Monoamine Oxidase Inhibitors

Selective Serotonin Reuptake
  Inhibitors
Atypical Antidepressants
Antidepressants for Children and
  Older Adults
- **Antimanic Medications (Mood**
  Stabilizers)
  Side Effects of Lithium
  Antipsychotic Agents
  Anticonvulsants
  Antidepressants

Key Terms

- **Abnormal Involuntary Movement Scale (AIMS)**
- **agranulocytosis**
- **akathisia**
- **anhidrosis**
- **anticholinergic**
- **anxiolytic**
- **cognitive dysfunctions**
- **contact dermatitis**
- **drug holiday**
- **dysphagia**
- **dystonia**
- **emotional dysfunction**
- **extrapyramidal side effects (EPS)**

- **monoamine oxidase inhibitors (MAOIs)**
- **neuroleptic malignant syndrome (NMS)**
- **neurovegetative dysfunction**
- **orthostatic hypotension**
- **paradoxical side effects**
- **parkinsonism**
- **photosensitivity**
- **postural or orthostatic hypotension**
- **sedation**
- **selective serotonin reuptake inhibitors (SSRIs)**
- **serotonin syndrome**
- **tardive dyskinesia**
- **urticaria**

Objectives

Upon completing this chapter, the student will be able to:

1. Identify two changes that occurred in the life of psychiatric clients as a result of the development of Thorazine.

Objectives—cont'd

2. Discuss symptoms most likely to improve with antipsychotic drugs.
3. Choose four major side effects of antipsychotic drugs and describe the nursing intervention for each.
4. Explain the role of anticholinergic drugs in treating EPS.
5. Identify the two expected effects of anxiolytics.
6. Explain why side effects of antidepressants may deter medication compliance.
7. Summarize main food restrictions with MAOIs.
8. Identify two positive differences that have popularized SSRIs.
9. Identify one difference in children and older adults regarding metabolism of medication.
10. Discuss how to prevent lithium toxicity.

Psychopharmacology is the study of medications used to reduce or control symptoms of mental disorders. Reduction and/or control of symptoms permits the client to function more effectively and be more responsive to psychotherapies. Medications are classified according to their intended effect on the patient. They include antipsychotics, anticholinergics, anxiolytics, antidepressants, and antimanic medications. Medications within each classification have approximately the same action, effectiveness, side effects, and nursing considerations. The nurse should review medications in a drug book before administering them so he or she can identify specific considerations for each client.

Reality Check

The safety steps for administering medications apply to all clients. What additional precautions do you foresee in administering medications to clients who are mentally ill? *Clue:* Think of what you have learned about behaviors related to specific disorders.

ANTIPSYCHOTIC MEDICATIONS

Antipsychotic medications were originally called *major tranquilizers* because the effect on the client's psychosis was thought to be secondary to a calming or sedating effect. Reduction of psychotic symptoms by antipsychotic drugs is now recognized, especially in schizophrenia, schizoaffective disorders, mood disorders, and cognitive disorders. In all of the disorders, the *positive* (outward, serious) symptoms are most likely to improve; the *negative* (not outward but very serious) symptoms are least likely to improve. Table 22–1 compares positive and negative symptoms.

Table 22–1	Positive and Negative Psychotic Symptoms
Positive Symptoms (Most Likely to Improve)	**Negative Symptoms (Least Likely to Improve)**
Hyperactivity, combativeness, agitation, hostility, acute hallucinations, irritability, negativism, acute delusions, insomnia, anorexia, poor personal care, uncooperativeness, paranoid ideas, thinking disorder, withdrawal, autistic behavior	Blunted affect, apathy, decreased memory, disorientation, retardation, limited insight, limited judgment, lack of motivation, anhedonia, grandiosity, anxiety, tension, somatic complaints

Common Antipsychotic Medications

Laborit, a surgeon in Paris, first noted that chlorpromazine (Thorazine) had a calming effect on preoperative clients. He urged psychiatrist colleagues to give chlorpromazine to their clients with schizophrenia and mania. The effect of symptom reduction was dramatic. Use of the drug spread, changing care in psychiatric hospitals throughout Paris and Europe.

Thorazine was first used in North America in 1954. Reduction and control of psychotic symptoms for many clients made possible the change from custodial to therapeutic programs. It also led to discharge from hospitals and return to community living (deinstitutionalization). Thorazine and other common antipsychotic medications are listed in Table 22–2.

Uses for Antipsychotic Medications

Antipsychotic medications produce a calming effect in most patients within a short period of time. Reduction in acute psychotic symptoms and behavioral control takes 1 to 5 days. About 6 weeks is needed for maximum improvement. Table 22–3 shows uses of antipsychotics for various disorders.

Side Effects

Antipsychotic medications as a classification are considered safe and effective. However, side effects can and do occur. Sometimes medications are chosen for a specific side effect. For example, a sedating side effect may be beneficial for a client who is unable to sleep because of a manic episode, severe depression, or pathological suspiciousness.

Extrapyramidal Side Effects

Antipsychotic drugs, with the exception of newer antipsychotic drugs that include clozapine, are associated with neurological side effects. Because these drugs affect brain structures that control body movement but not the structures known as the *pyramidal tract,* the side effects are known as **extrapyramidal side effects (EPS).** All extrapyramidal side effects involve muscle control.

The most common EPS include dystonia, parkinsonism, and akathisia. Table 22–4 describes these side effects and the appropriate interventions.

Tardive syndromes are dystonias that may occur after prolonged therapy and often persist after antipsychotic drugs are stopped (months up to 2 or more years). The most common of these is tardive dyskinesia (Table 22–5). The **Abnormal Involuntary Movement Scale (AIMS)** includes an examination procedure and a way to document findings regarding possible tardive dyskinesia. Areas examined include facial and oral movements, extremity movements, trunk movements, global judgments, and dental status (Raynor, 1998, p. 82).

Table 22–2	Common Antipsychotic Medications		
Classification	**Trade Name**	**Generic Name**	**Route**
Phenothiazines	Thorazine	Chlorpromazine	Oral, IM
	Prolixin	Fluphenazine	Oral, IM, depot
	Stelazine	Trifluoperazine	Oral, IM
	Trilafon	Perphenazine	Oral, IM
	Mellaril	Thioridazine	Oral
Butyrophenone	Haldol	Haloperidol	Oral, IM, depot
Thioxanthene	Navane	Thiothixene	Oral, IM
Dihydroindolone	Moban	Molindone	Oral
Dibenzoxazepine	Loxitane	Loxapine	Oral, IM
Benzisoxazole	Risperdal	Risperidone	Oral

Table 22–3 Select Uses for Antipsychotic Medications

Disorder	Select Uses
Schizophrenia and schizo-affective disorder	Positive outcome related to early intervention
Major depression with psychotic features	Used when antidepressants are ineffective against psychotic symptoms; antipsychotic medication is used to treat hallucinations and delusions
Mania	Reduces/controls manic symptoms and behaviors quickly compared with manic medication; once therapeutic blood level of manic medication is attained, antipsychotic medication is decreased or discontinued
Cognitive disorders (elderly)	Reduces/controls symptoms such as agitation and suspiciousness secondary to cognitive mental syndrome; medications most often used are low-dose, high-potency medications such as Haldol, Prolixin, Navane, and Risperdal
Substance-related disorders	Psychotic symptoms are often time limited in substance-related disorders; antipsychotic medications are used only if severe suffering or dangerous behavior occurs (for example, stimulant abuse)
Borderline personality disorder	Reduces hallucinations and delusions, but also *reduces seizure threshold* if in withdrawal; benzodiazepines (anxiolytics) are used instead in withdrawal
Tourette's disorder	Stress-induced, temporary psychotic symptoms may be reduced by antipsychotic medication; severe, disabling motor and vocal tics may be reduced with medication (usually Haldol)

Table 22–4 Extrapyramidal Side Effects and Related Interventions

EPS	Special Features	Intervention
Dystonia is characterized by bizarre, painful muscle contractions; it usually involves head and neck muscles, sometimes trunk and lower extremities	• Onset takes 1 to 5 days • Younger males are especially vulnerable • Examples: torticollis, contractures of tongue, trismus, oculogyric crisis (eyes roll back involuntarily)	• Antiparkinson drugs are given with antipsychotic drug to prevent EPS *or* • Treat EPS when symptoms appear *or* • Discontinue medication
Parkinsonism is characterized by tremors, rigidity, masked facies, "pill rolling" motion of fingers, shuffling gait	• Onset takes 5 to 30 days • Initial symptom is often a decrease in normal arm swing and reduced facial expression • Older clients with history of Parkinson's or receiving high-potency antipsychotic drugs are most susceptible	• Symptoms may decrease with time *or* • Treat with antiparkinson drug (levodopa is not effective) *or* • Discontinue medication
Akathisia is characterized by motor restlessness; client paces constantly or moves legs while sitting	• Onset takes 4 to 72 days • Akathisia is the most common EPS • Women are especially vulnerable	• Determine whether effect is caused by psychosis or medication; if caused by psychotic symptoms, cease when distracted • Intervention is the same as for other EPS

Table 22–5	Tardive Dyskinesia and Related Interventions	
	Special Features	**Intervention**
Tardive dyskinesia (TD) is characterized by bizarre movements of lips, tongue and cheeks (lip smacking, sucking, puckering); sometimes involuntary movement of fingers, toes, and trunk is involved	• Usually late-occurring • Clients with cognitive mental illness (often elderly), mood disorder, or sensitive to other EPS are especially vulnerable • Originally thought to be irreversible; symptoms may continue, stabilize, improve, or remit	• Discontinue antipsychotic drug; antiparkinson and other drugs for symptom relief • Check tongue regularly for vermiform (worm-like) movement; this is often the first sign of TD

Anticholinergic Side Effects

Another group of side effects of antipsychotic medications are **anticholinergic,** or drying, effects, including dry mouth, dysphagia, postural hypotension, urinary hesitancy or retention, constipation, and anhidrosis. Anticholinergic drying effects are felt throughout the body. Table 22–6 discusses these side effects and related interventions.

Additional anticholinergic side effects include the following:

• *Dry eyes:* The client may need additional artificial tears to relieve discomfort. Contact lenses may have to be replaced with glasses temporarily.
• *Dry skin:* Switching from an "institutional" soap to a soap plus oil and lotion is helpful.
• *Nasal congestion:* Often mistaken for a cold; the client should avoid administering cold remedies, which increase the drying effect.
• *Inhibited ejaculation:* This is both an anticholinergic and an endocrine problem. Changing to a different antipsychotic drug usually relieves the problem.

Allergic Side Effects

Another important group of side effects are the allergic side effects. They include *urticaria, photosensitivity,* and *contact dermatitis.* Table 22–7 describes these effects and lists appropriate interventions.

Agranulocytosis is an acute blood *dyscrasia* (disorder in which blood cells or platelets are affected). It seems to be an allergic response that occurs during the first 6 weeks to 6 months of treatment. It rarely results from any other antipsychotic medication other than clozapine. (About 1% of clients taking clozapine develop agranulocytosis.) Clients receiving clozapine have weekly blood tests. The condition is reversible if medication is stopped. The client needs immediate medical attention when diagnosed because agranulocytosis can be fatal. Nurses need to be alert to early symptoms, including profound weakness, high fever, chills, rapid and weak pulse, sore throat, dysphagia, and pharyngeal, buccal, or rectal ulcerations.

Neuroleptic Malignant Syndrome

Neuroleptic malignant syndrome (NMS) is an uncommon, but important, side effect that includes severe muscle rigidity, hyperthermia, tachycardia, and changing levels of consciousness. Presenting symptoms often include muscle rigidity and elevated temperature. Improved recognition of symptoms has reduced the former mortality rate of 20% to 30%. Antipsychotic drugs should be discontinued when NMS is present. Supportive and symptomatic treatment are standard and make include the following:

- Administering antiparkinson drugs for EPS
- Correcting fluid and electrolytic imbalance
- Treating fever
- Managing hypotension or hypertension

- Administering other medications as needed
- Intensive medical monitoring as needed

Other Side Effects

Other side effects may also occur in clients who are taking antipsychotic medications. Table 22–8

Table 22–6	Anticholinergic Side Effects of Antipsychotic Medications	
Anticholinergic Side Effects	**Special Features**	**Intervention**
Dry mouth characterized by "mouth full of cotton" sensation	• Common • Usually mild and temporary	• Rinse mouth • Sips of water • Chewing sugarless gum or saliva-stimulating gum such as "Quench" • Frequent oral hygiene • Paste adhesive for dentures • Sip of water before taking pills
Dysphagia is characterized by inability to swallow and may lead to choking or silent aspiration	• Client lets liquids such as milk run off his or her mouth (corners of mouth are often first clue)	• Supervise mealtime: solids and semi-solids are often easier to swallow
Postural or orthostatic hypotension characterized by a sudden drop in blood pressure when going from reclining to standing position	• May result in fall or injury, especially among older adults • Often related to poor hydration	• Instruct client to sit up slowly, dangle legs a few minutes before getting up • Lay down for a specified time after receiving antipsychotic medication by intramuscular injection; client often jumps up: be prepared to make a catch
Urinary hesitancy and retention characterized by delay in starting stream or inability to void	• Males affected	• Reduce dose or change to different medication
Constipation characterized by inability to defecate, leading to impaction	• Especially older adults • Clients on clozapine are at serious risk if constipation progresses to paralytic ileus	• Monitor toileting, especially during acute psychotic phase: client may not be aware of own physical discomfort • Mild laxatives and stool softeners • Increase water, juices, fruits, vegetables, bran; increase fluids when giving bran so bran does not increase constipation
Anhidrosis characterized by inability to perspire	• Uncommon • Perspiration is a natural cooling mechanism; disruption may result in heat stroke	• Be alert to red, hot, dry skin and complaint of discomfort • Remove client to cooler area; same first aid as for heat stroke

Table 22–7	Allergic Side Effects of Antipsychotic Medications	

Allergic Side Effects	Special Features	Intervention
Urticaria characterized by a generalized rash	Usually mild	Dermatological lotion may provide relief Lower dosage Change medication
Photosensitivity characterized by sunburning rapidly and severely	Associated with Thorazine (phenothiazine)	Sunscreen factor 15 or higher is helpful Long sleeves, wide-brimmed hat Advise to stay indoors until body adjusts
Contact dermatitis characterized by rash at areas of contact *Client:* mucous membranes of mouth and mouth corners *Nurse:* hands from contact with medication on outside of bottle	Related to direct contact with liquid antipsychotic medication	Dilute medication Take through straw Nurse should clean outside of bottle and wear rubber gloves if necessary

describes these side effects and related interventions.

Compliance

Approximately 60% of clients discontinue their antipsychotic medication. One reason seems to be that, although the client is free of psychotic symptoms, he or she continues to experience some residual side effects. Because the antipsychotic agents are long-acting, the antipsychotic effect remains and the side effects disappear first. By the time symptoms of the illness reappear, the client does not connect them with discontinuing medication. In 1966, Ayd, a psychiatrist, introduced a **drug holiday** concept for chronically mentally ill clients in his care. His "never-on-Sunday" policy provided an intermittent drug-free schedule that helped relieve side effects. It proved to be safe and effective. He added days off and varied them.

Long-acting intramuscular (IM) forms of some antipsychotic drugs are available for extended passes and long-term maintenance of clients with disorders such as chronic schizophrenia. For ex-

ample, fluphenazine decanoate (Prolixin) and haloperidol decanoate (Haldol) can be given every 1 to 6 weeks; Prolixin enanthate can be given every 2 weeks or as ordered by the psychiatrist. These are partial solutions being used by some psychiatrists who work with chronically ill clients. The result is often greater compliance. The client has some sense of control of his or her own life. The client feels he or she is improving and is not dependent on daily dosing.

Future Implications

Clozapine and other new atypical antipsychotic agents are proving to be effective for some clients who have not responded to other antipsychotic drugs. They also appear to target negative symptoms, including blunted affect and emotional withdrawal. At this time, it is anticipated that clients will not experience the serious neurological side effects sometimes associated with the older antipsychotic drugs. The atypical antipsychotic agents include clozapine, risperidone, and the more recently released Seroquel, sertindole, olanzapine, and ziprasidone.

ANTICHOLINERGIC MEDICATIONS

Sometimes antiparkinson drugs are ordered along with antipsychotic medication to prevent EPS. Some psychiatrists prefer to wait and see if EPS develops. EPS can be treated in most clients. Cogentin, Artane, and Benadryl are the most commonly used agents. Levodopa does not relieve drug-induced parkinsonism.

The anticholinergic medications have their own side effects. These include drying symptoms such as blurred vision, dry mouth, constipation, and urinary retention. There is also some evidence that they may cause memory loss. This side effect is reversed when the medication is discontinued.

Additional medications used to relieve EPS of antipsychotic medications include amantadine (Symmetrel) for parkinsonism and propranolol (Inderal) for akathisia. They may be given to-

Table 22–8	Other Side Effects of Antipsychotic Medications	
Other Side Effects	**Special Features**	**Intervention**
Ocular changes characterized by blurred vision and difficulty focusing	Difficulty reading or participating in games Usually mild	Instruct client to focus longer on object at which he or she is looking
Seizures occur because of a lowered seizure threshold	5% of clients taking clozapine for a year experience seizures	Antipsychotic medications should be used with caution, if at all, during alcohol withdrawal
Endocrine (hormonal) side effects characterized by symptoms that mimic pregnancy in women and sexual disorders in men	Women may experience breast enlargement, lactation, amenorrhea (lack of menses), weight gain, falsely positive pregnancy test Men may experience inhibited ejaculation and decreased libido	Include questions as part of regular data collection Change to a different antipsychotic medication
Water intoxication characterized by excessive oral ingestion of water; potentially serious	May be related to attempts to relieve dry mouth or inappropriate secretion of antidiuretic hormone	Be alert to client water intake and symptoms of water intoxication Signs/symptoms include: increased bounding pulse, increased blood pressure, increased shallow respirations, pale cool skin, headache, visual disturbance, muscle weakness, diarrhea, vomiting
Paradoxical side effects characterized by the client experiencing the reverse of expected effect	Client may appear more psychotic after administration of antipsychotic medication	Avoid giving an additional PRN antipsychotic drug; request assistance in data collection from psychiatric nurse practitioner

gether with anticholinergic drugs (Marder, 1997, p. 1580).

ANXIOLYTIC (ANTIANXIETY) MEDICATIONS

Anxiolytics are drugs that are used to treat anxiety. Historically, sedatives were used for this purpose. During the 19th century, opiates, alcohol, and bromides were drugs of choice. After barbiturates were developed, they were considered superior to the drugs that had been available previously. Barbiturates were effective, but in doses high enough to relieve anxiety they were sedating. The therapeutic index was narrow, with a lethal dose not much higher than the therapeutic dose. They were also addicting. Considered the "gentile woman's secret," barbiturates were also lethal in higher doses—a potential for suicide. The effectiveness of barbiturates, their prolonged action, and their low cost made use attractive.

The first modern anxiolytic was meprobamate (Equanil, Miltown). It was effective, but like the barbiturates, it proved to be both highly and easily addicting. Meprobamate was followed by hydroxyzine (Atarax, Vistaril), an antihistamine. Highly sedating, they proved to be of limited value in relieving anxiety. Chlordiazepoxide (Librium) became available in 1961, followed by diazepam (Valium) in 1964. Both were considered safe and effective anxiolytics, relieving anxiety and muscle tension (Jenkusky, Reeves, and Uhlenhuth, 1997, p. 1640).

Traditional Anxiolytics

Benzodiazepines, buspirone, and beta-blockers are considered traditional anxiolytics. Table 22–9 lists the trade and generic names of several common anxiolytics in these categories. The factors taken into consideration when determining which medication to use for a specific client include the following:

- Current symptoms
- Previous history
- Medications used previously and their effect

Table 22–9	Common Anxiolytics	
Category	**Trade Name**	**Generic Name**
Benzodiazepines	Ativan	lorazepam
	Centrax	prazepam
	Klonopin	clonazepam
	Librium	chlordiazepoxide
	Paxipam	halazepam
	Serax	oxazepam
	Tranxene	clorazepate
	Valium	diazepam
	Xanax	alprazolam
Azapirone	BuSpar	buspirone
Beta-blockers	Inderal	propranolol
	Tenormin	atenolol

- Presence of other illness, including psychiatric illness

Table 22–10 reviews some of the major characteristics and uses for traditional anxiolytics.

Benzodiazepines

As the major category of anxiolytics, benzodiazepines differ from antipsychotic drugs in significant ways. For example, benzodiazepines lack antipsychotic activity, no matter how large the dose. They also lack antiemetic activity and do not have significant anticholinergic side effects. Consequently, clients tend to prefer these agents because they relieve the uncomfortable anxiety and muscular tension, usually without producing significant side effects. Ideally, these medications are used to relieve high levels of anxiety and tension. The client is left with sufficient anxiety to motivate seeking a solution to the actual problem(s). The benzodiazepines are effective and useful medications when used properly.

These medications also have an anticonvulsive action. They are useful during alcohol detoxification in preventing or decreasing the intensity of end-stage withdrawal symptoms. Benzodiazepines are central nervous system (CNS) depressants. A benzodiazepine taken with alcohol, barbiturates, narcotics, or other CNS depressants can result in a combined effect greater than the sum of the effects of the two individual drugs. The combination affects the client as though he or she ingested a larger amount of CNS depressants. Some people accidentally overdose by taking two CNS depressants concurrently.

Side effects. The most common side effects of benzodiazepines are drowsiness, fatigue, and ataxia. Confusion is a significant side effect among the elderly. Occasionally, paradoxical behavioral changes occur. The person becomes agitated, hostile, or irritable. Sleep patterns can be disturbed by the onset of nightmares. Depression is a rare effect, as are blood dyscrasias, jaundice, skin rash, hypotension, slurred speech, and blurred vision (Pennebaker, 1995, pp. 565–566).

The most common problems, although less common than originally thought, continue to be drug dependence and abuse. This insidious effect is often caused when the client increases dosages on his or her own in an attempt to use the drug as a solution to difficulties. Clients may develop a psychic or a physical dependence, with the psychic dependence being most common.

Clients with a psychic dependence feel they need to have the medication to function. They do not experience physical effects from drug withdrawal. Physical effects from drug withdrawal are usually related to long-term high doses. However, these effects have occurred with usual therapeutic doses. Therefore gradual tapering from the medication is recommended. With long-acting drugs such as Valium, withdrawal symptoms may be delayed for days. These symptoms may be misinterpreted as anxiety. Withdrawal symptoms include insomnia, diaphoresis, nausea, irritability, twitching, and convulsions.

Table 22–10	Use of Traditional Anxiolytics		
Category	**Characteristics**	**Possible Use**	**Psychiatric Disorder**
Benzodiazepines (e.g., Ativan, Klonopin, Librium, Valium, Xanax)	Rapid onset (days), relatively safe, low interaction with other medications except CNS depressants (example: alcohol), lack of tolerance for anxiolytic effect, tolerance development for sedating effect. Taper off slowly to prevent rebound or withdrawal symptoms. *Concern:* dependence and abuse potential	Acute and chronic anxiety, anticonvulsant, muscle relaxant, anti-aggression, sedative	Generalized anxiety disorder. Panic disorder. Social phobia. Obsessive-compulsive disorder. Alcohol withdrawal
Buspirone (BuSpar)	Delayed response (weeks), lacks sedating effect, psychomotor impairment, dependence, withdrawal effect, and abuse potential; no interaction with alcohol	Relieve anxiety	Generalized anxiety disorder with depressive symptoms. High anxiety related to stopping smoking. Chronic anxiety unrelated to acute stress
Beta-blockers (Inderal, Tenormin)	Reduces palpitations, tachycardia, tremor, sweating	Peripheral manifestations of anxiety	Performance anxiety (form of social phobia)

ANTIDEPRESSANT MEDICATIONS

Antidepressants were first developed in the 1950s—accidentally. The drug was iproniazid, a monoamine oxidase inhibitor (MAOI). (See the discussion of MAOIs later in this chapter.) Researchers were seeking an improved treatment for tuberculosis. They noticed the mental stimulation and mood change in clients taking iproniazid. However, the serious side effects, including hypertensive crisis resulting in stroke, limited its use.

Imipramine (Tofranil) was developed from chlorpromazine (Thorazine). Researchers were disappointed in the lack of antipsychotic effect until they noted the antidepressant effect on clients. Furthermore, clients did not have the serious side effects seen with iproniazid. Tofranil has become the drug against which all new antidepressants are measured.

According to Keller and Boland (1997, p. 1608), all antidepressants are about equally effective in treating depression. Antidepressants are also useful in treating severe anxiety disorders and some medical disorders. Table 22–11 lists examples of antidepressants that are commonly prescribed.

Antidepressants are chosen for specific clients based on how the client's brain functioning is affected by the illness. Depression can cause dysfunction on three levels: neurovegetative, emotional, and cognitive functioning (Keller and Boland, 1997, p. 1608).

- **Neurovegetative dysfunction** (problem with sleeping or appetite) can cause hypersomnia or insomnia and anorexia or overeating. It can also cause a decrease in energy levels and libido.
- **Emotional dysfunction** includes a blunted or flat affect, anxiety, irritability, and apathy.
- **Cognitive dysfunction** can cause disinterest, feelings of low self-worth, poor health, and feelings of helplessness or hopelessness. The client may also present with poor concentration, a short attention span, and sometimes symptoms associated with dementia.

Table 22–11	Common Antidepressants	
Classification	**Trade Name**	**Generic Name**
TCAs	Anafranil	clomipramine
	Elavil	amitriptyline
	Sinequan	doxepin
	Tofranil	imipramine
	Norpramin	desipramine
	Pamelor	nortriptyline
	Vivactil	protriptyline
MAOIs	Marplan	isocarboxazid
	Nardil	phenelzine
	Parnate	tranylcypromine
SSRIs	Paxil	paroxetine
	Prozac	fluoxetine
	Zoloft	sertraline
	Luvox	fluvoxamine
Atypical	Asendin	amoxapine
	Desyrel	trazodone
	Ludiomil	maprotiline
	Wellbutrin	bupropion
	Effexor	venlafaxine hydrochloride

Tricyclic Antidepressants

Tricyclics (TCAs) are the most familiar antidepressants. Tofranil belongs to this category. The TCAs are considered safe and effective when used as directed. The key to success is related to treatment with enough of the right drug for a sufficient period of time. This often includes a long-term maintenance dose.

The onset of the antidepressant effect of TCAs takes approximately 2 to 4 weeks. It may take more than 4 weeks to determine the optimum dose.

Side Effects

Side effects of tricyclics can appear within 24 hours. The body usually builds a tolerance to the side effects within a week or so. Some clients continue to experience the side effects throughout the course of treatment. Initially, however, many clients experience both the depression and side effects. This causes them to question the appropriateness of their treatment.

Major side effects resulting from TCAs fall into three general categories:

- Anticholinergic effects, including dry mouth, constipation, dilation of the pupils, urinary hesitancy or retention, loss of accommodation of the lens of the eye, tachycardia, and, in high doses, delirium
- **Orthostatic hypotension** (sudden blood pressure drop when arising quickly, which can result in serious falls, especially among the elderly)
- **Sedation** (drowsiness); the client may appear to be asleep, but will respond when addressed

Infrequent side effects include the following:

- Activation of mania
- Visual hallucinations and delusions
- Blood dyscrasias
- Allergic dermatitis
- Photosensitivity
- Gastrointestinal symptoms
- Muscle tremors

TCAs also lower the seizure threshold. The rate of seizures is higher in the client with an existing seizure disorder. Ways of dealing with potentially annoying side effects are included in the section on antipsychotic medication.

TCAs, with the exception of Vivactil, are often ordered as a single dose at bedtime. This allows the largest portion of the side effects to occur while the client is asleep. A sedating side effect may even promote sleep. The dosage is individualized according to the client's needs and reaction to the medication. Overdose of these medications can cause cardiac toxicity, which can be lethal.

The nurse needs to work closely with the client during the onset of medication therapy to explain the action of the medication, the expected time of onset, the body's adjustment to side effects, and effective management of the side effects that remain. An ever-present danger in early antidepressant therapy is suicide. The client receiving medication is able to channel energy to formulate and implement a suicide plan before his or her depression improves significantly.

TCAs are approximately 70% effective in treating acute depression, preventing relapse (in maintenance dosages), and treating other depressive syndromes. These include bipolar depression, atypical depression, and dysthymic disorders. TCAs are also useful in treating most panic disorders, obsessive-compulsive disorders (Anafranil), bulimia-nervosa (Tofranil, Norpramin) and enuresis (Tofranil).

Monoamine Oxidase Inhibitors

Another group of antidepressants are the **monoamine oxidase inhibitors (MAOIs).** *Oxidase* is an enzyme that breaks down monoamine transmitters at many places in the body, including the intestine. MAOIs inhibit the oxidase enzyme, which in turn increases the availability of these transmitters, improving message transmission in the brain.

Clients who are receiving an MAOI (Marplan, Nardil, Parnate) need to be cautioned about ingesting products that would cause a significant additional supply of monoamines. Some foods contain significant amounts of *tyramine,* a monoamine that affects blood pressure. Large amounts of tyramine can lead to a hypertensive crisis (an extreme elevation of blood pressure), leading to rupture of blood vessels and resulting in a cerebrovascular accident (stroke). The client needs instruction on foods to avoid, what may be consumed in small amounts, useful substitutes, and drugs to avoid. Unnecessarily harsh diet restrictions may cause the client to give up an MAOI even if it is an effective treatment.

Table 22–12 lists examples of foods to avoid and those that can be ingested in small amounts. A client on an MAOI will need further instruction. A general rule is to be wary of anything that is smoked, aged, pickled, or overripe. Some drugs, prescribed or over-the-counter (OTC), may cause reactions when combined with an MAOI. Clients are instructed to tell their physicians that they are taking an MAOI. They are further instructed to read labels and seek assistance from the pharmacist when choosing an OTC drug. Box 22–1 lists drugs to avoid while a client is taking an MAOI.

A marked hypertensive crisis usually presents a headache at the base of the skull, a stiff neck, and a pounding heart. Less frequent symptoms include nausea, vomiting, and dilated pupils. A client should assume a possible crisis and seek help immediately because a hypertensive crisis can lead to death.

Selective Serotonin Reuptake Inhibitors

The **selective serotonin reuptake inhibitors (SSRIs)** are the newest category of antidepressants. Their focus on the neurotransmitter *serotonin* makes them more specific in action. Many

people recognize the more common drug names, including Prozac, Zoloft, and Paxil.

The SSRIs take approximately 1 to 3 weeks for onset. They remain in the system longer than other antidepressants. For this reason, a 6-week clearance period is required when client therapy changes from an SSRI to an MAOI. Clients wait at least 2 weeks after discontinuing an MAOI to begin taking an SSRI (Pennebaker, 1995, p. 555).

Side Effects

Side effects for SSRIs are different from those with TCAs or MAOIs. For example, SSRIs do not seem to increase the appetite and carbohydrate craving as do TCAs and MAOIs. The most common side

Table 22–12	Avoiding Side Effects When Taking MAOIs		
Must Be Avoided	**Small Amounts**	**Useful Substitutions**	
Most cheese and cheese products	Sour cream, yogurt, unless stored too long	Cream cheese, cottage cheese, ricotta cheese	
Fermented meats (examples: sausage, salami, pepperoni)			
Aged meat (reaction with as little as 2–3 days of aging)		Fresh meats (caution in restaurants: meat may not be fresh)	
Liver (avoid paté and other prepared dishes—chicken liver is very high in tyramine)		Fresh beef liver	
Smoked or pickled herring		Fresh fish	
Caviar	Avocado (avoid if overripe)	Most vegetables	
Broad bean pods (examples: Italian beans, fava beans)	Banana (avoid if overripe; peeling has highest tyramine)	Most fruits	
Sauerkraut			
Yeast extract (examples: brewer's yeast, "Marmite," some packaged soups)		Baked yeast breads	
Chianti wines (and possibly some other red wines)	Beers and ales (small amount only)	Other wines and alcoholic drinks in small amounts only	
Vermouth			
Any food that causes an unusual effect	Soy sauce	There continues to be a question about caffeine-containing foods, canned figs, game, meat extract, and raisins	

BOX 22–1	Examples of Drugs to Avoid Combining With MAOIs

- Phenylethylamine compounds (e.g., amphetamines, phenylpropanolamine, ephedrine, phenylephrine [Neo-Synephrine], and related stimulants)
- Decongestants (e.g., many over-the-counter cough, cold, and allergy medications contain tyramine)
- Bronchodilators (e.g., Isuprel, Dey-Dose)
- Demerol (meperidine)
- Darvon (propoxyphene)
- Lomotil (diphenoxylate hydrochloride with atropine)
- Simultaneous use with TCAs and SSRIs
- Sympathomimetic agents (e.g., epinephrine [adrenalin], Sus-Phrine, Bronkaid, AsthmaHaler, Bronitin, Medihaler Epi, EpiPen, Levophed)

effects include restlessness, insomnia, nausea, diarrhea, headache, dizziness, dry mouth, and tremor. Males may experience delayed ejaculation. Clients seem to have limited cardiovascular side effects. There is no additive effect with alcohol and other CNS depressants. SSRIs are also safer in case of an overdose (Pennebaker, 1995, p. 555).

Serotonin syndrome is a potentially serious side effect. It is related specifically to combining an SSRI with other serotonin antagonists or taking an SSRI too soon after another drug has been discontinued. Examples of potentially harmful combinations include the following:

- MAOIs (Marplan, Nardil, Parnate)
- L-Tryptophan
- Lithium
- Carbamazepine (Epitol, Tegretol, Mazepine, APO-carbamazepine)
- Pentazocine (Talwin)

Symptoms of serotonin syndrome include abdominal pain, diarrhea, sweating, elevated temperature, rapid heartbeat, elevated blood pressure, irritability, agitation, seizures, and delirium. The most serious cases of serotonin syndrome can include coma, cardiovascular shock, and death.

Uses

SSRIs are useful in treating acute depression and preventing relapse. They also are of value with other depressive syndromes, including bipolar depression, atypical depression, and dysthymic disorder.

Other disorders that may be treated using SSRIs include obsessive-compulsive disorders (Zoloft, Prozac) and bulimia-nervosa (Prozac). SSRIs have also been used to treat panic disorder, obesity (Prozac), substance abuse, impulsivity, anger associated with personality disorders, and pain syndromes.

Atypical Antidepressants

Atypical antidepressants are those that do not fit in other classifications. Trazodone (Desyrel) is used frequently with older clients for its antidepressant and sedating effect. It is also useful for reducing behavioral problems associated with dementia. It works as a catalyst for weaning clients off benzodiazepines and other sedating drugs. One important side effect of trazodone is orthostatic hypotension. Clients need instruction on how to get up slowly to prevent falls. Blood pressure should also be monitored.

Bupropion (Wellbutrin) is used for its antidepressant effect and also for treating attention-deficit disorder in both adults and children. Seizure potential must be assessed before treatment, because the drug lowers the seizure threshold. Use of bupropion is contraindicated in clients who have seizure disorders.

Antidepressants for Children and Older Adults

TCAs are prescribed with caution for children and older adults because of a report of cardiac arrests in a small number of children taking desipramine (Norpramin) (Nolen-Hoksema, 1997). SSRIs are better tolerated than TCAs and have become the drugs of choice for children and adolescents. MAOIs are seldom used with children and adolescents because of dietary restrictions (Colson, 1998, p. 923).

An interesting anatomical feature is that a child's liver is actually larger in proportion to the child's size than that of an adult so children may need a larger dose of medication because of the liver's ability to metabolize the drug rapidly. In contrast, an older adult's liver is slower to metabolize and detoxify substances. The amount of medication needed to attain the needed effect and prevent toxicity is smaller. Use of TCAs with anticholinergic side effects (such as Elavil) may be difficult for the elderly. Side effects such as confusion, dizziness, drowsiness, and orthostatic hypotension can cause multiple problems, including an increased risk of falling.

ANTIMANIC MEDICATIONS (MOOD STABILIZERS)

Lithium is the mainstay of treatment in both phases of bipolar disorder (Bauer 1997, p. 980). Lithium is approximately 80% effective. It especially targets symptoms of elation, grandiosity, flight of ideas, irritability, manipulativeness, and anxiety. Clients who cycle rapidly, abuse substances, or have mixed episodes do not respond as favorably as other clients.

Lithium was first determined to be effective in the treatment of manic disorder in the late 1940s. However, it was not approved for use in the United States until the 1970s because of deaths related to lithium intoxication. The deaths occurred during the time that lithium chloride was being used as a salt substitute.

The therapeutic window (range for maximum effectiveness) for lithium is narrow because of concerns for toxicity. Although toxicity is severe, lithium can be used safely if the serum lithium level is monitored regularly. To get an accurate reading, the blood sample is drawn 12 hours after the last dose of lithium. The best time for sampling is in the morning. The morning dose is held until blood is drawn. Once lithium therapy has begun, the serum level is usually monitored three times a week, or as ordered by the physician, until the client's illness is stabilized. A serum level of 1.2 to 1.5 milliequivalents per liter (mEq/L) is considered therapeutic for most clients, although sensitivity to lithium varies (Gelenburg, Hopkins, Delgado, 1997, p. 1588). The risk of toxicity increases above 2 mEq/L. Once the client's condition is stabilized, medication is reduced to bring the serum level to 0.8 to 1.2 mEq/L for maintenance. While on maintenance dose, clients should be monitored weekly at first, and later monthly.

Even though treatment with lithium is 80% effective, approximately 60% of clients discontinue medications on their own. Clients frequently complain of "feeling low." Psychoeducation is often used along with medication to help achieve compliance.

Side Effects of Lithium

Nausea and fatigue are common side effects that can occur early in the therapy. Tremor, thirst, edema, and weight gain may be present throughout the therapy. Confusion is an important *toxic* side effect that is often missed because it is misinterpreted as an illness symptom. Other toxic symptoms include ataxia, impaired coordination, dizziness, headache, blurred vision, muscle weakness, and gastrointestinal symptoms. Untreated, lithium intoxication can lead to coma and death.

Impaired renal function, decreased sodium intake, and diuretic therapy provide a risk for toxicity. To prevent toxicity, it is important to understand the relationship between lithium and sodium. Lithium and sodium share similar chemical characteristics. The sites for absorption of both are in the kidneys, where some of each chemical is absorbed and some is excreted. As long as the sodium intake and output remain the same, the lithium absorption and excretion will be stable. However, anything that changes this balance will have an inverse effect on the lithium. For example, a low-salt diet or diuretics will result in more lithium absorption sites in the kidney. This can result in toxicity. More salt in the diet can result in fewer lithium absorption sites, and this can cause a return of manic symptoms. This points out the need for the client to know as much about his or her medication as possible. The client needs to take responsibility for seeing the physician for medication adjustment whenever he or she experiences a major lifestyle change or becomes ill, for example, with nausea and vomiting.

Antipsychotic Agents

Therapeutic effect from lithium takes about 2 to 3 weeks of therapy. Consequently, the client usually receives temporary treatment with an antipsychotic medication until the therapeutic blood level of lithium is obtained. The antipsychotic medication targets symptoms such as irritability, insomnia, and acute delusions. Sometimes the medication is chosen for its sedating side effect so that the client can rest. Longer-term use may include targeting co-morbid symptoms.

Anticonvulsants

Valproic acid (Depakene) and carbamazepine (Tegretol) are anticonvulsants with antimanic properties. They provide therapy alternatives not available before. Both lithium and Tegretol have been shown to have prophylactic properties as well.

Antidepressants

In some clients, bipolar depression does not respond to lithium because of characteristics such as the following (Gruenberg and Goldstein, 1997, p. 1007):

- Mood reactivity (mood response to external events)
- Reverse neurovegetative symptoms (increased appetite, weight gain, sleeping a lot, a heavy feeling)
- Interpersonal hypersensitivity (increased sensitivity to rejection)

In these cases, the bipolar depression may respond to MAOIs. Tofranil is sometimes used for maintenance therapy against depression. It does not seem to prevent mania.

SUMMARY

Thorazine, the first significant antipsychotic medication, was first used in North America in 1954.

EPS and anticholinergic side effects are the most common side effects with antipsychotic drugs. Anticholinergic drugs are prescribed to treat EPS side effects.

Nursing observation and intervention are key in assisting clients to deal with side effects and medication compliance. Tardive dyskinesia may or may not be permanent. Neuroleptic malignant syndrome is a rare but potentially fatal side effect.

Anxiolytic medications relieve anxiety and muscle tension. Limited side effects make anxiolytics attractive to the client. Because of anticonvulsant activity, use of anxiolytics has contributed to safety of withdrawal of alcohol.

Tofranil is the standard against which all antidepressants are measured. MAOIs are useful antidepressants, but they require food and medication restrictions. Antidepressants do not reduce psychotic symptoms. Side effects appear before reduction of depressive symptoms when taking antidepressants. Lethality with overdose or additive effect with alcohol and other CNS depressants is decreased in clients who are receiving SSRIs.

Children and older adults have different abilities to detoxify because of liver size and efficiency. Therefore age and the state of the liver are determining factors in drug dosage.

Lithium is the mainstay of treatment in bipolar disorders. Depakene and Tegretol, both anticonvulsants, have antimanic activity.

Critical Thinking Activities

For each drug classification listed below, review the major side effects, early signs, prevention when possible, and nursing intervention(s).

- Antipsychotic
- Anxiolytic
- Antidepressant
- TCA
- MAOI
- SSRI
- Antimanic

Review Questions

Multiple Choice—Choose the best answer to each question.

1. Which symptoms are most likely to improve with antipsychotic medications?
   a. Negative symptoms
   b. Affective symptoms
   c. Positive symptoms
   d. Somatic symptoms

2. What is meant by *extrapyramidal side effects?*
   a. Neurological side effects
   b. Drying effects
   c. Late-occurring effects
   d. Allergic side effects

3. What is an expected result of treatment with anxiolytics?
   a. Decrease mania
   b. Alleviate psychosis
   c. Improve depression
   d. Reduce anxiety

4. Which group of medications includes food and drug restrictions?
   a. TCAs
   b. SSRIs
   c. MAOIs
   d. EPS

5. How is lithium toxicity avoided?
   a. Frequent blood serum levels
   b. Providing a drug holiday
   c. Including supplementary salts
   d. Monitoring daily blood pressure

References

Bauer M: Bipolar disorders. In: Tasman A, Kay J, Lieberman J (eds): Psychiatry, vol 2. Philadelphia, WB Saunders Co, 1997.

Colson C: Children and adolescents. In: Varcarolis E (ed): Foundations of Psychiatric Mental Health Nursing, 3rd ed. Philadelphia, WB Saunders Co, 1998.

Gelenburg AJ, Hopkins HS, Delgado PL: Mood stabilizers. In: Tasman A, Kay J, Lieberman J (eds): Psychiatry, vol 2. Philadelphia, WB Saunders Co, 1997.

Gruenberg A, Goldstein R: Depressive disorders. In: Tasman A, Kay J, Lieberman J (eds): Psychiatry, vol 2. Philadelphia, WB Saunders Co, 1997.

Jenkusky SM, Reeves A, Uhlenhuth EH: Anxiolytic drugs. In: Tasman A, Kay J, Lieberman J (eds): Psychiatry, vol 2. Philadelphia, WB Saunders Co, 1997.

Keller MB, Boland RJ: Antidepressants. In: Tasman A, Kay J, Lieberman J (eds): Psychiatry, vol 2. Philadelphia, WB Saunders Co, 1997.

Marder SR: Antipsychotic drugs. In: Tasman A, Kay J, Lieberman J (eds): Psychiatry, vol 2. Philadelphia, WB Saunders Co, 1997.

Nolen-Hoksema S: Understanding Depression: A Seminar for Health Professionals. Duluth, Minn, April, 1997.

Pennebaker DF, Riley J: Psychopharmacological therapy. In: Antai-Otong D (ed): Psychiatric Nursing. Philadelphia, WB Saunders Co, 1995.

Raynor J: Psychobiology of mental disorders. In: Varcarolis EM: Foundations of Psychiatric Mental Health Nursing, 3rd ed. Philadelphia, WB Saunders Co, 1998.

TWENTY-THREE

Physical and Medical Therapies

Outline

Key Terms

- electroconvulsive therapy (ECT)
- light therapy
- psychosurgery
- topectomy
- transorbital lobotomy
- unilateral treatment

Objectives

Upon completing this chapter, the student will be able to:

1. Describe modern ECT safeguards for the client.
2. List two possible treatment uses for modern psychosurgery.
3. Discuss the use of light therapy by the person experiencing SAD.
4. Identify the illness for which insulin coma therapy was used.
5. Explain how hydrotherapy was used with an excited client.

Some physical/medical therapies were used long before psychotherapeutic medications were available. Of these, electroconvulsive therapy (ECT) and modernized psychosurgery continue to be utilized. Light therapy is a more recent addition. Insulin coma therapy and hydrotherapy are no longer used.

ELECTROCONVULSIVE THERAPY

Various methods of inducing convulsions to treat psychiatric disorders have been used since the 1500s. In 1938 an Italian psychiatrist, Cerletti, and a neurophysiologist, Bini, introduced **electroconvulsive therapy (ECT)**—convulsive therapy induced by electrical stimulation. Their first client, who had catatonia, began to speak after the first treatment. Use of this form of convulsive therapy spread throughout the world.

The use of ECT increased in the 1940s and early 1950s. It was thought to be especially worthwhile for clients with severe depression, acute mania, and acute schizophrenia.

Psychotherapeutic medication, starting with Thorazine in the early 1950s, was accepted as a replacement for ECT. Furthermore, fear and misunderstanding of ECT was supported by special interest groups, some movies, and media. Confusion and memory loss, both usually temporary, were presented as widespread and permanent. The electricity used to trigger a convulsion was presented as highly damaging to the brain. No mention was made of people returning to productive life after ECT, suicides that were averted, and lack of medication side effects.

ECT is once again being valued as a safe, effective therapy. Three factors have helped re-establish ECT as a suitable form of therapy (Rudorfer, Henry, and Sackeim, 1997, pp. 1535–1536):

First, critical limitations of psychopharmacology and other treatment approaches have been recognized, including a significant rate of treatment resistance in the major psychiatric disorders as well as medication toxicities. Second, a series of critical examinations of ECT by professional organizations around the world . . . have supported the important role of convulsive therapy in modern medicine. Finally, coincident with advances in the clinical science of ECT and with the personal testimonies to the benefits of convulsive therapy by a number of public figures, media accounts of this treatment have become notably more balanced in the last decade.

Modern Electroconvulsive Therapy

ECT procedures have changed. They now consist of the passage of a small, carefully controlled electrical current through electrodes on the head to the brain. Originally, electrodes were applied bilaterally (to both sides) on the frontal temporal areas. The change to **unilateral treatment** (treatment on one side) on the nondominant side (usually the right), has reduced memory loss and confusion. The electrodes are placed on the frontal temporal and parietal cortex areas (Fig 23–1). The option of bilateral placement of electrodes remains if the client's illness does not respond to unilateral treatment.

ECT is treated like a surgical procedure. Informed consent involves written consent by the client or through the court system. Consent may be withdrawn at any time and is good only for the treatment series. A new informed consent is needed in writing for another course of treatment or for maintenance therapy.

A physical evaluation before beginning ECT includes a thorough history and physical examination. Additional tests may be ordered according to agency protocol, the client's medical condition,

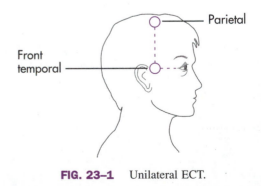

FIG. 23–1 Unilateral ECT.

the client's age, and the psychiatrist's discretion. Consultations with other specialists are requested if needed. The anesthesiologist also assesses a new client before the first treatment. At present the risk of serious complications is about 1 in 1000 patients. The risk of death is about 1 in 10,000 patients, which approximates the risk of general anesthesia for a minor surgical procedure (Rudorfer, Henry, and Sackeim, 1997, p. 1548).

The treatment is given in a specially equipped room or at the bedside. Treatments are usually in the morning with the client NPO after midnight. Nursing intervention includes preparing the client for ECT, monitoring after-treatment reorientation as needed, and posttreatment supervision. The client usually receives a drug, such as atropine, to reduce secretions about one-half hour before the ECT. Loose clothing is worn; jewelry, eyeglasses, dentures, and other prosthetic devices are removed. The client is reminded to void before the treatment. Once in the treatment room, the client receives a short-acting anesthetic, such as Pentothal, which quickly makes him or her unconscious. A muscle relaxant, such as succinylcholine (Anectine), reduces the external effects of the convulsion, preventing injury to the bones and joints.

The client is asleep during the procedure. He or she has no awareness of discomfort and does not feel the electrical current. The treatment produces a generalized convulsion of about 30 to 60 seconds. Sometimes an area such as the foot is "cuffed" with a sphygmomanometer cuff or tourniquet to prevent the muscle relaxant from entering the foot. This allows the therapist to monitor the convulsion in the "cuffed" area during the brief time that blood flow is interrupted to the foot. Contractions caused by the convulsion are barely, if at all, visible on the rest of the body. The best indicator is the pattern of brain waves on the electroencephalograph (EEG). The EEG is now a standard component of ECT devices. Heart rate, pulse, and oxygen saturation are also monitored, and an electrocardiogram (ECG) is performed. Monitoring of vital signs continues until the client is awake. The client is positioned on the side. Oxygen is given for 2 to 3 minutes. When the client is

fully awake and oriented (usually after about 20 minutes), the client is ready for breakfast.

Treatments are given two to three times per week. The number varies according to the needs of the client and the country in which it is given. The average course is 8 to 12 treatments. Amnesia is limited to a couple of weeks. Permanent memory loss is rare.

Effectiveness of ECT

The effectiveness rate for ECT is about 50%. In carefully selected clients, the rate is 70% to 90%. There is still a prevailing attitude of ECT as a treatment of last resort, after drug and other therapies have failed. The relapse rate of 80% is probably related to the same reason.

If a client has responded favorably to ECT in the past, chances of a future favorable response are good. Some psychiatrists incorporate an ECT maintenance regimen or follow-up with a maintenance psychotherapeutic drug and counseling.

Illnesses that seem especially responsive to ECT include the following:

- Severe depression with neurovegetative signs, psychosis, or suicidal behavior
- Acute mania
- Acute schizophrenia (early stage), schizophreniform and schizoaffective disorders, and catatonic and paranoid types of schizophrenia

PSYCHOSURGERY

Psychosurgery is actually surgery on the brain, not the psyche (Jenike, 1997, p. 1557). It is brain surgery that, in turn, has an effect on the client's psyche. The term *psychosurgery* continues to be a catch-all term for surgeries of years past, as well as modern sophisticated surgery.

Early Psychosurgeries

The first psychosurgery that reduced psychotic symptoms and destructive behaviors was performed in 1935 by Moniz and Lima of Portugal and was known as a *prefrontal lobotomy*. It consisted of severing the white-matter connections of the frontal lobe. The client's ability to perform activities of daily living was disrupted, and intensive training was needed after surgery for retraining. Numerous surgeries, up to 5000 per year, were performed as a way of controlling behavior. Monil received a Nobel prize in 1949 for his work on prefrontal lobotomy. However, not all facilities provided experienced staff to do the retraining. Numerous post-surgical clients remained in institutions permanently under custodial care.

Other psychosurgeries were introduced during this time. The **transorbital lobotomy** involved introducing a sharp object (originally an ice-pick) into the brain to sever the intended connections. It was performed in the doctor's office and lacked follow-up rehabilitation. It was also done in some state institutions without the client's permission. The procedure was abandoned because some clients developed personality problems.

The **topectomy** involved removing cortical material thought to be from the brain area related to the behaviors. It did not prove to be successful.

The advent of psychotherapeutic drugs in the 1950s provided a safer method of behavioral control. The calming effect was often referred to as a *chemical lobotomy*. Unlike the effect of the physical lobotomies, the calming effect of chemical lobotomy was not permanent.

Modern Psychosurgery

The modern psychosurgeries developed by neurosurgeons and psychiatrists in research centers are precise and use advanced methods, including magnetic resonance imaging (MRI). The neurosurgeons and psychiatrists use a variety of advanced techniques to create the lesions. They make the initial lesion as small as possible. If necessary, a second operation is performed to enlarge it. Like ECT, psychosurgery is usually not painful (Grebb, 1995, p. 2141). The surgery is named after the precise area of the brain involved. Surgery is followed with psychotherapy and psychotherapeutic medication as needed.

Client Considerations

Candidates for psychosurgery are chosen with great care. They must have a history of 5 or more years of chronic mental illness that has not responded to other therapies. The illness must cause the client to suffer and affect the client's family, social, and work situations. As a part of informed consent, the client must know the possible positive and negative effects of the procedure.

The age range for psychosurgery is generally over 25 years and under 65 years. Clients with organic mental disorder, delusional disorder, severe personality disorder, or serious substance abuse are not good candidates for psychosurgery.

Disorders Treatable by Psychosurgery

Clients who have severe depression and related obsessive-compulsive symptoms or obsessive-compulsive disorder have benefited from psycho-surgical treatment. Surgery has not been successful for treating schizophrenia. Non-psychiatric conditions that are not responsive to other treatments but have improved with psychosurgery include intractable epilepsy, chronic pain syndrome, and Parkinson's disease. Success is related to surgery on the involved areas of the brain.

Rate of Response

In carefully selected clients, modern psychosurgery has a 50% to 70% success rate. Improvement continues for years in some clients and may affect mental abilities, concentration, and intelligence. Negative effects for clients who do not improve may be depression and suicide, particularly in clients who saw the surgery as their last hope.

LIGHT THERAPY

Full-spectrum and bright white light are used to treat seasonal affective disorder (SAD). (See Chapter 13 for a more detailed discussion of SAD.) Bright white light is preferred by many therapists because it reduces the potentially harmful UV light to which the client is subjected (Light Therapy,

1997, p. 322). Light boxes of white light ranging in intensity from 2000 to 5000 lux are the most common form used. The client sits about 18 inches from the box and faces the light while doing tasks, without looking directly at the light. Sessions of 30 minutes to 2 hours usually bring improvement within a week or so. There is also some evidence that **light therapy** may be helpful in treating bulimia, delayed sleep phase syndrome (falling asleep late) and with shortening and regulating menstrual cycles. The effect is thought to be on the hypothalamus, the part of the endocrine system whose secretions govern bodily functions including blood pressure, temperature, respiration, digestion, sexual function, mood, the immune system, and body rhythms.

Reality Check

1. Name one or two currently popular over-the-counter products advertised as relieving symptoms of SAD or mild to moderate depression.
2. What scientific evidence does product advertising include to support its claim for relief of depression?

INSULIN COMA THERAPY

Insulin coma therapy, sometimes referred to as *insulin shock treatment,* was introduced by Sakelin in 1933 for the treatment of schizophrenia. The most common use was for clients with long-term schizophrenia.

The amount of insulin in the bloodstream determines the rate of oxidation of carbohydrates. Injection of large amounts of insulin into the body greatly reduces the sugar content of the blood, producing hypoglycemia. As the brain cells are deprived of glucose—their principal fuel—loss of consciousness and coma occurs.

Treatment involved administering small doses of insulin of about 10 to 15 units initially. The amount was increased during each day's treatment

until the desired depth of coma was obtained. With the development of psychotherapeutic medication, use of the cumbersome insulin coma therapy, which required skilled practitioners, declined rapidly. It is no longer used today.

PHYSIOTHERAPY

Two forms of physical treatments developed to treat mental illness were hydrotherapy (water therapy) and the cold, wet sheet pack. Both of these therapies were discontinued when psychotherapeutic drugs were introduced. Although neither is used today, a knowledge of their intent provides valuable background knowledge of therapy development.

Hydrotherapy

Before the introduction of psychotherapeutic medication, hydrotherapy was a common method of treating people with mental illness. Hydrotherapy consisted of a continuing, very warm water bath maintained at a constant temperature in a special tub. The treatment was soothing to an excited or agitated client. The client was continuously supervised by a calm, attentive staff person.

Cold, Wet Sheet Pack

A different version of hydrotherapy was the cold, wet sheet pack. The client was wrapped mummy-fashion in two wet sheets that had been thoroughly wrung out. Care was taken that no two skin surfaces touched and no pockets of air were left in the wrapping. When the entire body was suddenly cooled, the immediate action was for the cutaneous blood vessels to contract, resulting in a feeling of comfortable warmth, relaxation, and drowsiness. The client's condition, pulse, color, and general reaction were monitored on a regular basis by the staff person attending the client.

SUMMARY

Physical and medical therapies have evolved to become useful treatment methods for some forms of mental illness. ECT has again emerged as a viable therapy for selected psychiatric disorders. Modern psychosurgery targets the specific area of brain involved in a psychiatric or physical disorder. Some clients respond favorably to light therapy when experiencing SAD.

Insulin coma therapy was used before development of psychotherapeutic medications for clients with long-term schizophrenia. Physiotherapy, either as controlled very warm tub baths or cold, wet sheet packs, was used to calm excited clients before the development of psychotherapeutic drugs.

Critical Thinking Activities

1. Think about your personal reaction to ECT. Would you consider having it as a treatment if you were severely depressed? Explain why or why not. How does your conclusion affect the way you will answer a client's question about ECT?
2. Where could a light box for treatment of SAD be placed in the home to make it convenient to use while doing other tasks? Think of as many convenient places to use it as you can.

Review Questions

Multiple Choice—Choose the best answer to each question.

1. Which of the following reduces potential memory loss as a result of ECT?
   a. Placing electrodes bilaterally
   b. Placing electrodes unilaterally
   c. Using atropine 30 minutes before ECT
   d. Combining ECT with psychotherapeutic medication

2. What is one possible use for modern psychosurgery?
   a. Obsessive-compulsive disorder
   b. Organic mental disorder
   c. Delusional disorder
   d. Severe personality disorder

3. Which psychiatric disorder responds to light therapy?
   a. Substance abuse
   b. Dissociative disorders
   c. Conduct disorder
   d. Seasonal affective disorder

4. How did clients respond to physiotherapy?
   a. Energy was increased
   b. Agitation was reduced
   c. Disorientation was reduced
   d. Blood pressure was increased

5. What disorder responded most favorably to insulin coma therapy?
   a. Bulimia
   b. Major depression
   c. Long-term schizophrenia
   d. Chronic pain syndrome

References

Grebb JA: Psychosurgery. In: Kaplan H, Sadock B (eds): Comprehensive Textbook of Psychiatry, vol 2, 6th ed. Baltimore, Williams & Wilkins, 1995.

Jenike MA: Psychosurgery for obsessive-compulsive disorder. In: Tasman A, Kay J, Lieberman J (eds): Psychiatry, vol 2. Philadelphia, WB Saunders Co, 1997.

Light Therapy. *Alternative Therapy,* 1997, p. 322–323.

Rudorfer MV, Henry ME, Sackeim HA: Electroconvulsive therapy. In: Tasman A, Kay J, Lieberman J (eds): Psychiatry, vol 2. Philadelphia, WB Saunders Co, 1997.

Psychotherapies

Outline

- **Individual Psychotherapy**
    Long-Term Psychotherapy
    Short-Term Psychotherapy
- **Group Therapy**

- **Psychotherapy Groups**
    Structured Groups
- **Family Therapy**

Key Terms

- cognitive therapy (CT)
- cognitive behavioral therapy
- distorted thinking
- family therapy
- group therapy
- insight

- interpersonal psychotherapy (IPT)
- psychoanalytic therapy
- psychotherapy
- reality orientation
- scapegoat
- transference

Objectives

Upon completing this chapter, the student will be able to:

1. List three possible goals of psychotherapy.
2. Describe the nondirective role of the therapist in long-term psychotherapy.
3. Explain what is meant by "here-and-now" issues as a basis for short-term psycho-therapy.
4. Name three possible areas of focus for interpersonal psychotherapy.
5. List three distortions in thinking that are challenged during cognitive and cognitive-behavioral therapy.
6. Explain the therapist's role in supportive therapy.
7. Name the four phases of group therapy.
8. Summarize the guidelines for conducting group sessions.
9. Discuss the possible benefit of each structured group for people with cognitive im-pairment.
    - Socialization group
    - Problem-solving group

Objectives—cont'd

- Reminiscent group
- Reality-orientation group
- Remotivation group
- Sensory stimulation group
10. Explain the value of family therapy.

Psychotherapy, commonly referred to as *talk therapy,* is an all-inclusive term involving individual, group, and family therapies. Psychotherapy may be a primary therapy or a secondary therapy along with psychotherapeutic drugs or other physical or medical therapies. Some of the possible goals of psychotherapy include dealing with underlying issues, finding new ways of thinking, modifying behaviors, communicating effectively, and achieving education.

INDIVIDUAL PSYCHOTHERAPY

At one time, it was believed that emotional problems were caused by outside forces such as possession or punishment. After researchers recognized that emotional problems related to self rather than to external forces, psychotherapy became a reality. *Individual psychotherapy* assists clients in reaching goals by changing their thinking, feeling, and behavior.

Long-Term Psychotherapy

Freud is accepted as the father of psychoanalysis. His work on early interpersonal experiences and the influence of childhood memories became the basis for long-term therapy.

Psychoanalytic therapy involves intensive exploration of the inner self, including repressed memories. Psychoanalysts are psychiatrists specifically trained in this method. Therapy involves frequent contact and may take years. A therapy goal is to change bothersome personality characteristics that prevent the client from achieving personal goals.

The client responds to the therapist by **transference** (as though he or she is experiencing the early event). The therapist remains neutral in response. Through this process, the client develops an understanding of how these early events and relationships relate to current behavior, or **insight**. The insight provides the ability for change.

Various forms of long-term psychotherapy have evolved as theorists have modified, changed, or added to Freud's work. The modern version involves one to two sessions per week for approximately 6 months to 3 years.

Short-Term Psychotherapy

Several factors have influenced the development of short-term therapies, including the following:

- The cost of intensive, long-term psychotherapy
- Limits on insurance coverage for therapy
- Research on interventions
- The modern need for a quick fix

However, both long-term and short-term psychotherapies continue to be considered viable therapies. Client need for and response to available therapies varies.

The various forms of short-term psychotherapy, also known as *time-limited* or *brief* psychotherapy, share the following common characteristics:

- *Time is limited,* averaging about 12 to 20 sessions. Length and frequency of sessions vary according to need. Time limits may lessen the perception of helplessness.
- *A participating therapist* is involved in redirection, offering suggestions, and giving assignments. Trained therapists include psychiatrists, psychologists, social workers, master's-prepared psychiatric nurses, nurse practitioners, and clinical nurse specialists. All receive specialized training in the type of therapy involved.
- *Limited treatment focus* avoids getting off the

path of set goals. Therapy targets particular symptoms or a narrow aspect of personal character.

Short-term psychotherapy may not be suitable for some clients, including most who are psychotic, overtly suicidal or acting out, highly anxious, cognitively impaired, or extremely dependent. Clients who respond most favorably are motivated, focused, and able to enter into a time-limited, goal-directed therapeutic relationship.

Interpersonal Psychotherapy

Hildegarde Peplau, a nurse theorist, developed **interpersonal psychotherapy (IPT)** for nursing based on the theories of Sullivan. It focused on the significance of interpersonal relationships in human development. Later, IPT was developed in the 1970s as a therapy for people with nonpsychotic depression; studies showed the connection between interpersonal stressors and depression.

ITP is problem-focused. According to Swartz and Markowitz (1997, p. 1408), "One of the four interpersonal areas—grief, role dispute, role transition, or interpersonal deficits—serves as the explicitly agreed-on focus of treatment." Depression is presented to the client as a medical disorder. The therapist links the current interpersonal problems to the depression with IPT as the treatment of choice. IPT does not focus on past problems or issues. All of the therapy relates to the "here-and-now." Psychotherapeutic medications may be included with IPT as needed.

Cognitive Therapy

Cognitive Therapy (CT) is based on Beck's theory that a person's thoughts drive his or her mood or behavior. "A depressed person experiences 'automatic negative thoughts' that cause or perpetuate depression. Cognitive therapy attempts to change this pattern through the use of homework assignments and exercises to help patients to identify, test the validity of, and challenge these maladaptive assumptions" (Swartz and Markowitz, 1997, p. 1410).

The client's distorted thinking shapes his or her view of self and the world. Examples of **distorted thinking** include:

- *All-or-none thinking:* Everything is interpreted as black or white, good or bad
- *Overgeneralization:* A single event is interpreted as a part of a larger pattern of negative events
- *Mental filter:* Focuses on the negative aspects of a situation
- *Disqualifies the positive:* Brushes off positive events, comments, and experiences
- *Jumps to conclusions:* Assumes that something negative is happening
- *"Should" statements:* Puts constant demands on self of what he or she "should be" or "should do"
- *Emotional reasoning:* Assumes that negative emotions reflect reality
- *Personalization:* Accepts everything as being his or her fault (Nolen-Hoksema, 1997 workshop)

The therapist plays an active role in cognitive therapy. He or she helps the client detect the negative thoughts, learn how to challenge the thoughts, and replace the negative thoughts with positive ones.

Cognitive Behavioral Therapy

Cognitive behavioral therapy (CBT) is a combination of CT and behavior therapy. Both have been used separately to treat depression. Behavioral therapy uses action-oriented interventions to modify behavior (see Chapter 25). Integrating CT with behavioral therapy teaches the client new problem-solving skills and new behavioral skills for dealing with his or her environment. These therapies have also been useful in dealing with some anxiety disorders, eating disorders, sexual disorders, and substance abuse disorders.

Supportive Therapy

Supportive therapy often assists in maintaining a client within the community. Therapy may be short-term to deal with specific problems, or long-term on an as-needed basis. "Supportive therapy involves the therapist becoming a sort of role model or parent figure for the patient in a supportive or understanding manner. As such, the therapist helps the patient maintain the best level of functioning" (Carson and Arnold, 1996, p. 379). A client who has experienced successful relationships is most likely to benefit. The therapist uses a variety of therapeutic techniques, depending on the client's presenting problem(s). The therapist is actively involved, and a positive client-therapist relationship is an important part of the therapy.

Clients likely to benefit from supportive therapy often have poor interpersonal skills, poor problem-solving skills, inappropriate affect, or poor impulse control. If stressors are recent, a limited number of sessions may be needed. Clients with chronic mental illness may need more frequent sessions for an extended period. Some clients with bipolar disorder have responded favorably to combined client education and psychotherapeutic medication.

Client education involves the psychiatrist or psychiatric nurse therapist and client in a teacher/student mode and includes the following:

- Facts about his or her illness
- Role of psychotherapeutic medication or other treatment
- Maintenance therapy to prevent reoccurrence of symptoms
- Client's role in preventing relapse

GROUP THERAPY

Groups are a part of living, and the primary group is the family. Attitudes and behaviors develop within the family toward people who have something in common. These attitudes and behaviors influence each family member's future success in groups.

Group therapy is a regular, structured meeting between two or more people. The purpose of group psychotherapy is to reach each client's health goals. The group format allows clients to interact as peers in addition to their interaction with the therapist. As a result, group psychotherapy is an important form of treatment for clients who have interpersonal problems (Carson and Arnold, 1996, p. 390).

Since World War II, group therapy has been a popular form of treatment with mentally ill clients. Psychotropic medication, introduced in the 1950s, made clients more receptive to this form of treatment. With some of the observable symptoms under control, clients were able to share experiences and provide feedback to group members. Group therapy has also become a cost-effective way of treating several clients at the same time.

Psychotherapy Groups

Groups led by professional therapists—psychiatrists, psychologists, psychiatric social workers, master's-prepared psychiatric nurse therapists, clinical nurse specialists, or nurse practitioners—include the psychodynamic, action-oriented, and interpersonal counterparts of individual psychotherapies. Knowledge of psychological theories and group process is essential. Therapists function in a *nondirective role* (avoid giving specific advice and direction) in psychodynamic groups. These groups focus on feelings and the dynamics that affect current functioning. The insight gained becomes the basis for change.

Groups should include at least five, and no more than ten, clients to provide needed interaction and attention. Members are in groups because of their similarities rather than their differences. Clients can relate to each other's problems and lose the sense of being "the only one." Contact and involvement between clients outside of the group setting is strongly discouraged. Some groups are "closed groups" meaning no one may join the group once it has started. In "open groups," members join and leave without restriction.

Groups pass through the following chronological phases:

- *Preinteraction:* Pregroup interview to present goals, purpose, format, and expectations and determine makeup of group.
- *Engagement (orientation):* Testing of therapist and group members; outline of goals, rules, and roles. Premature disclosure is discouraged,

boundaries are set, and the group agrees on the contract length and time.

- *Working:* Real work takes place. Clients learn group trust by risking honesty and confronting each other negatively as necessary. It is a time of increased self-disclosure and in-depth exploration of problems.
- *Termination:* Mixed emotions such as anger, sadness, rejection, sense of loneliness, abandonment, retesting of the therapist, satisfaction with goal attainment and loss of group support. Clients need time to process their responses. It is important for the therapist and members to "stick with" their original contract.

Each phase requires clients to complete more complex tasks. The termination phase, as the culmination of the group's work, is especially important (Carson and Arnold, 1996, p. 396).

Structured Groups

The group work described in the remainder of this section focuses on structured groups that deal with concrete issues. These groups are led by a wide spectrum of health providers and are effective with confused and disoriented clients. Box 24–1 lists reasons for forming structured groups.

Various types of structured groups can be formed, depending on client needs. The most common types of groups are:

- Socialization
- Problem-solving
- Reminiscent
- Reality orientation
- Sensory stimulation

Socialization Groups

A *socialization group* focuses on concrete and realistic aspects of the person and his or her environment. The group's goals are to stimulate the participants to begin thinking about things outside themselves. It provides them with an opportunity to talk about these things freely and promotes personal interaction between leader and client, as well as among clients. Clients chosen for this group are those whose contact with reality is

BOX 24–1	Reasons for Group Work

Structured groups provide clients with an opportunity to do the following:

- Practice alternative ways of dealing with negative feelings in a nonjudgmental, protective environment
- Gain a sense of belonging and acceptance
- Give as well as receive, increasing self-confidence
- Engage in self-disclosure and realize that others have similar feelings and problems
- Interact with others, developing greater interpersonal effectiveness
- Gain some understanding of his or her feelings
- Engage in positive reinforcement and hope for improvement
- Develop a feeling of community with others, thus decreasing the feeling of loneliness
- Realize how his or her behavior impacts knowledge and affects others through peer feedback
- Transfer what is learned in the group to other situations, such as home, work, or an alternative living situation

tenuous, who have difficulty using their intellectual faculties, and who have difficulty interacting or socializing with others.

The group leader is directive with the members of this group. He or she sets the stage for the group theme and draws group members into the discussion. The group leader needs to prepare in advance. Suggested techniques include the following:

- Topic ideas will be most successful if they bear some relation to group members' actual interests. The group leader can get some clues for topics by talking to clients before the session. Talking to other staff and family members and checking charts regarding previous interests and occupations may be helpful. Holidays, sports, hobbies, work, weather conditions, and pets are possible topics for beginning discussion.
- Props, such as colorful pictures, maps, plants, tools, or a pet, when permitted, can stimulate conversation. Props, like topics, are limited only by the leader's imagination. Clients can be

assigned to bring one prop of importance to them to a meeting.

- Questions and statements by the leader may be helpful in stimulating conversation. These might include questions such as:

What is the funniest thing that ever happened to you?

If you could be an animal, what kind would it be, and why?

The holiday I remember most is _____ because _____ .

The first thing I remember while growing up was _____ .

The quality I value most about me is _____ .

The physical arrangement of the room must lend itself to conversation. Arranging the chairs in a circle encourages the clients to have some physical contact with each other and places them in a position to observe others. Juice and light snacks available at the beginning of the session helps to break the ice.

Problem-Solving Groups

The problem-solving process can be part of all groups, but it can also be the main focus of a group. If this is the case, the *problem-solving group* is open-ended and is concerned primarily with the teaching, demonstration, and implementation of the problem-solving process.

The leader of this group works to establish a nonthreatening and trusting environment by explaining the group's purposes. Explanation of the problem-solving technique, owning one's own problem, directing questions to other clients for their input, and supporting each other's strengths are part of the orientation. The leader models the desired process and behavior. For example, the leader might give verbal praise, nodding and smiling when someone makes a contribution to the group. The leader also guides the group away from any lengthy confrontation with one client.

Criteria for selecting clients to participate in a problem-solving group include a willingness to participate, the ability to verbalize, an awareness of problems, and the ability to use one's intellectual faculties. Group size ranges from eight to ten

members, with a circular seating arrangement. The problem-solving techniques used in the group include the following:

- Isolating and defining the problem through open discussion, role playing, and exercises in communicating and establishing relationships.
- Gathering information about the defined problem through open discussion.
- Exploring methods to solve the problem, including open discussion, and role playing. Feedback from group members can offer possible solutions. A problem always has at least four or five solutions.
- Trying the selected method. The participant must try to implement the selected method. This can be done by assigning the task to be completed by the next meeting.
- Evaluating whether the selected method solved the problem in a reasonably satisfactory way.

Reminiscent Groups

A *reminiscent group* supports the wisdom of the aged. Sometimes older people who, in their mid-life had well-developed creative ability, are unable to continue at that level. This may be related to confinement at home or in a facility. Reminiscing provides an opportunity for memory stimulation and a sense of belonging to a group. This, in turn, may stimulate the person to use his or her creative talents once again.

The membership of a reminiscent group is limited to five or six clients. Usually these groups are held for about 10 sessions, each 1 hour in length. It is important that the group leader approach each potential group member individually and invite that person to attend meetings to talk about the past. The leader must express interest in learning about each member's history. Also, each member is told who the other members will be, since each person must be free to make his or her own decision about attending. As with all groups, the leader begins with introductions. Sometimes relaxation exercises, music, and snacks are ways of increasing verbal responsiveness. Additional ways to begin reminiscing include the following:

- Each member can locate his or her birthplace on a map. Mark the place with a map pin and his or her name. Have the member tell the group whatever he or she can remember related to birthplace.
- Other possible topics/themes include members' hobbies, jobs, celebration of certain holidays, favorite bands, singers, radio shows, movie stars, cars, inventions, completing old sayings, and word synonyms or antonyms.
- Use props, such as bright visual aids, selected pictures, picture books, old newspapers, and old tools or farm equipment.

Termination can sometimes be difficult in reminiscent groups because of the many personal memories that have been shared.

Reality Orientation Groups

Reality orientation is a way to improve the quality of care for clients who are confused or, more specifically, disoriented to time, place, things, and person. Causes for the impairment vary and may include cognitive impairment resulting from arteriosclerosis, head injury, stroke, sensory deprivation, overmedication, or drug or alcohol use. Clients with long-term, chronic mental illness who are disoriented also benefit from reality orientation.

Reality orientation must be followed through on a 24-hour-a-day basis to be effective. Consequently, it involves all staff—total involvement makes success possible. The techniques are simple and can be learned by any staff person who has demonstrated skill and patience in working with confused clients. Reality orientation is different from reality therapy, a psychotherapy facilitated by a professional therapist. Reality therapy focuses on here-and-now issues and presumes that unhappiness is the result—not the cause—of irresponsibility. The major emphasis in reality therapy is on rewriting life scripts, self-discipline, and personal responsibility. As with all therapies, reality orientation is effective with some, not all, clients.

Reality orientation begins immediately on rising. When the client is awakened, he or she is addressed by name, oriented to time and day, and told at what time breakfast will be served. The client continues to be addressed by name throughout the day. He or she is reoriented to all aspects of care and scheduling during the day, evening, and night shifts.

The reality board, an established part of most units with confused clients, is a helpful tool for the client. It helps the client remember information, such as where he or she is, the day of the week, date, and year. Additional information, such as the weather, next holiday, and next meal, are often included. Staff must immediately reward current responses with verbal praise, a touch, or a smile, both on the unit and during group sessions.

Planned group sessions are held daily for 30 minutes, preferably at the same time each day. Sessions held in the same room each time provide consistency. The room itself must be pleasant, with plenty of light and table space. A basic group is limited to three or four very confused clients.

Ideally, the group has both a leader and a co-leader. Reality materials, such as a chalk board, felt board, large clock, and calendar are essential props. Additional materials, such as jigsaw puzzles, maps, adult picture books, and plastic fruit, vegetables, and flowers can be obtained from thrift stores. The use of these materials is limited only by the imagination. One way is to have clients associate an object with its name, which appears in large letters, such as matching an apple to the word APPLE.

At the beginning of each session, the client should review information already on the chalk board, including the following:

The place is _____
The time is _____
The day of the week is _____
The date is _____
The weather is _____
The next holiday is _____
The next meal is _____

When the client learns the simple information offered in the basic group, he or she is moved into the advanced group, made up of eight to ten members. Memory games that are not too difficult—those at a sixth-grade or lower level are suggested—are excellent for stimulating recall and concentration. A somewhat more advanced version of the questions asked in the basic group is useful. The group content should be varied enough so as not to become boring, but not so much as to be confusing. The advanced group sessions can also include grooming, physical exercise, and sensory training.

A trial period of 2 months is necessary to evaluate participants' progress. If at the end of that time the client shows no progress, it is best to discontinue his or her involvement in group sessions. The client can be readmitted to the group at a later date. Groups are evaluated monthly and changes are made when indicated.

The attitude of the leader and all staff is most important during attainment of the desired goals. Clients must not be embarrassed or singled out because of their confusion. Directions are given in simple, short sentences and delivered in clear, distinct tones on an adult level. Information may be repeated as often as necessary. Clients need extra time for response. The leader's expectant manner supports the expectation that the client will respond if given adequate time. Consistency in the routine, once it is established, is essential.

Remotivation Groups

A remotivation group provides a way to stimulate clients who are no longer involved in the present or the future. This structured group is based on reality. The objective materials used by the leader are intended to stimulate discussion about present or future issues.

A remotivation group is limited to 15 members who are willing to participate in a structured format. The suggested number of sessions is 12, meeting once or twice a week for 30 minutes to 1 hour. Each session involves five basic steps that relate to a topic:

- Introductions and getting acquainted
- A member reads, out loud, an article or poem related to the topic
- The topic is developed using questions, visual aids, and props

- Members are directed to think about work in relation to themselves
- Members are thanked for attending and participating, and plans are made for the next session

Box 24–2 is an example of a remotivation group session.

Sensory Stimulation Groups

Throughout the life cycle, sensory stimulation continues to be a significant aspect of the growth process. Most people are able to meet this need because they participate in many activities in the outside world. It is the person who is unable to

---

BOX 24–2	**Example of a Remotivation Session**

The topic for the session, which was determined at the end of the previous session, is "The Potato."

Step One

The members introduce themselves to one another. The leader comments on positive aspects of the members' appearance and dress.

Step Two

One of the group members is asked to read the rhyme, "One Potato, Two Potato, Three Potato, Four."

Step Three

The leader asks the members of the group if they know how a potato grows. As members discuss a potato's growth, a real potato is passed around the group. Members are asked to describe the various kinds of potatoes. While this is going on, one member is asked to pass a dish of potato chips around the circle.

Step Four

A discussion begins about the work involved in preparing potatoes, from the garden to the market. Members are asked if they have ever been involved in similar work activity.

Step Five

The leader thanks group members for attending, and together they plan the topic for the next session, which they decide will be an animal, namely, "The Pig."

move about in the outside world because of illness or age who experiences sensory deprivation and requires sensory stimulation.

A *sensory stimulation group* is small, with no more than six members. Members are seated in a tight circle so that their knees or arms are close to the person on each side. The leader can easily reach out and touch the members without getting out of his or her chair. The leader relates to the group members with warmth and supportiveness, explaining that the purpose of the group is to stimulate their senses. Focusing on one sense during each session will maximize the stimulation in that area. Each session is about 30 minutes long.

Props than can be used for sensory stimulation include the following:

- *Sight props:* Clocks, calendars, bright colors, pictures, mirrors, windows, houseplants, flowers.
- *Sound props:* Meaningful conversation, singing, music, children's voices; choices of radio, stereo, TV, piano, tambourine.
- *Touch props:* Back rub, massage, holding hands, feeling different textures. A bag with pieces of various materials, such as velvet, fur, burlap, silk, and corduroy, can be passed around the group. Each member closes his or her eyes, reaches into the bag, and tries to identify the materials.
- *Smell props:* Varied and appetizing foods, perfume and cologne, powder, flowers, and spices. Each person in the group smells each item, then tells the group what he or she thinks the item is. Praise is given for the correct answer. If the answer was incorrect, have the person smell the item again, repeat its name, and receive reinforcement for saying it correctly.
- *Taste props:* Varied and appetizing foods, especially fresh fruits; good oral hygiene; varied fluids.
- *Internal stimulation props:* Exercise, walking, stretching, movement therapy, relaxation therapy, dancing.

The nurse can retard the progression of deterioration in the elderly client by intervening with sensory exercises.

Reality Check

Psychotherapeutic and structured groups have many similarities. Which of the following statements apply to both types of groups?

_____ 1. Selection of clients is based on certain criteria, such as similar problems, similar ability in verbal expression, emotional level, and similar or varied interests.

_____ 2. Group size is based on group goals; if clients are confused and disoriented, six to eight clients is the maximum.

_____ 3. Select comfortable surroundings; a permanent meeting place free from distraction is desirable.

_____ 4. Acquaint oneself with clients before the group begins.

_____ 5. Briefly describe the group's purpose/ goals at the beginning of the first session.

_____ 6. Have clients introduce themselves to each other.

_____ 7. Establish a nonthreatening and trusting climate with a statement such as, "If you don't want to contribute, that's all right."

_____ 8. Allow group members to perform tasks, such as arranging chairs, gathering materials, or whatever they can do. A small, close circle promotes intimacy and cohesiveness.

_____ 9. Relate to group members with warmth and supportiveness. The leader's attitude is contagious.

_____ 10. Use verbal praise, nodding and smiling to reinforce contributions from group members.

_____ 11. Encourage group members to reinforce one another's strengths.

_____ 12. Make reluctant clients feel that their ideas are wanted and needed by incorporating their contributions into the discussion.

_____ 13. Prevent talkative clients from dominating the group without feeling rejected.

_____ 14. Be patient and wait for group members to break the silence.

_____ 15. Encourage group members to direct questions to each other rather than to the leader.

_____ 16. Give power to the group by allowing them to make decisions after areas of choice have been clarified.

_____ 17. Provide for the safety of group members; guide the group away from any lengthy attack on one member.

_____ 18. Keep discussion and activity moving.

_____ 19. Listen for themes in the group and reinforce them so that all members can be involved.

_____ 20. From time to time, summarize what has been said and ask for clarification.

_____ 21. Stimulate the group by varying techniques and format such as role playing, films, and guest leaders. Group members should participate in selecting activities.

FAMILY THERAPY

Family therapy is systems theory from physics, applied to human behavior. The family is viewed as a system, with subsystems, boundaries, rules, alignment, and power. Changes within the family system affect the environment and behavior of others within the family.

Often a child becomes the **scapegoat** who acts out the dysfunction in a family and brings the family into therapy. In a sense, it is the child's behavior that keeps the family together. As long as the child is the identified problem (sick one), the rest of the family is able to function. If the child's behavior improves, it creates a shift within the system, and behavior of others is affected (Lala, 1994, p. 150).

Family therapy is based on a nonmedical model and is facilitated by specially trained family therapists. Types of family therapy include the following (Carson and Arnold, 1996, p. 473):

- *Individual family therapy:* Each family member has a therapist. The family comes together periodically to deal with family issues.

- *Couples therapy:* Married or unmarried couples deal with relationship issues.
- *Conjoint family therapy:* Entire nuclear family is involved.
- *Multiple-family group therapy:* Several families with similar issues meet as a group.
- *Multiple-impact therapy:* Similar to multiple-family group therapy, but is an intense short-term encounter (weekend or week) that focuses on a specific problem or issue.
- *Network therapy:* Takes place within the community. Anyone connected or interested in the crisis is invited. Network therapy involves professionals, community members, family, friends. A long-term network of support may emerge for the family who had the crisis.

SUMMARY

All therapy involves the team effort. The nurse plays a major role in this team effort.

Psychotherapy is facilitated by professional, trained therapists. Long-term psychotherapy often deals with childhood experiences that have influenced current difficulties. The therapist plays a nondirective role. Insight (personal discovery) developed by the client becomes the basis for change. Short-term psychotherapy focuses on "here-and-now" issues that are creating current problems. The therapist may be directive, as in cognitive and cognitive-behavioral therapy.

Psychotherapy groups go through four basic phases: preinteraction, engagement, working, and termination. Structured groups include socialization, problem-solving, reminiscent, reality orientation, remotivation, and sensory stimulation groups. These groups are frequently of value for people with cognitive impairment. They are facilitated by a variety of knowledgeable staff.

Family therapy is based on systems theory. The family is a system in which anyone's shift in behavior causes a change in others. The "sick" one, usually a child, is the symptom-bearer for the family and brings the family to therapy. Therapy assists the dysfunctional family with moving from a closed system into an open system with open, honest, communication.

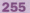

Critical Thinking Activities

Think about a structured group that you would like to co-facilitate.

1. Write a plan for co-facilitating the group.
2. Which clients would you choose to be part of the group? What is your rationale for the choice of clients?
3. What inexpensive, reusable props would you make to use with clients?
4. What is your most important reminder to yourself regarding this particular group?

Review Questions

Multiple Choice—Choose the best answer to each question.

1. What is meant by "here and now" issues?
   a. Issues that are here today and gone tomorrow
   b. Current issues that are causing distress
   c. Issues related to childhood trauma
   d. Issues that cause long-term confusion and disorientation
2. Which is an example of distortion in thinking that can be challenged during cognitive therapy?
   a. "Should" statements
   b. Cognitive impairment
   c. Disorientation to time, place, thing, person
   d. Interpersonal problems
3. Which phase of group therapy focuses on self-disclosure and exploration of problems?
   a. Preinteraction
   b. Engagement
   c. Working
   d. Termination
4. Which of the following is a possible benefit of a structured group for people with cognitive impairment?
   a. Deal with repressed memories
   b. Quick fix for "here and now" issues
   c. Opportunity for sense of belongingness and acceptance
   d. Deal with family dysfunctions
5. Which therapy involves a directive, action-oriented therapist?
   a. Psychodynamic therapy
   b. Psychoanalytic therapy
   c. Family therapy
   d. CT and CBT

References

Carson VB, Arnold EN: Family therapy. In: Mental Health Nursing: The Nurse-Patient Journey. Philadelphia, WB Saunders Co, 1966.

Lala CM: Communication within groups. In: Varcarolis EM (ed): Foundations of Psychiatric Mental Health Nursing, 2nd ed. Philadelphia, WB Saunders Co, 1994.

Nolen-Hoksema S: Understanding Depression: A Seminar for Health Professionals. Duluth, Minn, April, 1997.

Swartz HA, Markowitz JC: Time-limited psychotherapy. In: Tasman A, Kay J, Lieberman JA (eds): Psychiatry, vol 2. Philadelphia, WB Saunders Co, 1997.

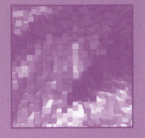

Behavior Management

Outline

- **Positive Approaches Using Behavior Principles**
    - Increasing Behavior: Positive Reinforcement
    - Increasing Behavior: Shaping
    - Reducing Behavior: Extinction
    - Reducing Behavior: Reinforcing Alternative Behavior

- **Aversive Approaches Using Behavior Principles**
    - Reducing Behavior: Time-Out
    - Reducing Behavior: Response Cost
    - Increasing Behavior: Escape

Key Terms

- behavior management
- behavior principle
- behavior procedure
- consequence
- escape
- extinction

- negative reinforcement
- positive reinforcement
- Premack Principle
- response cost
- shaping
- time-out

Objectives

Upon completing this chapter, the student will be able to:
1. Define four positive behavior management approaches.
2. Give an example for each defined behavior management approach.
3. Identify the key points in implementing positive reinforcement.
4. State a circumstance in which an aversive approach may be needed.
5. List criteria for developing and evaluating a behavior program.

Behavior management is the application of behavior principles to modify behavior (Slater, Weickgenant, and Dimsdale, 1997, p. 1506). These principles can be applied systematically to reinstate, increase, maintain, teach, or decrease the behavior of people in short- or long-term health care facilities.

The behavior principles applied in behavior management are based on the following:

- Behavior change focuses on the here and now. Developmental history, intelligence, and other factors are considered important; however, primary emphasis is on what the person is doing in his or her current environment.
- There is a search for lawful relationships in behavior, with an emphasis on identifying what factors are currently maintaining the problem behavior.
- The focus is on changing the problem behavior. Behaviors are defined in terms that are observable, measurable, and precise.

Table 25–1	Events and Consequences	
Specific Condition	**What a Person Does**
Hears a funny joke	Laughs
Feels something in his or her throat	Coughs
Eats a big meal	Secretes gastric juice
Receives a pay raise	Jumps up and down

- There is an emphasis on the person, not on groups of people. Behavior management programs are custom-fit to the unique problems of each client.
- There is an ongoing process in which behavioral objectives are progressively reanalyzed as time passes.
- Methods can be designed so that clients have input into the decision-making process, and informed consent is obtained before initiating the program. When needed, guardians or relatives can approve the approaches and goals.

One of the greatest advantages to using behavior change techniques is the results that occur. Clearly identifiable changes in behavior can be accomplished using the principles described in this chapter. Box 25–1 lists criteria for developing and evaluating a behavior program.

A **behavior procedure** is the application of behavior principles to bring about behavior change. A **behavior principle** is a rule describing the relationship between what a person does and a specific condition. Table 25–1 shows this relationship. The examples in the table—laughing, coughing, secreting gastric juices, and jumping up and down—all follow a certain behavior or event. What follows a behavior is called a **consequence**.

Behavior principles used to change behavior include both positive and negative approaches. In each case, the goal of the approach is to increase good behavior or decrease poor behavior. One major advantage of a behavioral approach is that it can be applied easily and rapidly, leading to behavior change.

BOX 25–1	Criteria for Developing and Evaluating a Behavior Program

The following criteria can be used as a checklist when developing a program and as a means to evaluate an existing program:

1. Is the behavior to be changed (target behavior) clearly specified?
2. Does the program provide for immediate reinforcement?
3. Does the program outline small steps to attain the desired behavior?
4. Does reinforcement occur frequently and in small amounts?
5. Does the program call for and reinforce accomplishment rather than obedience?
6. Is the performance of the desired behavior reinforced *after* its occurrence?
7. Is the program for modifying the behavior positive?
8. Is the program for modifying the behavior mutually negotiated, if possible?

POSITIVE APPROACHES USING BEHAVIOR PRINCIPLES

The single most important factor causing human behavior may be the consequence of that behavior. Because of their backgrounds, many people connect consequence with punishment. It is important to note that other consequences are readily available. Consequences can be good or reinforcing, bad or punishing, or neutral (things remain the same). A positive behavioral approach focuses primarily on consequences that are good or positively reinforcing. The following are everyday examples of what people will do for positive consequences:

- Work for money
- Take shelter for protection from cold weather
- Study for good grades
- Wait for a speeding car to pass to avoid being hit
- Save for retirement
- Swim to prevent drowning

Increasing Behavior: Positive Reinforcement

We learn from the effects of our behavior. If a client repeatedly experiences some pleasant effect immediately after a particular behavior, he or she tends to repeat that behavior. A client is more likely to assist the nurse with an activity if after the activity the nurse comments, "Thanks so much; I really appreciate your help." The next time the nurse begins the same activity, it is likely that the client will return to assist. This is known as the *principle of positive reinforcement*. In **positive reinforcement,** when a stimulus (object or event) follows a behavior, the strength or rate of that behavior increases or remains constant.

Effects of Positive Reinforcement

The only way to tell whether a consequence is reinforcing is to observe its effects on the behavior that follows. This is a critical point, because consequences that are reinforcing for one person may not be effective, positive reinforcers for another. Some people would walk a mile for a piece of candy; others would not take the candy if it were given to them free of charge. The nurse or therapist cannot proclaim something to be a reinforcer; it is determined by the rate of response, or its effect on the behavior that follows. A consequence is a positive reinforcer only if it maintains or increases the behavior it follows.

Reality Check

Mary has just completed making her bed, a task she rarely completes unassisted. The nurse gives her a graham cracker as a reinforcer. The next day Mary does not make her bed. The nurse then states to Mary, "If you help me make your bed, you can have a graham cracker." Still, Mary only observes.

Is the graham cracker a reward proclaimed by the nurse or a reinforcer? Explain your reasoning.

Determining Positive Reinforcers

The following techniques can be used to discover possible reinforcers for a specific client:

- Ask the client what he or she enjoys doing
- Observe what the client does in his or her leisure time
- Observe what available activities or outings a client attends
- Observe with whom the client talks
- Offer a pair of reinforcers and observe which one the client selects
- Ask the client to fill out a reinforcer survey (a list of events, activities, edibles, etc.)

Table 25–2 presents a short list of possible no-cost or low-cost positive reinforcers.

Consequences may not be the single most important factor causing behavior. Social reinforcers, as listed above, are also very important consequences that maintain behavior. Any contact with a person has an important effect on his or her behavior.

The only time a person may believe that he or she is noticed is when either doing something

Table 25–2	Positive Reinforcers	
Social	**Activity**	**Material/Edible**
Kind word	Housekeeping tasks	Magazines
Hug	Mending	Letters
Friendly smile	Collating papers	Clothes
Nod	Running errands	Hobby supplies
Wink	Setting tables	Work displayed
Pat on back	Assisting with groups	Certificates
Hand shake	Serving nourishments	Ribbons
Coffee with supervisor	Movement games	Stickers
Phone call	Reading	Cosmetics
	Hobbies	Beverages
	Window shopping	Gum/candy/cookies
	Free community events	

wrong or not doing anything at all. For example, the nurse may say:

- "Come on, eat just a spoonful. Let's eat all our food if we want to stay good and healthy."
- "Let's go now. Come on, let's not be late; let's go."
- "I've told you the last six times I responded to your call bell, don't ring the bell for every little thing. I told you I make rounds every half-hour; that's when I can answer any questions."
- "Now comb your hair. Every day I have to remind you to comb your hair; don't you want to look pretty?"

Staff are often puzzled with recurring problem behaviors such as those reflected in the statements above. What can be done to change problem behaviors? First, the target behavior—the behavior to be changed—must be identified. This is done in precise, observable, and measurable terms. Then the consequences that follow the target behavior must be identified. The above examples could be illustrated as shown in Table 25–3.

The coaxing, assisting, and answering are forms of attention or social reinforcement. Attention can be a very powerful reinforcer; therefore the attention may be maintaining the very behavior you

are attempting to eliminate. Positive reinforcement can maintain both desirable and undesirable behavior.

If positive reinforcement is maintaining an undesirable behavior, the nurse should change strategies. Because attention can be a reinforcer, observing a client performing a desirable behavior should be a cue to respond (e.g., by saying "Thanks" or "That's great"). Now attention is focused on praising accomplishment and reinforcing achievement. A quick compliment, a timely nod, or an appreciative word are small investments that may have large payoffs. Table 25–4 lists key points in using positive reinforcement effectively.

Table 25–3	Problem Behavior and Its Consequences
Problem Behavior	**Consequence**
Eating small amounts of food during meals	Coaxing/assisting
Going to an activity late	Coaxing
Frequent use of call bell	Answering call bell
Uncombed hair	Coaxing

Table 25–4	Using Positive Reinforcement Effectively
Immediacy	Positive reinforcement must immediately follow the desired behavior. The faster a reinforcer is given after the behavior, the more effective it will be. The client learns which behavior is being reinforced. The nurse who comments on how well the client eats during mealtime (while he or she is actually eating) will reinforce the client more effectively than the nurse who waits until afternoon rounds to compliment the client.
Consistency	Positive reinforcement must be delivered consistently by all staff across all shifts. The client learns which behaviors lead to reinforcement and which do not. Behaviors to be reinforced and the reinforcement procedures should be clearly specified in the client's total plan of care.
Specific Praise	In certain cases, the delivery of positive reinforcement, especially in the form of praise, should be paired with the specific reason for its delivery. For example, rather then saying, "You did a good job," the nurse could say, "You did a good job filing the charts in the correct folders." Specific praise is focused on that aspect of the behavior that deserves it. Emphasis is on the behavior, not the person, which is important. Then, when praise is withheld for an undesirable behavior, the client learns that it is his or her behavior that is unacceptable, not him or her as an individual.
Deprivation	It is important to take into account the deprivation level of the reinforcer to be used. A client who is not thirsty is unlikely to do anything to obtain a drink. Crackers that are available three times a day at nourishment time may not be effective reinforcers at other times. Deprivation—how long it has been since the reinforcer was last delivered—plays an important role in ensuring reinforcer effectiveness.
Novelty	People find experiencing new objects or events reinforcing. Birthdays with wrapped packages testify to this! Some examples of novel reinforcers are a "surprise box" containing objects or slips of paper listing different activities, and a "job jar," which varies the order of daily tasks. Satiation, or "getting filled" on large amounts of one reinforcer, is not a concern when the nurse varies reinforcers and uses novel reinforcers.
Sampling	"Try it; you'll like it." Sometimes a person is unfamiliar with an object or has not experienced an event; therefore its potential reinforcing properties are unknown. Grocery stores give out free samples with the hope that customers will like the product and will purchase it. Sampling also helps discover possible reinforcers. Displaying a new magazine, starting a new activity, or teaching part of a new game are examples of reinforcer sampling. Once the person begins to enjoy an experience, it becomes a reinforcer for him or her.

The Premack Principle

A special form of positive reinforcement is the **Premack Principle**, often referred to as "Grandma's Rule." Grandma used to say, "Eat your vegetables before you can have your dessert." What Grandma was saying is that first you must do what you don't really want to do before you may do something you like to do.

Behaviors that a client already performs often can be used as reinforcement for behaviors that seldom occur. The Premack Principle utilizes only activities as reinforcers, thus providing nurses with a practical and convenient tool for behavior change.

Some other possible examples of the Premack Principle, or Grandma's Rule, include the following:

- "Take your meds; then you may have some recreation time."
- "Wash up, then go to the game room."
- "Clean off the work table before leaving."

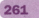

Table 25–4	Using Positive Reinforcement Effectively *Continued*
Contingencies	After the nurse identifies powerful, positive reinforcers, those same reinforcers can be utilized to bring about behavior change. "If you complete your exercise program, you can go to the lounge." "If you attend three in-house activities this week, you can go for a van ride on the weekend." These are "if . . . then" contingencies. If the client does a particular behavior, then he or she will receive reinforcement. If the client does not do the behavior, he or she will not receive the reinforcement. Reinforcement is contingent on the performance of a specific behavior.
Scheduling	When a nurse is trying to teach a client a new routine, the more often the client's behavior is reinforced, the better. The nurse may decide to teach a client to pick up after himself or herself. As part of the approach, the nurse may ask the client to put his or her dirty clothes in a hamper. Each time the client does so, the nurse may offer praise. When teaching a new behavior or reinstating a behavior, it is important to reinforce the behavior each time it occurs. This is called *continuous reinforcement*. After a behavior is fairly well-established by continuous reinforcement, the frequency of reinforcement can be reduced. Reinforcing some, but not all, responses is called an *intermittent schedule of reinforcement*. Intermittent reinforcement is most effective in maintaining behavior. Once the new routine is learned and dirty clothes are always being placed in the hamper, praise for performing this behavior can be delivered occasionally.
Tokens	There are times when it is simply not possible to deliver a reinforcer immediately. Using some tangible item can solve this problem and help bridge the delay between the behavior and the reinforcer. For example, money can "bridge the gap." It can be earned for a certain behavior, saved, then exchanged for a desired object or activity at a later time. In clinical settings, tokens can function as money. Tokens can be points, checks, slips of paper, chips, or other tangible items that can be accumulated and traded in. Token reinforcement systems are often used with people who do not respond to praise or attention. It is useful to pair praise with delivery of the token, so eventually the nurse can phase out the token and the behavior will be maintained with praise or social reinforcement alone. In health care facilities, tokens can be exchanged for a pass, a community activity, edibles, or whatever has an impact on the client's behavior.

- "Complete your assignment before break."
- "After five minutes of leg exercises, you can make your phone call."

Increasing Behavior: Shaping

As a ceramic pot must be shaped from a lump of clay, so a new behavior must be shaped from an existing behavior. **Shaping** is the procedure used to teach a complex behavior using small steps. It can aid nurses in teaching clients new behaviors that will promote independent functioning. This is done by reinforcing responses that approximate more and more the final, sought-after behavior. When a person fails to reach his or her goal, how many times has he or she given up? The reasons for these failures can, to a great extent, be attributed to attempting too large a task. Table 25–5 lists key points in using the shaping technique effectively.

Reducing Behavior: Extinction

The nurse may observe many undesirable or peculiar behaviors every day in the work setting, such as recurring physical complaints, temper tantrums, excessive office visits, nagging or begging, persistent questioning, peculiar talk, unusual gestures, and junk collecting. The nurse may be perplexed by such behaviors; these behaviors are often considered unaccountable. Are these behav-

Table 25–5	Using Shaping Effectively

Start at the client's current level of behavior	The nurse must work with the client at the client's level and shape his or her behavior from that point.
Break the complex behavior into small steps	By breaking the complex behavior into small steps, each succeeding step gets closer to the final behavioral goal; an example of breaking a complex behavior, such as washing, into small steps follows: • Pick up soap • Pick up washcloth • Soap washcloth • Wash face and neck • Wash stomach and chest • Wash arms • Wash thighs and genitals • Wash lower legs • Wash feet • Rinse • Dry
Reinforce successful completion of each step	Failure to complete a step suggests the need for smaller steps and more repetitive practice; reinforcement techniques should reinforce all previous steps
Prompting (once the behavior is learned, it is important to gradually phase out or remove the prompts so that constant reminders and suggestions are no long required)	Rather than waiting long lengths of time for a client to begin the next step in the shaping procedure, the nurse should prompt that step. There are at least three varieties of prompts. The use of prompts should progress from the least intrusive (verbal prompt) to the modeling prompt and, if required, to the physical guidance prompts (most intrusive). The following are examples of these three prompts: • Verbal prompt: "Pick up your spoon" • Modeling or demonstrating prompt: "Watch as I pick up my spoon; then pick up yours in exactly the same way" • Physical guidance prompt: The nurse places his or her hand on top of the client's hand and together they pick up the spoon (a physical guidance prompt is often combined with a verbal prompt)
Reaching the goal is not enough	It is crucial to strengthen the newly acquired behavior with positive reinforcement; once the behavior is firmly established, an approach can then be developed to maintain that behavior

iors unaccountable, or could they possibly be maintained by some form of consequence?

Situations arise in which a person would like to give a little extra attention or a small gift to make up for or get rid of an unpleasant behavior (e.g., pick up a child to silence a temper tantrum, dismiss a rowdy group, give a quarter to a person who lost his money). However, the attention of picking up the child may actually be a positive reinforcer for the temper tantrum behavior and may increase the probability of additional temper tantrums. Likewise, dismissing a rowdy group may be a strong reinforcer for some members of the group. In the same way, replacing the lost quarter could actually be reinforcing "careless" behavior. Consider another situation in which two people are arguing and one runs and tattles. The consequence is attention for the tattler. Throughout this chapter, attention has been touted as a very powerful positive reinforcer for some people. However, *a caregiver may accidentally reinforce the very behavior he or she would like to eliminate*. What can be done to change these problem behaviors?

Once the problem behavior has been identified, the consequences that follow that behavior must be identified. If attention is identified as the consequence, then attention must be discontinued for that particular behavior. **Extinction** is the discontinuation or withdrawal of positive reinforcement for a specific behavior. For example, Mrs. Jones is incontinent three or four times a day. When her incontinence is discovered, the nurse talks with her as she cleans her up and changes her clothing. The nurse talks with Mrs. Jones more when she is incontinent than when she is continent; therefore the attention (conversation with the nurse) could be the reinforcing consequence maintaining the incontinence. "Ignore the bad behavior" is easier said than done. Many techniques can be used in ignoring a behavior (using an extinction procedure), and if these techniques are not used carefully, the behavior may actually get worse. Table 25–6 lists key points in using the extinction technique effectively.

Extinction can be an effective method for reducing many undesirable behaviors; however, it is a procedure to use only when behaviors will not lead to physical harm or danger. When withholding reinforcement for an undesirable behavior is not possible, an alternative reduction technique should be used.

Reducing Behavior: Reinforcing Alternative Behavior

A client frequently stands at the nursing station when nurses are busy charting. If the client were attending the three o'clock activity available in the dayroom, he would not have the opportunity to stand at the nurse's station. Activity attendance thus conflicts with the client's standing at the station.

Another client spends the day isolated in her room. Having the client assist with setting up nourishments and running errands reinforces behaviors that are incompatible with social isolation. Encouraging those behaviors should decrease the amount of time the client spends alone.

A person cannot walk around with both hands over his or her ears and hold a portable radio at the same time, nor can a person lie on the floor and sit in a chair simultaneously. Reinforcing alternative behaviors and incompatible alternative behaviors are positive approaches to decrease problem behaviors. The nurse should use positive reinforcement for appropriate behavior, combined with extinction for inappropriate behavior.

AVERSIVE APPROACHES USING BEHAVIOR PRINCIPLES

Up to this point, the behavior principles introduced have been based on positive approaches to either increase or decrease behavior. The final three behavior principles are aversive or punitive approaches. There are two circumstances in which aversive approaches may be required because the effects of positive reinforcement procedures would likely be slower. These circumstances are:

- If the person exhibits overt, self-injurious behavior, or he or she is a danger to others, aversive approaches may be required
- If the person's behavior is so frequent (e.g., head banging) that there is little or no incompatible behavior to reinforce, aversive approaches may be required

Alternative positive procedures should always be considered before implementing procedures that involve the use of aversive stimuli. Legal, moral, and ethical issues must be considered, particularly as they relate to informed consent, institutional review, and continual program supervision. Aversive procedures should be reserved for serious maladaptive behaviors. Positive approaches have

Table 25–6	Using Extinction Effectively
Identify the positive reinforcers	Look at a situation from an objective, analytical standpoint (i.e., do not make judgments, do not question a person's intentions, do not blame anyone). Simply observe and record the specific consequences that follow a problem behavior. Once the reinforcing consequences have been identified, a behavior program can be developed. *Example:* After a thorough medical examination ruled out organic causes for Robert's persistent eye complaints, the nurse decided to use an extinction procedure. All complaints of sore eyes were ignored, although nurses were always on the alert for any possible changes in his eyes. Robert then sought out a peer who reassured him that his eyes were all right. From an objective standpoint, the attention Robert received from his peer was the reinforcer maintaining his complaining behavior.
Identify the specific conditions of extinction	State specifically when to ignore what behavior. For example, rather than "Ignore Robert when he complains," state "Each time Robert complains about sore eyes, the staff are to ignore this behavior (make no verbal comment or gesture)."
Communicate the procedure	Make certain that all staff are familiar with the procedure. It is also wise to include the clients who associate with Robert so they can ignore his eye complaints as well. Never assume that someone knows what technique is being used or what changes have been made in a program.
Ride the crest of the wave	Eliminating a behavior takes time; therefore the nurse must maintain the extinction procedure for a sufficient length of time before evaluating the results. It takes a lot of stamina to ignore a bothersome behavior and to decide not to give in. Once the nurse no longer allows the client to have his way, the nurse can look for a temporary increase in the behavior before it begins to decrease. When this happens, the nurse should remember the long-term payoff, and the effort will seem worthwhile.
Combine extinction with positive reinforcement	When ignoring one problem behavior, the nurse must ensure that all other appropriate behaviors receive abundant positive reinforcement. For example, in using an extinction procedure to decrease delusional talk, delusional talk is ignored and all neutral, appropriate talk is reinforced with attention. Under these conditions, delusional talk may drop to a very low level and appropriate talk may increase. It must be determined before initiating an extinction procedure whether sufficient reinforcement is available to a client for his or her appropriate behaviors. A well-structured daily environment filled with ample opportunity to receive reinforcement goes a long way in decreasing inappropriate, attention-seeking behaviors.

long-lasting results, have few side effects, and can be generalized to other appropriate behaviors.

Reducing Behavior: Time-Out

Time-out simply refers to time out from positive reinforcement. Either the person is removed from the reinforcing environment or the reinforcing environment is removed from the person for a certain length of time. These two forms of time-out are illustrated in Table 25–7.

In the first situation listed in the table, the dayroom is the reinforcer; in the second situation, the nurse is the reinforcer. As noted before, *time-out* means time out from positive reinforcement. Therefore it is important to identify all positive reinforcers accurately before initiating this procedure. Because time-out serves as an aversive approach, it is important to consider more positive approaches or reductive procedures before using time-out. Once it has been decided to use time-out, all staff should be trained in specific techniques for using the procedure accurately and effectively.

Reducing Behavior: Response Cost

Response cost is an aversive technique for reducing undesirable behavior by withdrawing specific positive reinforcers. Although response cost is minimally intrusive, it still remains an aversive procedure and, as such, it may generate escape or aggressive behavior. As with other aversive procedures, ethical and legal issues must be considered.

Table 25–7	Behaviors and Time-Out Consequences
Behavior	**Consequence**
Yelling in dayroom	Removal of client from dayroom for 15 minutes
Yelling in dayroom	Nurse leaves dayroom and client is left in a nonreinforcing environment

Table 25–8	Behavior and Consequences in Response Cost
Behavior	**Consequence**
Speeding	$80 fine
Late for work	Loss in salary
Fighting	Loss of phone privileges
Refusing to bathe	Loss of extra afternoon snack

Response cost may be used to reduce undesirable behavior temporarily while alternative behaviors are being strengthened. When combined with positive reinforcement for desirable behaviors, response cost can lead to dramatic results. Table 25–8 provides examples of response cost.

Increasing Behavior: Escape

The dialogue that follows demonstrates escape behavior. Note the nurse's response to the client's repeated requests.

Client: "Is it time for my bath?"
Nurse: "No. Your bath is scheduled in a half hour."
Client: "Can't I take my bath now? Can't I just start my bath?"
Nurse: "Oh, OK, I'll run your water early just this once."

Running the bath water helped the nurse escape from aversive nagging. The behavior of "giving in" has been strengthened because it turned off something aversive—the nagging. Escape behavior and avoidance together comprise what is called **negative reinforcement. Escape** behavior is the withdrawal from undesirable behavior in an attempt to end the behavior (Mertens, O'Brien, Lamberg, and Larsen, 1982, p. 144).

Escape behaviors are an everyday occurrence (e.g., moving away from a hot fire, turning off a loud alarm clock, coming in out of the cold, taking a verbal response "back," hallucinating if a problem cannot be handled, or responding to persistent questions). There is one "catch." With the principle of escape, escaping from something aversive may actually reinforce undesirable behavior. In the previous nurse/client scenario, the nurse has escaped from the nagging. However, in doing so, the nurse has actually reinforced (by giving in) the very behavior that was bothersome. The nurse has temporarily escaped from the aversive behavior; however, the client has learned, "If I keep nagging long enough, I can get my way." Eliminating problem behaviors maintained by negative reinforcement can be accomplished by combining extinction with reinforcement for alternative behaviors.

Reality Check

Ed, a 16-year-old who just received his driver's license, wanted to use the family car to take his friends for a ride. His mother said, "No." It was getting dark. Ed kept begging his mother for the car keys. He would not let up on his constant haranguing. Finally, in desperation, the mother gave Ed the keys.

1. What behavior approach did Ed's mother use?
2. What effect might the mother's approach have on Ed's continuing behavior?
3. What alternative approach could Ed's mother have used?

SUMMARY

Behavior management is the application of behavior principles to modify behavior. It focuses on the unique problems of the person in the here and now. Positive approaches using behavior principles include positive reinforcement, shaping, extinction, and reinforcing alternative behavior. Aversive approaches using behavior principles are time-out, response cost, and escape. In developing a behavior program, it is important to define clearly the behavior to be changed and the provisions for immediate positive reinforcement.

Critical Thinking Activities

1. Target a behavior that you would like to change. Keep track of the number of times the behavior occurs in a day and in a week. For example, you might keep track of eating between meals. Note what you are doing before you have the urge to eat. Then note what happens after you eat and the consequences of your eating (Woolsey and Arnold, 1996, p. 440).
2. Plan a behavioral program to teach a child a new skill using the positive approach of shaping.

Review Questions

Multiple Choice—Choose the best answer to each question.

1. A positive approach using behavior principles is
   a. reducing behavior: time-out.
   b. reducing behavior: extinction.
   c. reducing behavior: response cost.
   d. increasing behavior: escape.
2. A procedure used to teach a complex behavior by using small steps is
   a. sampling.
   b. satiation.
   c. prompting.
   d. shaping.
3. Staff encourage problem behaviors to continue by
   a. ignoring the problem behavior.
   b. focusing on the problem behavior.
   c. offering an alternative behavior.
   d. praising desirable behavior.
4. A key point in implementing positive reinforcement is
   a. immediacy.
   b. prompting.
   c. shaping.
   d. reward.
5. Aversive procedures are
   a. frequently used for undesirable behaviors.
   b. an effective means of decreasing undesirable behavior.

c. only for serious maladaptive behaviors.
d. free of legal, moral, and ethical issues.

References

Mertens G, O'Brien S, Lamberg P, Larsen S: Workbook for Behavioral Science Behaviorally Taught: A Personalized Text for Learning About A Science of Behavior. Lexington, Mass, Ginn Custom, 1982.

Slater MA, Weickgenant AL, Dimsdale JE: Behavioral medicine. In: Tasman A, Kay J, Lieberman JA (eds): *Psychiatry,* Vol. 2, Chapter 78. Philadelphia, WB Saunders Co., 1997.

Woolsey SF, Arnold EN: Behavioral Therapy. In Carson VB, Arnold EN (eds): Mental Health Nursing: The Nurse-Patient Journey. Philadelphia, WB Saunders Co, 1996.

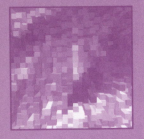

Relationship Between Physiological and Psychological Needs

Outline

- **Physical Care**
- **Nutrition**

- **Activities**
  Recreation
  Work Therapy

Key Terms

- **diversional activities**
- **leisure counseling**

- **recreation**
- **therapeutic activities**

Objectives

Upon completing this chapter, the student will be able to:

1. Explain the physical care required for clients with certain psychiatric disorders.
2. Describe the relation of nutrition to mental health.
3. Differentiate between diversional activities and therapeutic activities.
4. Identify factors to be considered in planning activities for a client.
5. Identify five basic goals of recreation as a therapeutic activity.
6. Explain the purpose of work therapy.

This chapter focuses on the many psychological needs that are met through physical care and activities for people with certain psychiatric disorders. The tables throughout the chapter provide suggestions on how these needs might be met. The challenge for nurses is to individualize these suggestions so that the unique goals of their client might be achieved.

PHYSICAL CARE

The client's physical care is threefold: (1) maintain reasonable health, (2) maintain physical safety, and (3) maintain social acceptability. The nurse's function varies depending on the client's mental and physical condition. At different times, it includes providing complete care, teaching the client how to do self care and, finally, occasionally reminding the client about the need for physical care. The data collection on the client at admission must include status of the client's nutrition, elimination, sleep and rest, grooming, and special problems.

The nurse's attitude in assisting or teaching the client about physical care sets the stage for client compliance. The client, no matter how psychotic, quickly senses whether the nurse is a respectful advocate who will assist with care until the client is able to care for himself or herself again. Table 26–1 emphasizes significant aspects of physical care for people with certain psychiatric disorders.

NUTRITION

Nutrition is an essential factor in the care of clients with a mental illness. They often have inadequate diets, eating too much or too little and not receiving the proper nutrients (Walsh and Carson, 1996, p. 496). Nurses need to understand some basic facts about nutrients and, more specifically, about the relationship between nutrition and emotional stress. There are six basic classifications of nutrients, each with its own function within the body. Table 26–2 identifies each nutrient and explains briefly the nutrient's function.

It is known that these nutrients affect not only physical health, but intellectual functioning as well. For example, several nutrients are highly involved in the functioning of the central nervous system (CNS). Severe protein deficiency during pregnancy can lead to mental retardation in the infant. Cretinism, characterized by severe mental retardation, is known to be related to severe iodine deficiency during pregnancy. Nutritional deficiencies during infancy and early childhood are related to learning disabilities. Although these relationships are clear-cut and based on scientific study, the relationship between nutritional deficiency and mental illness is not well-defined. It is generally accepted that well-nourished people are better able to cope with stress than those who are poorly nourished. Whether this applies to all forms of stress is unknown at this time. Some of the symptoms of nutritional deficiency are similar to symptoms of mental illness. Table 26–3 lists some related conditions.

This is not to imply that nutritional deficiencies cause mental illness. The Recommended Dietary Allowance (RDA) levels of nutrients are at this time considered to adequately meet the daily requirements. RDA continues to be the basis for determining a balanced diet for the client. However, the nurse must remember that the client's nutritional state and eating habits must be reviewed at the time of admission and attended to with the help of the dietary department. Eating habits leading to overnutrition or undernutrition may have changed for a number of reasons. Table 26–4 indicates briefly some of these changes and possible nutritional interventions.

ACTIVITIES

Activities are a significant part of the growth process. They provide a link between one's inner self and the external world. Activities help develop social skills and provide an outlet for self-expression. Emotional problems can inhibit or block this outlet for people with mental illness. There are two basic types of activities. **Diversional activities** are used to entertain or divert one's thoughts from stresses of life or to fill time. **Therapeutic activities** are used to attain a specific care plan goal or objective.

Table 26–1	Problems in Physical Care for Clients With Certain Psychiatric Disorders

Physical Care	Cognitive Disorder, Dementia
Nutrition	Sometimes client forgets that he or she has eaten. In late stages there is significant weight loss even with a good diet; client has to be fed.
Elimination	As illness progresses there is loss of bladder control; needs a specific schedule for bathroom care.
Sleep and rest	Client is confused and restless, with sleepiness and wandering.
Grooming	Needs assistance with all aspects of physical care.
Special problems	Safety is a concern of a client with a cognitive disorder; an identification bracelet should be worn.

Physical Care	Depressive Mood Disorder
Nutrition	May not eat or drink because of lack of appetite; feels undeserving or has somatic delusions regarding physical problems that he or she thinks make eating impossible. Sit with client; encourage and/or feed at first; needs small meals with dietary supplements and fluids.
Elimination	May forget to void; check for distended bladder. Take to bathroom regularly; remind to void. Check for constipation; monitor toileting. Increase water, juices, fruit, and activity.
Sleep and rest	Disturbed, unsatisfying sleep; may sleep too little or too much. Provide for a short nap daily but discourage long periods of bed rest during the day. A back rub at bedtime is relaxing and provides touch as well.
Grooming	Neglects appearance. Needs help with bathing, shampooing, setting hair, shaving, oral hygiene, nail care, foot care. Skin may be in poor condition because of poor food and liquid intake.
Special problems	Dehydration is always a concern with severe depression. Check for poor skin turgor, dry skin, scanty urine, thickened secretions. Check results of blood work and urinalysis. Immediate medical intervention may be needed.

Physical Care	Bipolar Mood Disorder
Nutrition	Too busy to eat or drink. May throw food. As likely to starve as a client who is depressed. Seat away from others. Serve finger foods that can be eaten on the run. Offer high-calorie liquids initially.
Elimination	Monitor elimination; may be too "busy" to toilet self.
Sleep and rest	Lack of sleep is a serious problem. Needs extra rest periods, soothing warm baths, quiet music, nonstimulating colors. Sit with client in a calming environment to promote rest.
Grooming	Needs a great deal of help. Too busy to groom self. Perspires profusely because of frantic activity. May experience skin breakdown. Frequently has minor cuts and bruises. Tends to "decorate" self. Uses too much make-up. Needs suggestions on more acceptable hygienic practices and clothing.
Special problems	Needs to be checked and monitored physically when acutely ill; blood work, urinalysis, vital signs, intake, and output need to be monitored.

Table 26–1	Problems in Physical Care for Clients With Certain Psychiatric Disorders *Continued*

Physical Care	**Schizophrenia Disorder, Catatonic Type**
Nutrition	May not eat or drink because of lack of interest. Severe regression may result in inability to eat or fear of eating. May need to be fed initially. Offer small amounts of fluids frequently between meals.
Elimination	May retain feces and urine. Needs regular reminding and monitoring.
Sleep and rest	Frequently disturbed; has difficulty sleeping or staying awake. Evaluate reason individually. For example, going to bed during the day may be a form of withdrawal that needs to be interrupted to support reality.
Grooming	Frequently will not initiate personal care. Responds to step-by-step directions on doing care. Check skin carefully since client may be unaware of injuries when very withdrawn. Difficulty making clothing choices; offer choice of two items.
Special problems	Lack of personal care may result in physical problems. Follow through on checking out abnormal physical signs. Decreased perception of pain stimuli, such as hot and cold, may lead to injuries. Needs additional supervision in bathing.

Physical Care	**Schizophrenia Disorder, Paranoid Type**
Nutrition	May not eat for fear of being poisoned. Let client prepare his or her own meal or serve food in closed containers. Allow client to taste food with utensil of choice, if requested.
Elimination	Usually not a problem unless related to lack of food and fluids related to delusions.
Sleep and rest	Disturbed because of fear of going to sleep or fear of sleeping in room with others. Have client sleep alone; if this does not work, consider hallway (check hospital rules before implementing). As one client remarked, "No one will dare hurt me with so many people around!"
Grooming	Usually not a problem. May be suspicious of nurse's attempt to help. Offer, but do not encourage vigorously. Will be more receptive when delusional pattern begins to subside.
Special problems	Tends to identify himself or herself as a staff person rather than as a client. Therefore implementing any physical care is a challenge.

Physical Care	**Anxiety Disorder**
Nutrition	Vomiting, fear of dishes or food, and lengthy rituals may prevent adequate intake of food and fluids. Advance reminder of mealtime will provide time to complete lengthy rituals.
Elimination	Check daily weight, intake, and output on client who is vomiting. Poor nutritional intake may affect elimination; monitor initially.
Sleep and rest	High anxiety, extensive rituals, somatic concerns may prevent adequate sleep and rest. Client needs advance reminder to complete rituals before bedtime. Use relaxation exercise at bedtime.
Grooming	May require total physical care and reminders at times. Paralysis may interfere with ability to do care. Frequently diaphoretic; check for skin breakdown.
Special problems	Rule out real physical problem without feeding the pathology. Check out physical problems when client is not complaining.

Table 26–2	Nutrients and Their Functions

Nutrient	Functions
Carbohydrates	Provide heat and energy; protect protein and assist in fat metabolism
Proteins	Build and repair tissue; assist body in resisting diseases; provide heat and energy; contribute to body secretions and fluids
Fats	Concentrated source of heat and energy; carry fat-soluble vitamins A, D, E, and K; aid in normal tissue functioning; provide feelings of satiety in the diet; reserve fuel supply; maintain body temperature by insulating; hold organs in place and prevent injury
Vitamins	Promote growth; aid in producing healthy tissue; resist infections; aid in vital body processes
Minerals	Necessary part of all cells and body fluids; form structural framework of body as part of bones and teeth; assist in acid-base balance and osmotic pressure; regulate metabolism of enzymes; assist in nerve impulse transmission
Water	Solvent that aids in softening and liquefying foods; regulates body temperature; transports nutrients and body secretions throughout the body; excretory agent adds bulk to intestinal tract; lubricant—moves parts of body surrounded with water to prevent friction and wear

Data from Williams SR: Basic Nutrition and Diet Therapy, 10th ed. Part I. St. Louis, Mosby, 1995, pp 26, 37, 49, 76, 113, 145.

In planning for therapeutic activities, the nurse collects data on the client's emotional and physical needs and his or her strengths and weaknesses. Knowledge of strengths, including old interests and successes, can be used to help the client cope with the present situation. Some considerations in planning activities include the following:

- The client should be involved, as much as possible, in selecting the activity
- The activity should utilize the client's strengths and abilities
- The activity should be of short duration to foster a feeling of accomplishment
- If possible, the selected activity should provide some new experiences for the client

Recreation

Recreation is a planned therapeutic activity that enables people with limitations to engage in recreational experiences. Some basic goals include the following:

Table 26–3	Symptoms of Nutritional Deficiency That Are Similar to Symptoms of Mental Illness

Nutrient	Symptoms of Deficiency
Vitamin B_1 (thiamin)	Depression, fatigue, nervous instability, Korsakoff's psychosis
Vitamin B_3 (niacin)	Depressive psychosis
Vitamin B_6 (pyridoxine)	Possible depression
Vitamin B_{12} (cobalamin)	Various psychiatric disorders
Folacin (folic acid)	Various psychiatric disorders
Pantothenic acid	Fatigue
Biotin (once known as vitamin H)	Rare, but increases depression, insomnia

Data from Peckenpaugh NJ, Poleman CM: Nutrition Essentials and Diet Therapy, 7th ed. Philadelphia, WB Saunders Co, 1995, pp 100–102.

Table 26–4	Some Potential Nutritional Problems With Certain Psychiatric Disorders and Nutritional Interventions	

Psychiatric Disorders	Potential Problem	Nutritional Intervention
Substance-related disorder (alcohol dependence)	Avitaminosis: May be malnourished (even though weight may not show it)	Additional vitamin B_6, B_{12}, thiamin, folic acid, niacin initially ordered by physician; may benefit from class on nutrition and alcohol consumption
	May experience dehydration because of the diuretic effect of alcohol	Needs additional liquids (fruit juice is especially good); responds to eating with peers after detoxification is complete
Anxiety disorder	May overeat or undereat or may have developed rigid eating pattern; faces problem of overnutrition or under-nutrition	Limit calories, or, if undereating, offer one food with one utensil at a time if client is having difficulty deciding what to eat
		Sit with client; may need food supplements initially and frequent, small meals throughout day
Depressive Mood Disorder	May overeat initially or undereat when severely depressed because he or she feels undeserving or because of somatic delusions of not being able to eat or of being very ill	Sit with client. Small servings do not seem as overwhelming. May use paper plates and plastic utensils initially; take utensils away when finished. May need to feed client initially or add food supplement until regular eating resumes.
	Faces problem of undernutrition and dehydration	
Bipolar mood disorder (manic episode)	Lack of time to eat or drink; faces problem of undernutrition and dehydration	Isolate client from others; sit with client if unable to sit still; walk with him or her
		Offer finger foods and sips of fluid frequently throughout the day

Table continued on following page

- Provide a nonthreatening and nondemanding environment
- Provide activities that are relaxing and without rigid guidelines and time frames
- Provide activities that will be enjoyable and self-satisfying
- Encourage social interaction and help decrease fear of contacting other people
- Decrease withdrawal tendencies
- Provide outlets for excess energy, physical tension, and negative feelings
- Promote socially acceptable behavior
- Develop skills, talents, and abilities so that the client can assume responsibility for his or her own recreation; these techniques become alternative ways of dealing with problems that were thought insoluble
- Increase self-confidence and feeling of self-worth
- Revitalize physical strength and mental awareness
- Provide for continuity of recreational activities so that clients may continue them in the community after discharge
- Provide a reality focus that is productive and constructive

Table 26–4	Some Potential Nutritional Problems With Certain Psychiatric Disorders and Nutritional Interventions *Continued*	
Psychiatric Disorders	**Potential Problem**	**Nutritional Intervention**
Schizophrenia disorder (paranoid type)	Concern that food may be poisoned; faces problem of undernutrition and dehydration	Provide choices of foods; allow client to serve self; use closed containers or taste food if requested by client
Schizophrenia disorder (catatonic type)	May experience delusions regarding food or lack interest in eating; check for dehydration and weight loss	May initially do better eating by self
Direct or fill one spoonful at a time if needed; may need planned dietary supplements and snacks until eating normally
Cognitive disorder (dementia)	May be confused or forgetful; faces problem of undernutrition and dehydration	Sit with client; offer direction; feed if necessary; use small spoonfuls; offer liquids in-between meals
Allow adequate chewing time; decreased saliva because of medication may hamper chewing and swallowing
Mental retardation and emotional disturbance	Depending on level of functioning, may stuff mouth with food; risk of choking; overeating may lead to vomiting
Steals food from other clients' plates	May have to offer one food with one utensil at a time
Teach client to place one hand on the lap while eating with the other
Sit with client; offer positive verbal reinforcement
Add one food at a time until client can deal with whole meal (this is a slow process; program must be followed faithfully to succeed)

Reality Check

Daryl, a 17-year-old, has a depressive mood disorder. He has been admitted to your unit, and you have been asked to help prepare a plan for his activity needs. What activities might you suggest? Why?

Leisure counseling involves classes on the effective use of leisure time. It focuses on recreational activities that can be performed throughout the life span. Examples include golf, swimming, running, jogging, and playing chess. Examples of activities not included are basketball and football.

These activities are performed during a limited period of life and require other people's involvement. Leisure activities are designed to help meet the client's maximum potential and functioning during leisure time. Recreational activities can be relaxing, enjoyable, and self-satisfying. By providing constructive outlets, the nurse can help revitalize a client's mental awareness.

Work Therapy

One of the basic needs a person has is to feel needed and worthwhile. One way of fulfilling this need is through work. Work provides structure, tasks, and goals. It gives the person a sense of being a contributing member of society. In addition, a by-product of work is earned income. Money provides people with an access to power, achievement, success, safety, and public recognition. The unemployed tend to lose their motivation to solve their problems. They may appear to have lost their skill and confidence in coping with reality.

Some psychiatric facilities have prevocational and sheltered work activities that prepare the client to work in the community. Work activities that are meaningful to the client need to be stressed. Clients are often placed in work programs because staff decide that the program will help them. Placing the client in a work program that is meaningless expends needless time and energy for both client and staff. The key is to find an environment in which the client will be motivated to work.

Employment

Staff frequently ask if it is worth the time and effort to involve clients in a rehabilitation program if employers will not hire them. Those familiar with vocational rehabilitation realize it is every rehabilitation facility's goal to place clients in the optimum working environment. Should the optimum working environment be competitive employment, then this becomes the goal. The idea is to secure a job that is meaningful to the client.

Clients are affected by long periods of inactivity. This allows them time to dwell on concerns of returning to work. The decision to return the client to a vocational setting is the result of a team decision that includes the client. The following questions are helpful in making this decision:

- Can the client handle the stress of a work setting caused by factors such as interactions with co-workers, working a specified number of hours, and following simple instructions? Clients who hear voices can learn to ignore the voices and continue to perform the work task.
- Has the client displayed appropriate judgment with regard to personal safety and medications?
- Has the client displayed appropriate grooming and hygiene?

Once these questions have been answered satisfactorily, the next step is to determine the client's replacement into the vocational setting. Movement into the vocational setting should be gradual to reduce the shock of transition from inactivity to work. To facilitate this, staff should know what the employer can offer regarding work positions, time expectations, and production standards.

Volunteer Work

Another possible avenue to pursue with the client is to seek out volunteer work. Volunteer work should not be minimized just because the client is not earning income. The activity in itself is important.

Volunteer work provides two opportunities for the client. First, meaningful volunteer work can be used as a stepping stone to competitive work. It provides all the components of competitive work, but with less stress. Often the work hours and days are more flexible, and the client can gradually regain self-confidence. The second benefit of volunteer work is perhaps more applicable to the client with serious mental illness who may never work. This meaningful experience can be beneficial because it provides an active way of stimulating the client. A question that often arises is whether the employer should be told that the client has had mental illness. The American with Disabilities Act (ADA) under Title I "makes it unlawful to discriminate against a qualified person with a disability in any aspect of employment" (Zuckerman, Debenham, and Moore, 1993, p. 16). It is recommended that the client explain to the employer that for a period of time he or she was experiencing difficulty but has been working to get his or her life in order. The client may go on to discuss job skills and accomplishments. Frequently the client's job performance is very good; it is the loneliness after work that tends to pull the client down. The client needs to get involved in activities outside of work, such as church groups, mental health support groups, YMCA, or bowling leagues. Table 26–5 suggests activities, recreation, and work for clients with certain psychiatric disorders. The material presented in this table and the tables

Text continued on page 280

Table 26–5 Suggested Activities, Recreation, and Work for Clients With Certain Psychiatric Disorders

Psychiatric Disorders	Activities	Recreation	Work
Anxiety disorder	Simple concrete task or simple game; painting, gardening, any activity that will get person outside himself or herself	Walking (allow client to pace); body contact sports (for aggressive urges; safety needs to be considered); jogging; active, physical, aerobic activity	Simple tasks with no more than three to four steps that can be learned quickly (e.g., kitchen tasks such as clearing and washing tables, sweeping or mopping floors, or outdoor work such as mowing lawn and weeding flowers; the client's expression of boredom may signal his or her readiness for more complex tasks
Depressive mood disorder	Simple tasks that can be finished, such as pouring a ceramic mold (client needs to experience success); activities of daily living (use simple but structured schedule)	Noncompetitive sports (provide outlets for anger, use up energy); jogging, running or walking briskly; achievement and success-oriented activities such as crafts, hobbies, service to others	Tasks that are helpful, such as folding laundry, cleaning ashtrays, emptying wastebaskets (client feels more worthy when a needed job is done); challenge client to complete one more task within a specific period of time; offer positive reinforcement after each achievement
Bipolar mood disorder (manic episode)	Noncompetitive activities that allow the use of energy and expression of feelings (e.g., tearing rags, writing and drawing, pounding on a leather belt); such activities should be *limited* and *changed frequently*; things that are simple and quickly done; activities of daily living (e.g., personal grooming)	Ball; badminton on one-to-one basis (for short periods of time); individual games that are physical and active	Housekeeping tasks, raking grass (large sweeping movements are good); it is helpful to have client work in an area away from distractions such as people walking through; use work goals interchangeably with the amount of money earned (e.g., the more the client accomplishes, the more money he or she earns)

Table 26–5	Suggested Activities, Recreation, and Work for Clients With Certain Psychiatric Disorders *Continued*		
Psychiatric Disorders	**Activities**	**Recreation**	**Work**
Schizophrenia disorder (paranoid type)	Noncompetitive, solitary, meaningful tasks that require some degree of concentration, such as jigsaw puzzles, crossword puzzles, Scrabble, leather tooling, and ceramics; through concentration, less time is available to focus on delusions; when client feels less threatened, bridge and chess are activities requiring more concentration	Avoid competitive, aggressive activities that involve close contact; provide outlets for anger, aggressive drives; client will experience success in groups when trust is established	Solitary occupations (e.g., interior decorating); client needs to organize and receive positive feedback; a task that requires concentration is desirable; after skill and confidence are gained, have client work with another client as a task trainer; develop a buddy system
Schizophrenia disorder (catatonic type)	Simple, concrete tasks in which client is actively involved, such as metal work and modeling clay (uses touch; gives client a chance to be creative); social activities to give client contact with others and reality; activity of daily living skills	Dancing; noncompetitive athletics; outings (e.g., picnics); hobby discussion groups	Simple work goals in 15- to 30-minute blocks of time; at the end of each block of time, praise for goals achieved and encourage appropriately; if client is hearing voices or otherwise losing touch with reality, interrupt process and reinforce reality; client needs continuous supervision and at first works best on a one-to-one basis
Childhood or adolescent disorder	*Child:* Play that is fun and recreational, such as storytelling, painting, poetry, or music *Adolescent:* Creative activities, such as leather work, painting	*Child:* Better to work with child on a one-to-one basis; give child a feeling of importance—put him or her in a role of leadership and assistance; establish a positive relationship with child	If old enough to work, the adolescent does best as an assistant to an adult worker; reinforce him or her no matter how small the achievement is; work suggestions include auto repair, kitchen work, making beds

Table continued on following page

Table 26–5   Suggested Activities, Recreation, and Work for Clients With Certain Psychiatric Disorders *Continued*

Psychiatric Disorders	Activities	Recreation	Work
Childhood or adolescent disorder–cont'd		*Adolescent:* Does better in groups; use gross motor activity to use up excess energy (e.g., sports, games)	
Antisocial personality disorder	Activities that enhance self-esteem and are expressive and creative but not too complicated; for example: making posters for a dance (this client tends to offer to do numerous tasks without following through; client needs supervision to make sure each task is completed)	Cooking, jogging, service groups, and projects for others	Initially place client away from other clients if seen as a source of distraction or friction; praise work that is well done, have client redo poor work, supervise closely to be sure tasks are completed; have client start with simple, boring tasks and progress to more difficult and interesting tasks; if acting out occurs, have client work on boring task; as behavior improves, again place him or her on more difficult, interesting task as reward for desired behavior
Cognitive disorder (dementia)	Group activities to increase feelings of belonging and self-worth; promote familiar, individual hobbies; activities need to be structured, requiring little time for completion and not much concentration; reality orientation as to time, place and, if necessary, person; reminiscent or life review activities	Concrete, repetitious crafts and projects that breed familiarization and comfort	Choose a task that builds on itself after a period of time; during the first part of the task, explain and demonstrate how the procedure should be done; then have client repeat the demonstration; this step may have to be repeated daily for several days, depending on the client; some clients will have to continue with the basic task indefinitely

Table 26–5	Suggested Activities, Recreation, and Work for Clients With Certain Psychiatric Disorders *Continued*		
Psychiatric Disorders	**Activities**	**Recreation**	**Work**
Substance-related disorder (alcohol dependence)	Group activities in which client uses his or her talents (e.g., involve client in planning social activities, encourage interaction with others)	Leisure counseling (*i.e.,* planned recreation for free time); leisure value clarification; introduction to and participation in recreational activities as an alternative to substance abuse; encourage responsibility for recreational activities	Insist that client complete work assignments; place on simple but meaningful work projects; a buddy system with another client who is displaying good work behaviors is effective; work behaviors gradually change and friendships are developed; any area of work can be appropriate; how the work is presented to the client is more significant than what the work actually is
Mental retardation and emotional disturbance	Simple activities at level of person's functioning; break activities into small steps with positive reinforcement after accomplishing each step; this is helpful in teaching self-help skills such as eating, dressing, brushing teeth; use adult pictures for coloring activity with adults	Recreational activities must be adapted to the client's level of functioning, such as walking, dancing, swimming, ball playing	Repetitive work assignments are ideal because these clients do not get bored; this type of work assignment is available in sheltered workshops (e.g., subcontracting work such as capsuling, making hammocks and bicycle brakes, unwrapping cheese, repackaging goods); in all of these jobs the client can experience success and be rewarded financially

on physical care and nutrition provide guidelines for client teaching in preparation for community reentry.

SUMMARY

Five areas of physiological and psychological needs of the client with certain psychiatric disorders are discussed. These include physical care, nutrition, activities, recreation, and work therapy.

Significant aspects in nutrition, elimination, sleep and rest, grooming, and special problems are highlighted for clients with certain psychiatric disorders.

The six basic classifications of nutrients and their functions are explained. Some of the symptoms of nutritional deficiency are similar to symptoms of mental illness.

Nutritional interventions are given for some potential nutritional problems that might occur with certain psychiatric disorders.

Basic goals for recreation as a therapeutic activity are listed.

Work therapy provides structure, tasks, and goals for the client, giving a feeling of self-worth.

Nurses are in an ideal position to teach clients knowledge and skills in physical care, nutrition, activities, recreation, and work for reentry into the community.

Critical Thinking Activities

1. Using information from Table 26-1 on physical care, determine the needs of a client with a psychiatric disorder in the areas of nutrition, elimination, sleep and rest, grooming, and special problems.
2. Using your creative talents, try some of the suggested activities in Table 26-5 with a client who has a specific psychiatric disorder. Evaluate the results of your intervention.
3. Use some of the suggested work tasks in Table 26-5 for a client with a specific psychiatric disorder. Does the work task help the client feel needed and worthwhile?

Review Questions

Multiple Choice—Choose the best answer to each question.

1. A therapeutic activity for a client is:
   a. one that is used to entertain.
   b. one that distracts from life stresses.
   c. one that has a specific care plan goal.
   d. one that is used to fill time.
2. An activity that would be included in leisure counseling is:
   a. Jogging
   b. Basketball
   c. Volleyball
   d. Football
3. Symptoms of depression, fatigue, and nervous instability are evidence of a possible deficiency in the following nutrient:
   a. Vitamin C
   b. Vitamin A
   c. Vitamin E
   d. Vitamin B_1
4. Volunteer work is:
   a. demeaning to a client with a mental illness.
   b. a stepping stone to competitive work.
   c. too stressful for a client with mental illness.
   d. meaningless in obtaining a regular job.
5. A *goal* in a client's physical care is to:
   a. provide all of the client's physical care.
   b. let the client do all of the care.
   c. have the client comply with requirements for care.
   d. maintain a client's physical safety.

References

Walsh M, Carson VB: Mind-body-spirit therapies. In: Carson VB, Arnold EN (eds): Mental Health Nursing The Nurse-Patient Journey. Philadelphia, WB Saunders Co, 1996.

Zuckerman D, Debenham K, Moore K: The ADA and People With Mental Illness: A Resource Manual For Employers. Part III. Washington, DC, American Bar Association and Alexandria, Vir, National Mental Health Association, 1993.

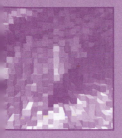
TWENTY-SEVEN

Enhancing Personal Strengths

Outline

- **Relaxation**
  Methods of Relaxation
  Choosing a Method of
    Relaxation
- **Imagery**

- **Touch**
  Hugging
  Using Touch
- **Music**
- **Humor**

Key Terms

- **humor**
- **imagery**

- **music therapy**
- **progressive relaxation**

Objectives

Upon completing this chapter, the student will be able to:

1. Describe the relaxation methods of Roon, Benson, and Jacobson.
2. Outline the use of imagery with a client experiencing anger.
3. List five ways of using touch in establishing contact with a client.
4. Identify six goals of a music therapy program.
5. Identify two positive uses of humor as it relates to the communication process.

In any setting, the nurse is faced with clients who feel overwhelmed by their response to stressful situations. A nurse can do more than just empathize with the client by learning some relaxation techniques. Practicing the suggested methods will enable the nurse to become a role model for the client.

It is the person's reaction to a situation, rather than the situation itself, that causes stress. People seem to do best with a moderate amount of stress in their lives. What constitutes moderate stress stimulation varies greatly from person to person. The nurse must keep this in mind while teaching clients to manage stressful situations in their lives wisely.

RELAXATION

Relaxation training is one way to manage stress. During a relaxed state, the heart slows down, the respiratory rate decreases, and the metabolism rate and blood pressure are lowered. Muscular tension decreases along with the physical responses to relaxation. The client feels refreshed and revitalized.

The nurse must know some basic information before considering relaxation training for the client. A relaxed state can affect the various systems of the body; therefore people on certain medications require medical monitoring. Sometimes medication can be decreased if relaxation is performed on a regular schedule. Clients who are psychotic have difficulty relaxing because of their inability to stay in contact with reality.

Methods of Relaxation

Many relaxation methods are available; the method taught must be tailored to the client's life style. This is important because the long-term goal is to have the client manage his or her own stress on a day-to-day basis. The object is to provide a tool that will induce relaxation. The purpose is not to cause the client to fall asleep, unless this is the reason for the relaxation. Table 27–1 presents methods of relaxation based on the work of Roon, Benson, and Jacobson. It is essential that the nurse

learn to relax himself or herself before attempting to help the client relax. It is further recommended that the nurse practice each exercise before introducing it to the client.

Choosing a Method of Relaxation

The following guidelines may be helpful in deciding with the client what the needs are. Also, the guidelines can assist in selecting the method best suited to meet those needs.

1. Obtain a database. Have the client record all high levels of stress for 2 or 3 days to help assess the stress pattern. Figure 27–1 shows a suggested format.
2. Explore with the client previous positive ways of dealing with stress. If possible, incorporate some of the information into a relaxation plan for the client. Remember that neither recreation nor sleep is synonymous with relaxation.
3. Ask the client how he or she visualizes relaxation occurring (i.e., head-to-toe or vice versa). If the client needs to learn **progressive relaxation** (relaxing muscle groups one at a time in a specific order), determine the order of relaxation according to this information.
4. Decide on a regular practice time. Some clients will want to start their day with a relaxation exercise. Others will want to end their day in this way. Short, on-the-spot relaxation exercises can be utilized as needed throughout the day. Overall relaxation training is accomplished most readily before meals or at least 2 hours after a meal. Food has a stimulant effect on the body. Caffeine-containing drinks, such as regular coffee and some soft drinks, are best avoided before the training session.

In a homogeneous group, it is often possible to simultaneously teach several clients with similar relaxation needs. The relaxation response can even be evoked during another activity such as jogging, swimming, knitting, or crocheting. The repetition of a focus may be the repetition of a word, sound, prayer, phrase, or muscular activity. The client needs reassurance in advance that distracting thoughts may occur. Instruct the client to simply let

Table 27–1	Relaxation Methods and Directions to Client

Originator and Synopsis of Method	Directions to Client
Roon: Applied Relaxation*	
Brief relaxation. This exercise prevents rush of thought. It can be used to promote sleep.	Part your lips slightly. Place the tip of the tongue behind the lower teeth. Keep it there without pressure for awhile. Continue with normal breathing.
Yawning. This is a one-minute tension-release exercise. The lungs expand; the back, jaw, mouth, and tongue relax. More oxygen comes into the system. Nice to do near an open window.	Drop your jaw gently until it feels large enough to take in a whole fruit. As you begin to yawn, it feels as though it will never end. As you yawn, you are taking in a deep breath. When the yawn ends, you feel relaxed, clear down into your stomach. Your lungs have expanded and your back begins to release its tension.
2-minute exercise. This exercise releases shoulder tension and is ideal for the client who will return to a job that requires hours of sitting.	Take a deep breath, hold it and raise your right shoulder. Gently roll it forward, up, back, and around in a complete circle. Exhale. Do the same thing with the left shoulder, always starting with a deep breath. Repeat for 2 minutes.
5-minute relaxation. This exercise relaxes aching eyes, neck, and shoulders.	Close your eyes gently. Tell yourself that your eyes are dropping forward out of their sockets. You see nothing at all except soft, soothing darkness. Let your head drop until your jaw is almost on your chest; let the hinges of your jaw relax. Take a deep breath and begin to rotate your head. Let it roll softly, first to the right, then to the left. Now exhale and rest.
Benson: Relaxation Response†	
This easy-to-learn technique has four components: • a quiet environment • a focus word or short phrase • a passive attitude • a comfortable position	*Step 1.* Pick a focus word or short phrase that's firmly rooted in your belief system. *Step 2.* Sit quietly in a comfortable position. *Step 3.* Close your eyes. *Step 4.* Relax your muscles. *Step 5.* Breathe slowly and naturally, and as you do, repeat your focus word, phrase, or prayer silently to yourself as you exhale. *Step 6.* Assume a passive attitude. Don't worry about how well you're doing. When other thoughts come to mind, simply say to yourself, "Oh, well," and gently return to the repetition. *Step 7.* Continue for 10 to 20 minutes. *Step 8.* Do not stand immediately. Continue sitting quietly for a minute or so, allowing other thoughts to return, then open your eyes and sit for another minute before rising. *Step 9.* Practice this technique once or twice daily.

Table continued on following page

Table 27–1	Relaxation Methods and Directions to Client *Continued*
Originator and Synopsis of Method	**Directions to Client**
Jacobson: Progressive Relaxation‡ ***Introductory exercise*** This exercise is useful for the very tense client. The nurse directs the client in relaxing skeletal muscles. This is a rather strenuous exercise and is best suited for someone in fairly good physical condition. Training is usually a half-hour to an hour, three to four times a week. The client is also encouraged to practice on his or her own. At no time does the nurse tell the client to stop thinking or to make his or her mind a blank. Directions include: • how to tense the various muscle groups • a reminder to be aware of the tension in each part of the body • direction to relax and to note the difference Demonstrate to the client how to relax and contract a muscle before beginning the exercise. An introductory exercise that teaches the client to recognize muscular tension is useful. No relaxing is attempted at this time. Ask the client what areas he or she noted as being tense. Both the right and left sides may be relaxed at the same time. If the client is very tense, do one side at a time, beginning with the left.	Have the client sit in a chair, close his or her eyes, and explore areas of tension in his or her body without attempting to relax. The following order is suggested: • left arm • right arm • left foot, leg, and thigh, then right • abdominal muscles • chest muscles • back and spine • shoulder muscles that move the shoulders forward • shoulder muscles that move the shoulders inward • shoulder muscles used in shrugging • muscles used in bending the head to the right, to the left, holding it stiffly • muscles for wrinkling the brow • frowning • closing eyelids tightly • with eyelids closed lightly, looking to the left, right, up, down, and forward • smiling, rounding the lips into an "O," sticking the tongue out and putting it back in • counting 1 to 10 • swallowing

the thoughts pass through and return to the repetition of the focus.

Reality Check

Try the method of progressive relaxation by Jacobsen. What effect does this technique have on your body? How can you use your experience with relaxation in working with the client?

IMAGERY

Imagery is another way of relaxing. The imagery presented here is not the guided imagery that requires a trained psychotherapist to deal with symbolic material that may emerge (Hill and Howlett, 1997, p. 139). The nervous system operates on imagery. Feelings and thoughts are pulled toward one's mental images. Personal images serve as self-fulfilling prophecies. Consider the image produced by "blue Monday" and "Thank God It's Friday!" Each image sets the tone for the day.

Images can be used for or against oneself. When a person is tired, the negative images seem to make the maximum impression. Therefore clients who picture themselves as failing to deal with their problems of daily living are apt to end up with trouble. It is possible, with selected clients, to encourage them to think about a time when they

Table 27–1	Relaxation Methods and Directions to Client *Continued*

Originator and Synopsis of Method	Directions to Client
Relaxation exercise Space directions for the relaxation exercise so that the client tenses each muscle for about 30 seconds, then relaxes the muscle group for about 60 seconds to experience the difference. Tell the client that different body sensations may be experienced as the body relaxes. Sensations of warmth, tingling, unusual heaviness or lightness are not unusual. Should the client feel uncomfortable, he or she can open his or her eyes, look around, and resume relaxing. The order of relaxation may be reversed to meet individual clients' needs.	Lie down with eyes closed, arms at the side, legs uncrossed. Take two or three deep breaths. Breathe deeply enough so that the abdomen rises while inhaling. For example: INHALE . . . EXHALE . . . Concentrate on your breathing for awhile and continue to breathe naturally throughout the exercise. Tense each of the muscle groups as directed. Note the tension. Relax when the word RELAX is said and note the difference. Ready? • point the feet and toes down (Note the areas of tension. Relax. Note the difference.) • point the toes up • straighten your legs out and lock the knees • dig your heels into the floor • tense the groin and buttock muscles at the same time • pull in the muscles of your stomach • push your shoulders down; keep your buttocks down and bring your chin to your chest • press your arms against your body • shrug your shoulders • bend your wrists up • make a fist • turn your head to the left • turn your head to the right • bring your chin to your chest • smile; make a tight "O" with your lips • close your jaw tightly • stick your tongue way out • frown and shut your eyes tightly • raise your eyebrows Continue to breath normally. Stay with the feeling. When you are ready to return to an alert state, count slowly from 1 to 10. Open your eyes when you are ready.

*Data from Roon K: Roon's New Way to Relax. New York, Greystone Press, 1961.
†From Benson H, Stark M: Timeless Healing: The Power and Biology of Belief. New York, Simon and Schuster, 1996, p 136. Copyright © 1996 by Herbert Benson, MD. Reprinted with permission.
‡Data from Jacobson E: Anxiety and Tension Control. Philadelphia, JB Lippincott Co, 1964.

Date	Time	Incident	Outcome	What Happened Before Incident

FIG. 27–1   Format for client stress level record.

have operated successfully. Using this experience, one can teach them how to change negative images into positive images of successful coping. Imagery has been used to stop smoking, control overeating, increase proficiency in sports, and enhance aspects of life. The nurse can use imagery to help the client move through anxiety-provoking situations.

Some clients are better at imaging than others. Some may see only shadowy figures, whereas others see vivid, Technicolor images. Images need not be particularly vivid to be effective. Mental pictures do seem to come more easily when the client is relaxed and free of distraction. After determining the goal with the client, the first step is to begin with a relaxation exercise suited to the client's needs. The second step is to follow with the imagery. Two or three breaths are helpful before the imagery. For example, the nurse may instruct the client to inhale, then exhale, pause, then repeat. Additional progressive relaxation may be needed by a very tense client.

At first, the nurse will have to guide the client through the relaxation and imagery to prevent the client from becoming sidetracked. When the human mind wanders, it often focuses on negative, unfinished business. The nurse's guidance gently pulls the mind away from the negative thoughts to focus on the imagery. In practicing imagery, it is important to take sufficient time to include enough detail to permit the client to "get into" the imagery. The nurse concludes the imagery by bringing the client to an alert state. When the client is ready, the nurse instructs him or her to count from 1 to 10 and continue to sit with eyes closed. When the client is ready, the nurse asks the client to open eyes and stretch. The client will need to continue sitting awhile longer before arising.

Clients must be reminded that if they experience anxiety anytime during the imagery, they need only to open their eyes. They can look around and reorient themselves to their surroundings. When satisfied, they may close their eyes and continue with the imagery. Some clients are comfortable with their eyes open during the entire process. They do not seem to have any problem visualizing the images suggested. Imagery, like any other technique, takes self-discipline; therefore it is recommended that the nurse plan with the client for daily practice sessions. An evaluation of the effectiveness of this technique is an integral part of the nurse's responsibility to the client.

Imagery is a useful tool for better living for the client. It can become an easy way for the client to develop some sense of control over response to problems of daily living. Table 27–2 includes several of the many ways in which imagery can be useful to a client.

TOUCH

Sometimes in the course of necessary care, touch is mechanical, a part of the job being done, and conveys no caring message. Some nurses use caring touch and are aware of it. Touch is a way of staying in contact, a way of supporting reality, and a way of reducing loneliness. Touching involves risk. It may be misunderstood by both the client and the nurse. Because it involves intimate space, it may be a threat. If the nurse is not sensitive as to how the client perceives him or her, touch may seem inappropriate and offensive to the client. On the other hand, no touch may be just as harmful. At

Table 27–2	Imagery As a Way of Dealing With Specific Situations

Situation	Imagery
Anger	Suggest that the client visualize the situation that helped create the angry feelings. Tell the client to see himself or herself as calm and in control, being able to get through the anger in a constructive way. Because anger often dies of neglect if it is not nurtured, the following new scripts are suggested. They are appropriate for the client to rehearse as he or she visualizes the original situation. Choose the appropriate script. Have the client rehearse it many times. • I do not like it when you treat me this way. • This problem does not belong to me and I do not have to feel angry just because you do. • I have other alternatives. I do not have to stay in this situation that frequently leaves me so angry. • I am clear-headed and intelligent. I am not going to fall apart and do something I will regret. • What am I doing to keep myself hooked into anger? • What am I getting out of being angry?
Anxiety	Have the client design a favorite scene and see himself or herself there, appropriately dressed (e.g., swimsuit). Have the client take time to look around and visualize the surroundings with great detail. Suggest that all the senses be used to experience the sight, sound, smell, touch, and taste available in the special hideaway. Have the client remain there for awhile and experience himself or herself as peaceful and calm. Remind the client that it is a safe place and that he or she can return there daily to rest. When the client is ready to leave, instruct him or her to take one look back, knowing that return can occur. Tell the client that he or she will continue to feel happy, relaxed, and peaceful on returning to continue with daily activities.
Interpersonal relationships	Suggest that the client visualize the person involved and rehearse the meeting with this person. Have the client visualize the meeting in great detail (e.g., surroundings, clothing). Imagine calmly speaking to and effectively answering questions presented by the person, even if he or she feels anxious inside. Have him or her visualize responding to both positive and negative statements, knowing that he or she will remain composed and confident. It is important to rehearse this scenario many times.
Sleeplessness	Have the client visualize a situation that he or she has experienced as boring or that he or she dislikes doing. Suggest that the client recreate the scene in great detail (e.g., relive the sights, sounds, smells that were part of the original situation).
Work skills	Have the client visualize awakening early enough to have time to groom appropriately. Have him or her imagine this preparation in detail. Have the client visualize sitting down to his or her favorite breakfast, being aware of how it looks, tastes, and smells so good! Have him or her see leaving for work, energetic and ready, and being aware of what his or her senses experience on the way. Have the client repeat several times, "I am smart and capable. I will do my best. If I need help, I will ask for it." Have the client visualize arriving at work; greeting other workers and the boss, if there; beginning work confidently and skillfully; knowing that if help is needed, he or she can ask for it without embarrassment; seeing the boss come in and hearing him or her say, "That's a fine job you're doing!" Have the client also visualize the boss saying, "Your work needs improvement." Then have the client see himself or herself remaining calm and saying to the boss, "I would like some information on how to do this work better."

times, words cannot reach the client, perhaps because of the client's inability to process information. The client may hide the need for touch because he or she feels it is inappropriate or childish. It has been suggested that one reason people may turn to drugs is to compensate for the lack of touch in their lives. Touch is the first tranquilizer the child experiences.

Sometimes touch is withheld out of fear of having it misinterpreted as a homosexual or heterosexual advance. Some clients make rules for themselves, such as, "If I don't touch someone of the opposite or same sex, it will be OK." Consequently, they may lavish their need to touch on pets.

Hugging

Hugging is a special form of touch. "Hugs generate warmth and affection, and nurture lasting bonds of friendship" (Smith, 1997). It has been shown that hugs relieve tension, improve blood flow, decrease stress, help self-esteem, promote good will, and are of value from birth to death. Deanna Edwards, a music therapist, sang about touching and hugging in her song "Folks Don't Kiss Old People Any More." The song begins "I still need the loving arms you put around me long ago, when you were just a little child of four" (Edwards, 1974).

Using Touch

The lack of touch and loneliness are thought to go together. Loneliness haunts the mentally ill; it is often described as the root of delusions. The client begins to fill his or her lonely time with fantasy. When there is insufficient human contact to balance the fantasy, the client may lose touch with what is real and what is fantasy.

Supporting the use of touch does not negate the importance of verbal communication. The nurse needs to recognize the need for a balance. Most nurses do not think of touch in a conscious manner. They may not be aware of their feelings about being touched and touching unless it has been brought to their attention. How then, can nurses learn the use of touch and make it part of their daily contact with the client? Box 27–1 offers several suggestions.

BOX 27–1 **Suggestions for Learning to Use Touch**

- Explore your own feelings about touch—your comfort level with touch and how you interpret touching—in both your personal and your professional life.
- Review Unit III on specific disorders, especially in relation to approaching the client. The different psychiatric disorders may influence the client's response to touch.
- Experiment with touch gradually if you are uncomfortable with it. For example: (a) extend your hand when meeting a new client, whether male or female; (b) place your hand on the client's shoulder when speaking to provide touch in a physically neutral area; (c) touch the client lightly when asking him or her to awaken.
- If you have been using touch in a mechanical fashion, become aware of how you touch and when.
- Develop a sense of your own body as you bathe, dress, or soothe an uncomfortable area. Because a great deal of personal touch is automatic, it takes effort to become consciously aware of when it occurs.
- Respect others' feelings about touch. Learn to tell when someone is in a mood to be touched or to be left alone.
- Remember that you have rights too and that you can say "No" to someone else's desire to touch.
- Discourage the use of touch to cling. Suggest an appropriate alternative, such as a warm handshake.
- Set limits on socially inappropriate touch by the client. Support touch that will be acceptable in the community.
- Be aware of and respect cultural differences. Some cultures are very comfortable with touching; others are offended by touching with anyone other than their loved ones.

MUSIC

Music has amazing power and is one of many ways to enhance the strengths of people. "Music, a universal language with many purposes, can be used in the health care setting to aid in stress reduction and anxiety" (Covington and Crosby, 1997, p. 37). Music allows each person to participate at his or her own level. **Music therapy** is the functional application of music toward the attainment of specific therapeutic goals. This medium, which is nonthreatening, can bring about positive changes in behavior. The following are some of the positive results of a music therapy program (Henschel, 1996):

- Social interaction is stimulated through music in a group activity.
- Exercise through body movement to music maintains good circulation and muscle tone.
- Gratification through creative activity, using music, can lead to a feeling of self-esteem.
- Contact with reality can be fostered through the use of music.
- Self-pity and somatic complaints decrease during music sessions.
- Development of a group feeling with a sense of well-being and satisfaction is promoted.
- Music encourages appropriate behaviors. People focus on the given task and tend to forget their inappropriate behaviors.
- Music provides structure. People can relate to the constant and steady beat when listening to or performing music.
- Attention span improves during music sessions. People focus on the music.

- Listening skills improve during a structured music session, with the opportunity to listen and express one's feelings.
- Emotional expression occurs through singing, dancing, facial expressions, or silence in a nonthreatening environment.
- Music improves cognitive skills. People increase their learning skills by implementing music, such as learning the alphabet by singing.

HUMOR

Humor is an essential part of human nature. Infants begin to smile and laugh during the first few months of life. "A sense of humor is both a perspective on life—a way of perceiving the world—and a behavior that expresses that perspective" (Wooten, 1996. p. 1). Joel Goodman, a full-time humor educator, refers to humor as moving "from 'grin and bear it' to 'grin and share it'" (1997, p. 108). **Humor** is an indirect form of communication that, despite the mirth that is conveyed in the concept, is serious business. The effectiveness of the use of humor is related to timing, spontaneity, and the sender's intent. Some of the positive effects of humor are described in Box 27–2.

Norman Cousins, in his *Anatomy of an Illness as Perceived by the Patient* (1979, pp. 82, 84), relates the part that humor played in the lives of Dr. Albert Schweitzer and Sigmund Freud. It was customary for Dr. Schweitzer to present an amusing story at mealtime when staff came together. This was a way of reducing the *effects* of the temperature, humidity, and tension. Freud believed that humor was an effective therapy in dealing with nervous tension.

Ways in which the nurse can assist the client in using humor include the following:

- Find out what makes the client laugh. What is the client's favorite joke?
- Have the client draw the present situation as a cartoon, exaggerating it so it is ridiculous. Some humor included into the situation may result in the client's ability to deal with it more effectively.

BOX 27–2   Positive Effects of Humor

- *The release of tension to relieve stress.* For example, on a busy psychiatric unit in a mental health center, a nurse commented, "As the Center Turns," parodying the soap opera "As the World Turns." This was just enough to break the tension in a rather stressful situation. Laughter and tension are incompatible. Laughter causes the muscles to relax. It is difficult to be anxious or tense when the muscles are limp. Research has shown that laughter also releases endorphins, the body's natural painkiller. Another effect of laughter is the increase of adrenaline in the brain, which stimulates alertness and memory and enhances learning and creativity (Robinson, 1991, p. 29).

- *An increase in understanding that helps clients gain a new perspective on problems and explore other situations.* For example, by blowing up an event to the point of ridiculousness, one can see irrational thinking. A child who breaks a lamp tells his mother that it broke because the table was in his way. The mother scolds the table for being in the way of the child; the child begins to laugh. He may think his mother is a little strange. However, he realizes at the same time how ridiculous his remark was and begins to assume responsibility for his behavior.

- *An outlet for expression that can improve communication and relationships.* For example, a client is obsessed with the delusional idea that she "is burning up"; however, she has quite a collection of jokes. Her delusional system can be interrupted by asking her to tell a joke; as a result, communication is improved.

- *A way trust can be achieved, thus enhancing self-confidence and understanding.* For example, a client who is mentally retarded uses a barrage of jokes in his relationship with staff. His jokes include the "knock-knock, who's there" sayings. Usually staff respond by indicating that they do not know the answer. The client receives great pleasure in giving the correct response to his jokes. In this way, he experiences a bond with staff, along with self-confidence and security.

- Share with the client whatever brings joy or laughter, such as a favorite book, record, picture, or story. The idea is to use these resources to get through the rough times.

- Offer a class on "Getting More SMILEAGE Out of Your Life." Such a class focuses on ways to use laughter in one's life. It helps develop a person's humor potential. Laughter is free, has no calories, no cholesterol, no preservatives, and no artificial ingredients.

Humor can be destructive and, if not used properly, can be a dangerous weapon. It is important to examine whose needs are being met with humor—the nurse's or the client's.

One type of humor is referred to as "gallows humor." It is used when people or groups are faced with dangerous or very stressful situations. These can include war, concentration camps, and life-and-death struggles. Freud's belief that humor helps relieve anxiety and helps a person change unpleasant feelings into pleasant ones may help explain the reason gallows humor helps in these situations (Robinson, 1991, p. 87). Gallows humor is often used to support one's own need; it can be helpful as a coping technique. A good example of the use of gallows humor was the well-known television series *M*A*S*H*. The staff's need for humor to survive difficult situations was demonstrated very clearly; however, the staff never put down or laughed at any patient. Rarely is harm done by laughing *with* someone. It is when we laugh *at* someone that we exclude that person from the network of understanding and support.

It is helpful for the nurse to assess the client's sense of humor. Included in the assessment are situations in which humor occurs and the frame of mind and emotional state at the time. Robinson addresses the use of humor in the total plan of care for the client as follows (1991, p. 212):

Humor is one communication tool, one mechanism for coping. . . . It is useful and therapeutic in the right situation and the right time. . . . What is important is to understand humor, to become skilled in recognizing when it is appropriate and beneficial and to encourage its use, not ignore it.

SUMMARY

Five ways to enhance personal strengths are relaxation, imagery, touch, music, and humor. Relaxation methods have been proposed by Roon, Benson, and Jacobson. Guidelines are listed to aid in deciding which relaxation technique will meet the client's needs.

Imagery can provide a way to deal with specific situations. The nurse can use imaging techniques to help the client move through anxiety-provoking situations.

Other ways to enhance personal strengths include the use of touch, music therapy, and humor. The nurse can learn to make touch a part of his or her contact with the client. Music therapy can have many positive results. Humor can release tension, increase understanding, be an outlet for expression, and develop trust.

Critical Thinking Activities

1. Apply one of the imagery techniques to a client who is experiencing anger, anxiety, or sleeplessness. Evaluate the result.
2. Try group singing with the clients on the unit to which you are assigned. First survey the group on familiar tunes so as many as possible can participate. What type of effect did the music have?
3. Write down a favorite joke or funny experience. How has the joke or experience relieved tension, anxiety, or embarrassment in your life?
4. How might you use your experience with humor in helping clients?

Review Questions

Multiple Choice—Choose the best answer to each question.

1. Benson's relaxation method includes
   a. a progressive relaxation of the body.
   b. a repetition of a focus word or short phrase.
   c. a one-minute yawning exercise.
   d. a gentle rolling of the shoulders.

2. In using imaging as a method of relaxation, the client needs to
   a. close his or her eyes.
   b. focus on negative images.
   c. have vivid images to be effective.
   d. feel relaxed and free of distraction.
3. When using touch, the nurse needs to realize that
   a. everyone enjoys being touched.
   b. touch is a mechanical gesture.
   c. touching involves risk.
   d. the nurse's comfort level is insignificant.
4. Music therapy can
   a. be too stimulating for clients.
   b. bring about positive change in behavior.
   c. foster somatic complaints in clients.
   d. provide too much structure for clients.
5. The nurse can assist the client in using humor by
   a. finding out what makes the client laugh.
   b. laughing at the client.
   c. using humor to meet self needs.
   d. learning to "grin and bear it."

References

Cousins N: Anatomy of an Illness as Perceived by the Patient. New York, WW Norton and Co, 1979.

Covington H, Crosby C: Music therapy as a nursing intervention. J Psychosoc Nurs 35(3):34–37, 1997.

Edwards DK: Peacebird, 1229 S. Santee Street, Los Angeles, CA 90015, Franciscan Communications Center, 1974.

Goodman J: Laughing Matters. 11(3):108, 1997.

Henschel H: If It's Music, It's Therapy!! Seminar, Green Bay, Wis, Spring 1996.

Hill S, Howlett H: Success in Practical, Nursing Personal and Vocational Issues, 3rd ed. Philadelphia, WB Saunders Co, 1997.

Robinson V: Humor and the Health Professions: The Therapeutic Use of Humor in Health Care, 2nd ed. Thorofare, NJ, Slack Inc, 1991.

Smith JW: Hugs to Encourage and Inspire. West Monroe, LA, Howard Publishing Co, Inc, 1997.

Wooten P: Compassionate Laughter: Jest for Your Health! Salt Lake City, Commune-A-Key Publishing, 1996.

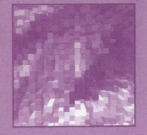

Managing Aggressive Behavior

Outline

- **Theories of Aggression**
  Instinct
  Drive
  Social Learning
  Biological
- **Causes of Aggression**
- **Verbal and Nonverbal Signs of Aggression**

- **Nurses' Reactions to Aggressive Behavior**
- **Therapeutic Interventions for Aggressive Behavior**
  Verbal and Nonverbal
  Physical
- **Restraint and Seclusion**

Key Terms

- aggression
- anger
- emotional honesty
- restraint
- seclusion

- setting limits
- talking down
- talking up
- verbal de-escalation

Objectives

Upon completing this chapter, the student will be able to:
1. Describe four theories of aggressive behavior.
2. Identify factors that may precipitate aggressive behavior in clients.
3. List verbal and nonverbal signs that are related to aggressive behavior.
4. Discuss the significance of the nurse's reaction to a client who is aggressive.
5. Describe two techniques for the verbal de-escalation of aggressive behavior.
6. Explain how nonverbal communication can help in calming a client who is aggressive.
7. Describe a nonharmful physical intervention technique for a:
   - wrist grab
   - clothing grab
   - hair grab
   - human bite
8. Identify the guidelines governing restraint and seclusion.

In addition to being a symptom of many psychiatric disorders, aggressive behavior is present in everyday life. It has become a common method of communication. The purpose of this chapter is to help the nurse understand what factors contribute to aggressive behavior. With knowledge of these factors, the nurse can use intervention techniques to prevent or decrease the behavior.

Aggression is an action, verbal or physical, and **anger** is an emotion. Aggression becomes a coping mechanism for dealing with the frustration and anxiety associated with not achieving a desired goal. The person feels that the only way a need can be fulfilled is through aggression. Figure 2-2 in Chapter 2 diagrams the process involved in goal achievement.

THEORIES OF AGGRESSION

Various theories try to explain the nature of human aggression. Examples include instinct, drive, social learning, and biological theories.

Instinct

Freud's theory of aggression is based on the instinct theory. He believed that the aggressive drive is at work in impulses to cause harm. It is present in the desire for control and power, in guilt and depression, and in the persecutory fears of people who are paranoid. He theorized that two forces—*life instinct* and *death instinct*—shape a person's activities and behavior (Inderbitzin and Levy, 1997, p. 406). However, the concept of a death instinct has largely been rejected.

Drive

The drive theory suggests that aggression is a natural internal drive that sometimes overflows into the environment. For example, frustration, which blocks an ongoing goal-directed behavior, can lead to arousal of the aggressive drive. This could lead to an attack against the person or object that is the cause of the frustration (Mays, 1997; Bauer and Hill, 1994, p. 610).

Social Learning

The theory of social learning views aggressive behavior as behavior learned through modeling or random activity. It is based on the concept "you are what you learn." Aggression or violent behavior is maintained through positive reinforcement. The following are examples of this theory (Bauer and Hill, 1994, p. 610):

- When adults in a home act aggressively toward each other, children incorporate this behavior as a way of responding to others
- Soldiers during war receive medals, promotions, and privileges for killing the enemy; gang members receive status and respect for following the gang code; and professional athletes reap financial rewards and fame for aggressive behavior required in their sport
- Activists often discover they receive more attention and media focus in movements to right perceived wrongs when they are involved in aggressive acts, even though their behavior might result in fines and jail sentences

Biological

A number of biological changes are associated with violence and aggression. Genetic studies show a compelling argument to support a role for heredity. Both genetic and environmental influences clearly exist.

Brain tumors, temporal lobe epilepsy, and cognitive disorders such as Alzheimer's disease can lead to aggressive behavior. The ingestion of mind-altering drugs, such as crack cocaine, PCP, and alcohol, is often closely linked to violent behaviors.

Neurotransmitters are chemicals that transmit impulses between nerve cells or neurons. No one neurotransmitter seems to regulate aggressive behavior. Regulation of one neurotransmitter system may reduce one kind of aggression and increase the occurrence of another. Some of the neurotransmitter actions are thought to be as follows (Mays, 1997):

- Acetylcholine facilitates aggressive behavior
- GABA and serotonin act as inhibitors
- Dopamine enhances fighting
- Norepinephrine may enhance fighting, but there is some question about this

CAUSES OF AGGRESSION

Certain factors in a person's life may be related to aggressive behavior. These possible determinants are broken down into the categories of personal, social, situational, and environmental (Table 28–1). When caring for a client who is subject to aggressive behavior, the nurse needs to collect data on these factors. Also, being aware of the client's reactions to the hospital environment may reduce the incidence of acting-out. Some situations that may precipitate outbursts include the following:

- Fears of being in the hospital, of possible loss of self-esteem, of bodily harm, and of a new experience
- Feelings of helplessness, when combined with the perception that nothing can be done to change an unacceptable situation
- Impersonal and rigid hospital routines, which may lead to renewed efforts to overcome obstacles to personal gratification
- The need to test external controls, to find the limits the situation will tolerate, and to be reassured of external control
- Threats by violation of personal space, especially within the limited environment of the hospital
- Boredom for clients seeking action and excitement

Certain psychiatric diagnostic groups show an increased possibility of becoming aggressive. The nurse should understand the following factors in dealing with clients with these diagnoses:

- *Acute psychosis:* Much of the behavior of a person who is acutely psychotic is based on internal, rather then environmental, stimuli. As a result, behavior is much less predictable and aggression always an increased possibility.
- *Impaired brain functioning:* Any person who shows impaired brain functioning is more likely to react with aggressive behavior in frustrating situations. These people also tend to have a more limited range of response options available.
- *Undercontrol:* Undercontrolled people often respond to minor frustrations with inappropriate aggressive behavior. If their internal controls developed early in the personality structure are rudimentary or lacking, they are unable to defer gratification.
- *Borderline personality disorders:* The borderline personality often decompensates under stress to more psychotic behavior. Unless the full extent of the decompensation is known through the treatment process, aggressive and unpredictable behavior may come as a surprise.
- *Substance-related disorders:* The person who is intoxicated is one of the most likely to become abusive and assaultive.

VERBAL AND NONVERBAL SIGNS OF AGGRESSION

Clients often give clues of increasing tension before an outburst of aggressive behavior. The nurse needs to be alert to behavior patterns and both verbal and nonverbal signs (Bauer and Hill, 1994, p. 613). Verbal clues include the following:

- False accusations
- Argumentative behavior (starting fights)
- Shouting or yelling
- Expressing intent to harm others (threatening)
- Disorientation to time, place, and person

Nonverbal signs of impending aggression include the following:

- Acting out hallucinations or delusions
- Increased motor activity (pacing, fidgeting)
- Irritability, agitation
- Rigid posture (clenched fists and jaw)
- Angry facial expression
- Responding to internal stimuli (voices)
- Staring or lack of eye contact

Table 28–1   Factors Related to Aggressive Behavior

Factor	Determinants	Comments

Personal	People may be prone to violence if they have:
	1. A previous history of violence
	2. A violent family background of abuse
	3. Certain mental disorders
	  • Psychosis (paranoid schizophrenia)
	  • Cognitive (Alzheimer's disease)
	  • Antisocial personality disorder
	  • Substance abuse
		Family violence is perhaps the single most treatable phenomenon responsible for violence in our society.
		
		Severity of pathology is more important than diagnosis. If perception is distorted or there is poor impulse control and confusion because of cognitive impairment, aggressive behavior is more likely.

Social	Frustration	Results in aggression when the frustration is intense or the cause is considered undeserved.
	Direct provocation from others	Physical abuse or verbal teasing are powerful triggers of aggressive behavior. Once aggression begins, escalation continues to the point that mild comments may initiate strong reactions.

	Exposure to aggressive models
	  • Relationships
	  • Television
	  • Films
		Attitudes, emotions, and overt behaviors are influenced by exposure to words and acts by others. The link between exposure to TV violence and aggression appears to be that new aggressive techniques are learned, inhibition is reduced, and the viewer is desensitized.

Situational	Heightened physiological arousal	Competitive activities, vigorous exercises, and exposure to arousal films under certain circumstances may enhance aggressive behavior if the person has a strong aggressive response tendency.
	Pain	May precipitate striking out at any available target, not those just associated with pain.
	Sexual arousal	Mildly erotic material may reduce aggressive level; strongly erotic material may enhance overt aggression.
Environmental	Air pollution	Exposure to noxious odors (chemical plants, other industries) may increase personal irritability and aggression. Involuntary exposure to cigarette smoke may increase aggression.
	Noise	Unpleasant noise may increase overt aggression in those with a strong tendency toward aggression.
	Crowding	Mixed results—under appropriate conditions, crowding may inhibit or increase the aggressive response.
	Heat	Does not appear directly related to violence. Reaction to heat is related to a combination of factors.

Data from Barron RA: Aggression. In Kaplan HI, Sadock BJ (eds): Comprehensive Textbook of Psychiatry, vol 1, 4th ed. Baltimore, Williams & Wilkins, 1985; Bauer B, Hill S: People who defend against anxiety through aggression toward others. In: Varcarolis EM (ed): Foundations of Psychiatric Mental Health Nursing, 2nd ed. Philadelphia, WB Saunders Co, 1994.

- Extremely quiet (unable to express feelings)
- Fear of losing control
- Fear of others

NURSES' REACTIONS TO AGGRESSIVE BEHAVIOR

Aggressive behavior in a client can be threatening to staff. Because of fear, staff members may tend to avoid the client. The avoidance by staff only causes more frustration for the potentially aggressive client. Staff members need to understand themselves—their physical limitations and emotional weaknesses. *By realizing that the aggressive behavior in clients is a response to a real or perceived situation, the nurse may avoid outbursts!*

A regular assessment of one's stressors is one way of identifying personal and work stresses. Questions that the nurse should ask include the following (Stevenson, 1991, pp. 6–7; Bauer and Hill, 1994, p. 615):

- Do I have problems in my home life that are affecting my work?
- What are my stresses at work?
- Are there particular clients or co-workers that bother me?
- Are personal issues in my life influencing my interactions with clients? (Sometimes a client can trigger an emotional response because of a similar incident in the nurse's life.)
- Am I tired?
- Am I afraid of the client?
- Am I trying to avoid the client?
- Do I think the client needs to be punished?
- What is my anxiety level?

Reality Check

1. How do your personal stresses affect your performance at work? What methods have you used to deal with this?
2. What techniques can you use to relate to a co-worker who upsets you?
3. What are some positive ways you could use to deal with your fear of a client?

It is important for the nurse to refrain from reacting solely on an emotional basis. If the nurse responds emotionally, then the client becomes lost because the nurse is busy taking care of his or her own needs. The client is very perceptive of the nurse's weak spots. When a client becomes disturbed, he or she attacks these weak areas. The behavior is similar to that of a child who acts out when the mother is not feeling well and is most vulnerable. Verbal attacks, such as name calling, need to be viewed in an objective way. They usually are not meant for the nurse personally, but for what he or she represents, such as authority or a disliked person in the client's life. It is helpful to have support group for staff in a psychiatric setting.

THERAPEUTIC INTERVENTIONS FOR AGGRESSIVE BEHAVIOR

Working effectively with an aggressive client is related to the nurse's own general attitude and behavior. The emphasis is always on *prevention* of aggressive and violent behavior.

Verbal and Nonverbal

Maier (1996) uses techniques of "talking down" and "talking up" in managing threatening behavior. He uses **talking down** to manage "hot threats" that are part of an escalating process. "Verbal abuse and verbal threats are the criteria that indicate that a patient is in an arousal pattern that will continue to escalate to physical aggression if effective interventions are not implemented" (Maier, 1996, p. 26). Another term used to describe talking down is "**verbal de-escalation.**" Again, the goal is to redirect the client toward a calmer state-of-being (Stevenson, 1991, p. 6). **Talking up** is used to manage "cold threats." People with personality disorders try to manipulate others through threats and praise to achieve a goal. The important way to handle this type of threatening behavior is to talk it up and share with staff what the client is trying to do (Maier, 1996, p. 28). For example, a client may have learned something very personal about the nurse that he or she does not want others to know. The nurse may have shared this information as a way of communicating understanding of the client's feelings. By informing the staff of what happened and talking it up, the nurse removes the threat of manipulation.

Nurses can employ many other verbal and nonverbal interventions to deal effectively with aggressive clients. Box 28–1 lists several appropriate interventions.

BOX 28–1	**Verbal and Nonverbal Nursing Interventions**

- Intervene immediately when the client needs controls or limits. This may mean just separating the client from what seems to be irritating him or her. If more than one client is involved in the disturbance, go to the client with the *power*; talk only to that client.
- Approach the client in a nonthreatening manner; allow physical space. When someone is emotionally disturbed, he or she needs more space. To trespass into one's space can be very threatening. Posture is important. Avoid threatening body language such as hands on hips, clenched fists, or hands folded across the chest.
- Speak slowly and calmly in a "normal" tone of voice; treat the client with respect—"What can I do to help you?" or "It seems that you are really upset about something; let's sit down and talk about what is bothering you."
- Refer *only* to yourself; not to supervisors, policies, or rules. Set limits; give directions in a voice that is firm, clear, and understanding. **Setting limits** provides a consistent set of expectations.
- Give three options to the client. The first two options offer the client a choice. Offering choices helps the client gain a sense of control. The third option is *not* a choice and *not* a threat. Always communicate in the first person. For example: "I cannot allow you to injure yourself, other clients, or me. I want you to go to your room until you can quiet down." or "I want you to help me fold the laundry." Do not get caught up in explaining who you are and why you are qualified, because then you begin losing control.
- Offer to sit and talk; offer food or drink. This provides for the basic needs of the client.
- Maintain the same physical level as the client. If the client sits down, sit down; if the client gets up, get up. This can prevent intimidation
and lessen the perception of a threatening posture.
- Attempt to discover the cause of the client's disturbance. The reason for the client's assaultiveness might have a very legitimate basis rather than being a distortion of reality.
- Provide appropriate diversion. Diversion can be a helpful technique in working with aggressive clients because of their short attention span. One of the best outlets for excess energy is strenuous noncompetitive activity.
- Communicate to the client that you accept him or her as a person, but that you do not approve of his or her behavior.
- Encourage the client to understand, control, and accept responsibility for his or her behavior. If you treat the client as though you expect him or her to be in control, the client is more likely to do so. Remind the client of the consequences of unacceptable behavior. Also, let the client know that he or she makes the decisions about behavior and therefore is responsible for those decisions.
- Reinforce positive behavior. Focusing on strengths increases the client's self-esteem, establishes trust, and increases feelings of security. The client is often unaware of his or her positive qualities because of the emphasis placed on the negative aspects of his or her behavior. Use positive reinforcement whenever possible.
- If medication is ordered, explain to the client about the medication in a short, simple, and clear manner. This information can help decrease the client's anxiety. Before giving medication, determine if extra staff will be needed. Sometimes the presence of extra staff provides security for the client as well as for staff.
- Highly structured surroundings with supportive and interpersonal measures can decrease aggressive behavior.

From Bauer B, Hill S: People who defend against anxiety through aggression toward others. In: Varcarolis EM (ed): Foundations of Psychiatric Mental Health Nursing, 2nd ed. Philadelphia, WB Saunders Co, 1994, p. 616.

Physical

When a client is assaultive and it is necessary to intervene physically, the following points are important to remember (Bauer and Hill, 1994, pp. 617–618):

- Before anything is to be accomplished physically, it must first be accomplished mentally. Mental rehearsal is used in many activities, such as sports and speaking before large groups. It is important to visualize successful management of the situation for it to become a reality. This can be done ahead of time by creating common situations in which physical aggression might occur. Then, the nurse should plan all possible strategies for handling these situations. In this way the nurse is being proactive. The nurse must *believe* in what he or she is doing!
- Defensive techniques are learned and therefore must be practiced until they become part of the nurse's automatic response to assault. This is important because physical assaults happen quickly. These techniques should be taught to the staff through in-service education.
- Don't try to be a hero. Get out of the way and get help, if possible.
- Maintain a firm base of support by placing one foot forward and angle the rear foot to the outside. This position helps maintain balance if suddenly pushed.
- Keep a proper distance from the client. Maintain eye contact and a relaxed posture with arms loose. The nurse's behavior should reflect **emotional honesty**. This means that the nurse's verbal and nonverbal communication send the same message. What he or she says is reflected in body language. Otherwise, the client receives double messages and can become more confused and agitated.
- If in a room, do not stand in a corner without a ready exit. At the same time, the client should be able to exit and not feel cornered, because this can be threatening.
- Always work against the weakest point of any

hold, using arms as levers (i.e., the area between the thumb and forefinger).
- Use arms and hands to protect the face and head; turn the thigh sideways to protect the groin area against a kick.

Specific physical techniques are described in Box 28–2. Again, a word of caution is necessary. Reading about physical management techniques alone is not enough. *They must be properly demonstrated and practiced.* Much of the success in using nonharmful physical intervention techniques is related to spontaneity, surprise, and teamwork within the hospital. It is hoped that by following the suggested verbal and nonverbal interventions, the nurse can avoid being assaulted and physical intervention will not be necessary (Foster, 1979; Bauer and Hill, 1994, pp. 618–619).

RESTRAINT AND SECLUSION

Restraint and seclusion are utilized only after less restrictive measures have proved ineffective to prevent the client from self harm or harming others. According to the *Comprehensive Accreditation Manual for Hospitals* (CAMH), **restraint** is "any method of physically restricting a person's freedom of movement, physical activity, or normal access to his or her body. In the context of these standards, *restraint* is considered involuntary use as either part of an approved protocol, or as indicated by individual orders." CAMH goes on to define **seclusion** as "the involuntary confinement of a person alone in a room where the person is physically prevented from leaving" (CAMH, 1996, p. TX–47).

The use of restraint and seclusion can result in serious consequences. Such measures can cause physical and psychological harm, resulting in loss of dignity and violation of the client's rights. Staff training on the correct use of restraint and seclusion and the protocol for implementation is essential.

CAMH (1996, p. TX–53) has listed several essential elements that govern how an organization uses restraint and seclusion in a way that is

| BOX 28–2 | **General Physical Intervention Techniques** |

To be effective, these techniques must be practiced by staff under qualified supervision. No technique is a guarantee that injury will be avoided.

- *Wrist or arm grabs:* The weak point of a wrist grab is between the client's thumb and fingers. The wrist can be removed by moving it against the thumb of the attacker's hand in a circular movement. This needs to be done quickly to be effective. However, evaluate the situation before implementing the wrist release. Sometimes a client grabs a wrist for support or to be close to someone. After a short time, the client may let go. If the client does not and the grip is bothersome, ask the client kindly to release his or her grip before implementing the technique.
- *Clothing grabs:* If a client grabs clothing, place one hand under and close to the grasping hand to keep the clothing against your body. With the heel of the other hand, push the client's grasping hand off in the direction of his or her knuckles. This technique will prevent clothing from being torn.
- *Hair grabs:* Note that the best defense is to be careful and not let the client grab your hair.

  Hair grab from front: When hair is grabbed, it is important to prevent pulling of the hair. This can best be done by interlocking your fingers over the attacker's hands and pressing down with the palms of your hands. Press on the backs of the attacker's hands, not the fingers. This alleviates pain from the hair grabbing and prohibits further pulling. Then step back into a crouching position with your head pointed toward the ground and your elbows pulled in. This forces the attacker to release his or her grip or lose balance.

  Hair grab from rear: Placement of hands should be the same as for the hair grab from the front. Step around as if to face the attacker, moving your upper body down so you are bent over at the waist. Facing the attacker, straighten up slowly, keeping the attacker's hand tight against your head.

  In both of these interventions, after the technique has been applied, squeeze the attacker's hands with the palms of your hands, forcing the release of the attacker's grip.
- *Human bites:* Human bites are dangerous. Because of the bacteria in the human mouth, broken skin should be treated immediately to prevent infection. As in the hair grab and clothing grab, do not pull away; instead, move into the attacker's mouth. Release can usually be obtained by placing the forefinger underneath the attacker's nose and pressing upward.

From Maxmen JS: Psychotrophic drugs: fast facts, New York, 1991, WW Norton & Co., Inc. Copyright © 1991 by Jerrold S. Maxmen. Reprinted by permission of WW Norton & Co, Inc.

appropriate to the people served. These elements include the following:

- Protection and preservation of client's rights, dignity, and well-being during use (i.e., explaining the need for restraint or seclusion)
- Restraint and seclusion based on the client's assessed needs
- Decisions made about least-restrictive methods
- Assurance of safe application and removal by competent staff
- Monitoring and reassessing the client during use
- Meeting the client's needs during use, such as food, hydration, toileting, skin care, and checking vital signs
- Limiting individual orders to licensed independent practitioners
- Time-limited orders
- Documentation in the medical record when restraint or seclusion clinical protocols are used or individual orders are written. This needs to include the exact behavior exhibited by the client that necessitated restraint and seclusion.

These essential elements ensure that the use of restraint and seclusion preserves and protects the client and his or her rights, dignity, and well-being. "Staff debriefing following an incident is crucial to discuss reactions to the use of restraints and seclusion and to plan for the use of alternative measures in the future" (Morales and Duphorne, 1995, p. 16).

SUMMARY

Aggression is a coping mechanism for dealing with frustration and anxiety related to not achieving the desired goal. Theories that attempt to explain the nature of human aggression include those based on instinct, drive, social learning, and biological theories. Factors related to aggressive behavior are personal, social, situational, and environmental. Also, a client's reaction to hospitalization can precipitate outbursts of violence.

Being aware of verbal and nonverbal signs of impending aggressive behavior can prevent a violent episode. Nurses need to understand themselves—their physical limitations and emotional weaknesses—to deal effectively with aggressive behavior. The emphasis is on *prevention* of aggressive and violent behavior. Verbal and nonverbal interventions can help redirect the client and hopefully avoid an aggressive episode. Specific physical intervention techniques are described for the wrist grab, clothing grab, hair grab, and human bites. Restraint and seclusion are only utilized after less-restrictive measures have proved ineffective.

Critical Thinking Activities

1. Think of real-life situations in which verbal and nonverbal communication do not agree. What are your reactions to these situations?
2. Review Table 28–1. Then describe the possible influences of television shows and films on the development of aggressive behavior.
3. What environmental conditions such as air pollution, noise, or heat have had an effect on your behavior or the behavior of others that you have observed?

Review Questions

Multiple Choice—Choose the best answer to each question.

1. A theory of human aggression that is based on the concept "you are what you learn" is
   a. instinct theory.
   b. drive theory.
   c. social learning theory.
   d. biological theory.
2. Which of the following is a nonverbal sign that is related to aggressive behavior?
   a. False accusations, argumentative
   b. Angry facial expression
   c. Expressing intent to harm
   d. Disorientation to time, place, person
3. A nurse might increase aggressive behavior in a client by
   a. responding in an objective way.
   b. setting limits.
   c. being sensitive.
   d. responding emotionally.
4. A technique for verbal de-escalation of aggressive behavior is
   a. talking up.
   b. speaking in a loud, firm voice.
   c. explaining the rules of the hospital.
   d. talking down.
5. An essential element that governs the use of restraint and seclusion is
   a. the needs of staff.
   b. time-limited orders.
   c. security of staff.
   d. PRN orders.

References

Bauer B, Hill S: People who defend against anxiety through aggression towards others. In: Varcarolis EM (ed): Foundations of Psychiatric Mental Health Nursing, 2nd ed. Philadelphia, WB Saunders Co, 1994.

Comprehensive Accreditation Manual for Hospitals (CAMH): The Official Handbook. Oakbrook Terrace, Ill, Joint Commission on Accreditation of Healthcare Organizations, 1996.

Foster R: Gentle Self Defense Workshop. Lawrence, Kan, Camelot Behavioral Systems, 1979.

Inderbitzin LB, Levy ST: Psychoanalytic theories. In: Tasman A, Kay J, Lieberman JA: (eds): Psychiatry, vol 1. Philadelphia, WB Saunders Co, 1997.

Maier GJ: Managing threatening behavior: the role of talk down and talk up. J Psychosoc Nurs 34(6):25–30, 1996.

Mays D: Violence and Aggression Paper. Principled Approaches for Managing Aggressive Behavior in Adult and Adolescent Clients Conference. Green Bay, Wis, 1997.

Morales E, Duphorne PL: Least restrictive measures: alternatives to four-point restraints and seclusion. J Psychosoc Nurs 33(10):13–16, 1995.

Stevenson S: Heading off violence with verbal de-escalation. J Psychosoc Nurs 29(9):6–10, 1991.

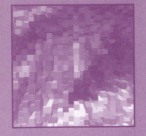

TWENTY-NINE

Community Reentry

Outline

- **Community Treatment**
    Philosophy of Community Mental Health Care Service
    Goals of Community Mental Health Care Service
    Services Provided in a Community Mental Health Program
- **Consumer Mental Health Movement**
    Early Mental Health Consumer Groups
    The Federal Community Support Program
- **Self-Help and Support Groups**
- **Role of the Nurse**

Key Terms

- adult family home
- advocacy
- alternative living settings
- Community Support Program (CSP)
- crisis facility
- empowerment
- group homes
- life skills training
- mental health consumers
- self-help group
- support group
- supportive apartment living

Objectives

Upon completing this chapter, the student will be able to:
1. Define the philosophy of community mental health care service.
2. List the goals of community mental health care service.
3. Name six classes that can be a part of life skills training.
4. Describe three alternative living settings.
5. Identify two principles for the organization of the consumer mental health movement.
6. Describe what self-help groups can do for mental health consumers.
7. Name three well-known self-help groups.
8. Define a resource for self-help groups for mental health consumers.
9. Describe the role of the nurse in the consumer mental health movement.

COMMUNITY TREATMENT

Community mental health centers (CMHC), which developed as a result of the Mental Retardation Facilities and Community Mental Health Centers Construction Act of 1963, are required to provide outpatient services. However, clients in the community need to seek out these services at the mental health center. This chapter focuses on the advances that have been made in treating clients with mental illness in the community setting and what mental health consumers have done to help themselves.

Many of the changes in community mental health care are related to the **Community Support Program (CSP).** This program, launched by the National Institute of Mental Health in 1978, established a focal point for responsibility within each state mental health authority for the care and treatment of people with severe mental illness. (Interagency Council on the Homeless, 1992, p. 16). Community Support Programs have various names, such as Community Support Systems (CSS), Community Treatment Program (CTP), or Program for Assertive Community Treatment (PACT). Whatever the name of the program, it offers a team approach to meeting the needs of people with serious or chronic mental illness who live in the community.

Philosophy of Community Mental Health Care Service

One philosophy of community mental health care service expresses the following (Brown County Human Services Community Treatment Program, Green Bay, WI, 1998):

- All clients have nondiscriminatory access to a comprehensive range of quality services.
- The highest priority is to provide services that are unavailable or inaccessible elsewhere in the community.
- A personalized and holistic service approach aimed at maintaining or improving functioning is cost effective.

- Working with agencies to improve systems interaction and build on existing resources is essential in providing effective mental health services to the community.
- All people need to be treated with dignity and respect.
- Regular program evaluation is essential in ensuring that the services offered are needed and are having a positive impact on individual clients and the community.
- Public participation in planning and evaluation increase the potential for quality services.
- The organization will be sensitive and responsive to the needs of the employees, provide an atmosphere of open communication, and actively encourage personal and professional growth.

Goals of Community Mental Health Care Service

The goals of community mental health care service are similar to those of other forms of community medical services, and include the following:

- Reduce the need for inpatient care among clients served
- Assist the clients in increasing personal independence
- Assist the clients in maintaining or improving their quality of life
- Assist the clients in proper utilization of community resources
- Increase usage of services on an outpatient/community basis for the targeted populations

Services Provided in a Community Mental Health Program

The needs of people with long-term mental illness who live in the community center around learning the life skills that are necessary to function in their environment. They need help with medication management, financial tasks, housing, employment, recreational activities, and health care. They also need an abundance of emotional support. Figure 29–1 is a model of a community treatment

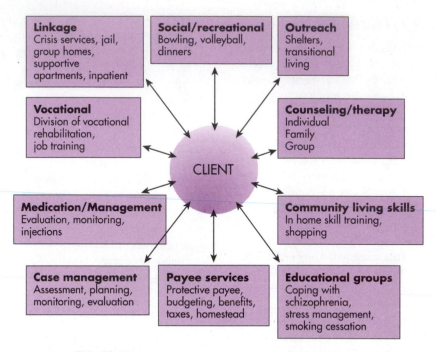

Linkage
Crisis services, jail, group homes, supportive apartments, inpatient

Social/recreational
Bowling, volleyball, dinners

Outreach
Shelters, transitional living

Vocational
Division of vocational rehabilitation, job training

Counseling/therapy
Individual Family Group

CLIENT

Medication/Management
Evaluation, monitoring, injections

Community living skills
In home skill training, shopping

Case management
Assessment, planning, monitoring, evaluation

Payee services
Protective payee, budgeting, benefits, taxes, homestead

Educational groups
Coping with schizophrenia, stress management, smoking cessation

FIG. 29–1 Model of a Community Treatment Program.

program depicting the numerous services that may be offered.

Life Skills Training

Life skills training can be developed as an educational program. Consumers and/or clients register for classes that cover specific subjects. These classes usually are 1 hour in length and are offered once a week over a specified period of time. Examples of topics and content suitable for life skill classes are shown in Table 29–1.

There are many other classes that can be included in life skills training such as Personal Hygiene, Human Sexuality, Nutrition, Introduction to the World of Literature, Crafts, Computer Skills, and Disabilities Awareness (N.E.W. Curative Rehabilitation, Inc., Green Bay, Wis, 1997). The nurse is an important member of the team in helping the mental health client and/or consumer develop, maintain, and improve life skills.

Alternative Living Settings

The goal of **alternative living settings** is normalization of clients. These settings provide an opportunity for clients to achieve independence while providing support and training (Gilkison, Neathery, 1995, p. 535). The types of alternative living settings range from crisis shelters to adult family care.

- A **crisis facility** provides a safe environment to people as an alternative to inpatient care. Such a facility is used by people in crisis situations and by those who are in need of a structured setting for a longer period of time to stabilize their condition. This is cost-effective care, but even more importantly, it is less traumatic for the individual than acute care hospitalization. Crisis facilities make transition back to a client's previous living situation much easier.
- **Group homes** are sometimes called *community-based residential facilities (CBRFs)*. These

Table 29–1 Contents of Life Skill Classes

Life Skill Class Topic	Topics for Discussion
Stress management	Main source of stress
	Symptoms of stress
	Healthy and unhealthy stress
	How stress affects you personally
	Reducing stress
	Preventing unhealthy stress
	Coping with stress you cannot control
Anger management	Anger and the mind
	How to cope with anger
	• positive ways of expressing anger
	• mental skills for controlling anger
	• using humor to decrease anger
	The power and importance of forgiveness
Improving your self-esteem	What is self-esteem?
	How does your self-esteem affect the way you live?
	What are common effects of low self-esteem?
	How do your emotions affect your self-esteem?
	How can you have more control of your emotions?
	Where does negative thinking come from?
	How can you decrease negative thinking?
	How can you develop a more positive attitude about yourself?
Assertive communication	How to talk so that people will listen
	How to be assertive, not aggressive
	The importance of communicating your ideas, feelings, and needs
	How to use "I" messages effectively
	What is the difference between what is said and what is heard?
	How to communicate in uncomfortable situations
	How to communicate socially
	Doing reality checks with yourself and others
World of work	Work values, interests, abilities, and goals
	Job-seeking skills
	Filling out job applications
	Developing a resume
	Interviewing
	Dealing with disability issues
	Job-keeping skills
Money management	Receipts
	Paying bills
	Carrying identification
	Safekeeping of cash on hand
	Making change/money value
	Saving for large purchases
	Understanding paychecks
	Understanding credit and interest
	Understanding SSI/SSA
	Checking/savings account
	Understanding insurance
	Banking skills
	Weekly budget and monthly budgets
	Following a budget

Table continued on following page

| Table 29–1 | Contents of Life Skill Classes *Continued* |

Life Skill Class Topic	Topics for Discussion
Using community resources	How would you locate commonly used services such as:
	• housing allowance, such as rental assistance
	• health department
	• library
	• city transit
	• Social Security office
	• city hall
	• legal aid
	• post office
	• hospital
	• bank
	• Department of Motor Vehicles
	How would you find a place to live in the community?
	What things do you need to consider when renting a place to live?
	How will you get from one place to another?
	What types of financial services are in your community?
	What types of legal services are in your community?
	What are your personal responsibilities as a citizen of your community?
Housekeeping	Housekeeping basics
	• dusting and vacuuming
	• checking for spoiled food
	• cleaning/organizing cupboards
	• defrosting/cleaning refrigerator
	• bed linens/towels
	• trash disposal
	• cleaning stove and oven
	• insect control
	• purchasing cleaning supplies
	Dealing with clutter
	Grocery shopping
	• making a list
	• reading labels
	• using coupons
	• courtesy while shopping
	• requesting assistance
	• bagging groceries
	• storing purchases
	Small appliance shopping (coffee pot, toaster, iron)
	• safety hazards
	• guarantees and warranties
Medical management	Clear information about prescribed medications (name of drug and possible side effects)
	Reason for prescribing medication; benefits of the drug
	Importance of taking medication as directed
	What to do if undesirable side effects occur
	Organization of a system for taking medication
	Possible reaction if medication is suddenly discontinued

Table 29–1	Contents of Life Skill Classes *Continued*

Life Skill Class Topic	Topics for Discussion
Laughter is the best medicine	Ways to bring humor into your life
	Laughing for the health of it
	Developing your humor potential
Problem solving	What are the general ways to go about solving a problem?
	How can you identify the real problem?
	How do you select the most appropriate solution to a problem?
	What to do if you do not get the desired outcome
	How important is assertiveness in problem solving?

From N.E.W. Curative Rehabilitation, Inc., Green Bay, Wis.

homes are for people who need supervision, care, and service in addition to board and room. They do not need a hospital or nursing home setting. Group homes provide a living environment that is as homelike as possible and is the least restrictive of each resident's freedom. The care and services provided encourage each resident to move toward functional independence in daily living or to continue functioning at the highest possible level.

- **Supportive apartment living** refers to individual apartments or cooperative apartments that are contracted or owned by a private or public mental health agency. These settings enable clients to maintain independence and responsibility through paying rent and housekeeping. At the same time, on-site supervision provides structure and counseling (Gilkison, Neathery, 1995, p. 536).
- **Adult family home** is a residence in which care and maintenance above the level of room and board, but not including nursing care, are provided to one or two residents by a person whose primary domicile is that residence. (Some states certify three- or four-bed adult family homes.)

All alternative living arrangements supervised through a community mental health care program have to meet governmental guidelines regarding fire codes, food service, staff supervision, and client rights.

Reality Check

> Carol Reed, a 30-year-old woman, has been in and out of acute care hospitalization. She was readmitted because she does not take her medication consistently. During her most recent admission, she has been stabilized once again on her medication.
>
> 1. What type of living arrangement in the community would provide the best supervision for Carol so that she would remain on her medication?
> 2. What educational program could you provide for Carol so that she would remain on her medication?

CONSUMER MENTAL HEALTH MOVEMENT

An early organizer of the consumer mental health movement was Judi Chamberlain. She published a book, *On Our Own: Patient-Controlled Alternatives to the Mental Health System* (1979). She is the founder of the U.S. National Association of Psychiatric Survivors. Other terms used to define former psychiatric patients are ex-patients or **mental health consumers**.

Early Mental Health Consumer Groups

The mental health consumer movement began in the 1970s. The major organizing principles of this movement were self-definition and self-determination. These motivations are similar to those behind the women's and gay liberation movements. Usually, nonpatients were excluded from mental health consumer groups. One reason given is that consumer perceptions about "mental illness" were opposed to those of the general public and of many mental health professionals (Chamberlain, 1990, p. 325 [79]). Mental health consumers needed to share and examine their own experiences, realizing that they had much to give each other. "As peers, we can offer this support, knowing that although we may be the ones giving help today, tomorrow we may need that help, and the people we comfort today may then be our comforters" (Chamberlain, 1995, p. 40).

The early consumer mental health groups formed on the east and west coasts. It took longer for local groups to develop nationwide because of lack of funding and the low income of members. Two means of communication were the annual conference on Human Rights and Psychiatric Oppression, held annually from 1973 to 1985, and the publication *Madness Network News* (which ceased publication in 1986). The latter became "the voice of the American ex-patient point of view" (Chamberlain, 1990, p. 327 [81]).

The heart of the consumer mental health movement is at the local level. The number of groups has continued to grow. Members realize that through organization they can bring about change. One example of a program run by mental health consumers is "The Gathering Place" in Green Bay, Wisconsin. It "is founded on the concept of 'consumer empowerment' in which mental health consumers pursue their own recovery and rebuild their lives through consumer-run programs and the friendship and support and understanding of peers" (Gathered News, January 1998, p. 1). "The Gathering Place" publishes a monthly newsletter listing

their activities. Some of these activities include expressive arts therapy, basic computer skills class, monthly speakers, recreation, educational videos, and the BRIDGES education course. The acronym BRIDGES stands for "**B**uilding **R**ecovery of Individual **D**reams & **G**oals through **E**ducation & **S**upport" (Tennessee Mental Health Consumers Association et al, brochure).

The Federal Community Support Program

The federal Community Support Program began funding consumer conferences with "Alternatives '85." These conferences are designed by and for mental health consumers. They have continued with increasing attendance each year. In addition, the consumer mental health movement has developed alliances with other disability groups. Together, these alliances have become a powerful force for legal change. The American with Disabilities Act (ADA) of 1990 is an example of the results of their lobbying for civil rights for the disabled. "Whether group members call themselves clients, consumers, ex-patients, users, or psychiatric survivors, groups throughout the world are united by the goals of self-determination and full citizenship rights for their members" (Chamberlain, 1990, p. 336 [90]). In 1998, the National Mental Health Association titled their National Conference "Consumers and Mental Health Associations Coming Together in '98: United in Leadership." They offered scholarships to consumers to attend the conference.

SELF-HELP AND SUPPORT GROUPS

In 1974, before the Community Support Program began, one of the authors became involved in a Social Therapeutic Club for mental health consumers living in the community. A group of students whom the author was supervising had to do a "change project" for one of their classes. They wanted to set up an aftercare program for discharged clients with mental illness. There was nothing available at this time for these clients. The author functioned as a volunteer, with the students making all of the arrangements for location and transportation. No money was available except through donations. The local Mental Health Association provided the rent for the facility that was used. The group met once a week on Tuesday evening for 2 hours. It was called the "Tuesday Night Happening" (TNH). All participants, including volunteers, were members of the club and carried a membership card. A typical evening attendance was from 15 to 20 people. The program had three main areas of focus: socialization skills, physical activity outlets, and problem-solving techniques (Bauer, 1980, p. 1).

The consumer mental health movement led to the development of self-help groups. A **self-help group** is a group of people who meet to work on one specific problem area which they all have in common. The focus is on learning ways to get control of their lives by dealing with their problem(s). It is through self-help groups that mental health consumers become empowered. **Empowerment** means that members become active and have a political, social, and cultural voice in matters that concern their cause. Members take on an **advocacy** role by representing the needs of clients on committees and boards (Chamberlain, 1990, p. 330 [84]). Some well-known self-help groups include the following:

- *Alcoholics Anonymous (AA):* This group is a fellowship of men and women who share their experience, faith, and hope with each other to help others with an alcohol problem achieve sobriety. The members of the group follow the 12-step program of recovery.
- *Al-Anon:* This is a group for family members of people who have a problem with alcoholism. The emphasis is on helping the family cope with the individual who has the alcohol problem.
- *National Alliance for the Mentally Ill (NAMI):* This organization is for relatives and friends of people with mental illness. Members receive support through sharing their experiences and promoting educational programs and literature.
- *National Depressive and Manic-Depressive Association (Mood Disorders):* This group pro-

vides mutual support to people coping with depressive and manic-depressive illness. Mutual encouragement helps members overcome the isolation and loneliness that accompany depression.
- *Recovery, Inc.:* This is a self-help group for people with nervous symptoms and fears. The recovery method is a system of techniques for controlling behavior and changing attitudes toward those symptoms and fears.

Another type of group that is helpful to people with mental illness is the **support group**. In such a group people meet to talk about how to cope with a specific problem or illness. These groups are often facilitated by professionals and are for people and/or families who are experiencing the problem. The major focus is on sharing feelings and helping one another accept hardships that cannot be changed.

Information on where self-help groups are located and how to contact them can be obtained from the National Mental Health Consumers' Self-Help Clearinghouse. This is a national technical assistance center funded by the Federal Center for Mental Health Services of the Substance Abuse and Mental Health Services Administration. "The Clearinghouse promotes consumer/survivor participation in planning, providing, and evaluating mental health and community support services and provides technical assistance and information to consumer/survivors interested in developing self-help services and advocating to make traditional services more consumer-oriented." (National Mental Health Consumers' Self-Help Clearinghouse, 1997).

ROLE OF THE NURSE

One of the important functions of the nurse in the consumer mental health movement is that of an advocate. The nurse needs to support and respect mental health consumers in their struggle for independence and empowerment. Nurses can develop a meaningful self-help partnership. This can be done by understanding the history of the mental health consumer movement and coordinating services among other community agencies involved with the client. They must be willing to go beyond their titles and appreciate the mutual benefits of a social, collective approach based on true equality between people working together (Emerick, 1990, p. 406). This is a positive way to bring about change and reduce stigma.

SUMMARY

The Community Support Program, launched by the National Institute of Mental Health in 1978, provided for community care and treatment of people with severe mental illness. A philosophy of community mental health care service provides all clients with nondiscriminatory access to a comprehensive range of quality services. Goals of a community mental health program are to assist clients in increasing personal independence and quality of life, thereby reducing the need for inpatient care.

Services provided in a community mental health program include case management, social/recreational activities, life skills training, medication management, vocational skills, counseling/therapy, and alternative living settings. Topics for life skills training include stress management, improving self-esteem, assertive communication, anger management, world of work, money management, using community resources, housekeeping, laughter, medication management, and problem solving. Alternative living settings in the community include the crisis facility, group homes, supportive apartment living, and adult family home.

Two major organizing principles of the consumer mental health movement are self-definition and self-determination. The consumer mental health movement led to the development of self-help groups. Through self-help groups, mental health consumers became empowered and took on an advocacy role. Some well-known self-help groups include AA, Al-Anon, National Alliance on Mental Illness, National Depressive and Manic-Depressive Association, and Recovery, Inc. A list

of self-help groups for mental health consumers can be obtained from the National Mental Health Consumers' Self-Help Clearinghouse.

The role of the nurse in the consumer mental health movement is that of an advocate. By understanding the history of the mental health consumer movement, nurses can help coordinate services among other community agencies involved with the client.

Critical Thinking Activities

1. Visit a group home for people with mental illness. Evaluate the life skills that the people are learning to help enable them to live in the community.
2. Plan a life skills course that you could offer people who are seriously mentally ill and living in the community.
3. Attend a self-help group for mental health consumers. How do members of the self-help group support one another? How does this support help the members advocate their rights?
4. How could you become an advocate for mental health consumers?
5. You are an employer interviewing a mental health consumer for a job. What do you consider when making a decision? How might the person feel?

Review Questions

Multiple Choice—Choose the best answer to each question.

1. An alternative living arrangement that enables the client to maintain independence and responsibility through paying rent and housekeeping is
   a. a group home.
   b. an adult family home.
   c. supportive apartment living.
   d. a crisis facility.
2. A life skill training class that helps a client understand credit and interest is
   a. assertive communication.
   b. using community resources.

c. medical management.

d. money management.

3. One of the *most* important functions of the nurse in the consumer mental health movement is

a. education.

b. advocacy.

c. independency.

d. problem solving.

4. A goal of a community mental health care service is to

a. assist clients in improving quality of life.

b. increase usage of inpatient services.

c. assist clients in personal dependence.

d. assist clients in utilization of inpatient resources.

5. A self-help group that focuses on family members of people who are mentally ill is

a. the National Depressive and Manic-Depressive Association.

b. Alcoholics Anonymous.

c. the National Alliance for the Mentally Ill.

d. Recovery, Inc.

References

Bauer B: The psychiatric nurse as a volunteer: a way to effect change. Free Association, 7(2):1–2, 1980.

Brown County Human Services Community Treatment Program, Green Bay, Wis, 1998.

Chamberlain J: On Our Own: Patient-controlled Alternatives to the Mental Health System. New York, McGraw-Hill, 1979.

Chamberlain J: Rehabilitating ourselves: the psychiatric survivor movement. Int J Mental Health 24(1):39–46, 1995.

Chamberlain J: The ex-patients' movement: where we've been and where we're going. J Mind Behav 11(3&4):323(77)–336(90), 1990.

Emerick RE: Self-help groups for former patients: relations with mental health professionals. Hospital and Community Psychiatry 41(4):401–407. 1990.

Gathered News. Green Bay, Wis, The Gathering Place, 1998.

Gilkison JR, Neathery MB: Mental health in the home and community. In: Antai-Otong D (ed): Psychiatric Nursing Biological and Behavioral Concepts. Philadelphia, WB Saunders Co, 1995.

Interagency Council on the Homeless: Report of the Federal Task Force on Homelessness and Severe Mental Illness: Outcasts on Main Street. Washington, DC, Interagency Council on the Homeless, 1992.

National Mental Health Consumers' Self-Help Clearinghouse, 1211 Chestnut St., Suite 1000, Philadelphia, PA 19107-9395, 1997.

N.E.W. Curative Rehabilitation, Inc. Life Skills Program. Green Bay, Wis, 1997.

Tennessee Mental Health Consumers' Association, Tennessee Alliance for the Mentally Ill, Tennessee Department of Mental Health: BRIDGES brochure. Nashville, Tenn, 1997.

Behaviors That Challenge the Nurse

Outline

- **Specific Behaviors That Can Present Problems**
  Aggression, Physical
  Aggression, Verbal
  Angry Feelings, Inappropriate Expression Of
  Blaming
  Delusions That Interfere With Functioning
  Demanding
  Denial
  Disrobing
  Distressful Behavior That Interferes With Functioning
  Eating, Refusal
  Forgetfulness Resulting From a Cognitive Disorder
  Guilty Feelings, Inappropriate Use Of
  Hallucinations That Interfere With Functioning
  Helplessness
  Hoarding
  Ideas of Reference That Interfere With Functioning

  Illusions That Interfere With Functioning
  Impulsiveness
  Inability to Follow Directions
  Indecisiveness
  Institutionalized Behavior
  Loneliness, Feelings of, That Interfere With Functioning
  Manipulation, Destructive
  Masturbation in Public Places
  Misidentification That Interferes With Functioning
  Nocturnal Wandering
  Nonassertiveness
  Noncompliance
  Physical Symptoms, Inappropriate Use Of
  Seclusiveness That Interferes With Functioning
  Sexual Acting Out
  Sleep, Unsatisfied
  Tattling
  Temper Tantrums
  Worry, Inappropriate Expression Of

Key Term

- community reentry goal

Objectives

Upon completing this chapter, the student will be able to:
1. Explain, in his or her own words, three core approaches that underlie all of the suggested interventions.
2. Identify one intervention and rationale for each behavior listed.

This chapter is a resource for dealing with behaviors that challenge the nurse. The reason for presenting the behaviors in the chosen format—Behavior Problem, Goals, Interventions, and Rationale—is to give the nurse guidelines for dealing with the specific behavior. For each client, the nurse must individualize interventions based on the client's specific behaviors. For ease in locating specific behaviors, the behaviors are listed in table format in alphabetical order.

Three core approaches underlie all of the suggested interventions. They are:

1. Help the client identify the problem behavior by using statements such as, "By the way, you have been pacing; something seems to be bothering you!"

2. Accept the client as a person without sanctioning the behavior. For example, "You have some good ideas, but I don't approve of your shouting them at me."

3. Explore alternatives and possible consequences for dealing with problem behaviors. For example, "From my observations, the way that you are displaying your anger is getting you into difficulty. Let's talk about other, more acceptable ways that you can deal with your angry feelings."

The new **community reentry goal** speaks to treatment that continues in a variety of community settings. Today, clients have short hospital stays with transfer to other facilities to complete treatment.

Specific Behaviors That Can Present Problems

AGGRESSION, PHYSICAL

GOAL 1: Will verbalize signs that indicate impending loss of control.

Intervention	Rationale
Look for signs of mounting tension and interrupt by acknowledging the situation. ("I can tell you are irritated.")	The key is prevention—early intervention can prevent total loss of control.
Show genuine concern.	Shows you are working with him or her. (This is not a power issue.)
Listen and encourage client to speak. ("Go on.") Do not impose your viewpoint.	May have a genuine complaint that can be addressed.
Give client a role in solving the problem. "What would you like us to do?"	Support client ability to take responsibility.
Set limits on angry behavior. ("I would like you to calm down so that I do not have to call for help." or "You do not want to hurt me.")	Parameters provide sense of safety (someone is in charge).

Continued

AGGRESSION, PHYSICAL—cont'd

GOAL 2: Will inform staff that he or she is losing control.

Intervention	Rationale
Basic guidelines include the following:	
• Attitude (calm, friendly, sincere).	Reduces anxiety.
• A good-natured sense of humor may get client over a rough spot.	
Do not irritate client. Postpone treatment or routine until client is more stable. If an emergency, give client brief explanation, perform treatment quickly with sufficient help, and back off.	Emergency is an exception in which prompt action is needed.
Avoid becoming defensive or angry yourself. Avoid arguments.	Defensiveness and anger excites client.
Provide enough space. Keep the client away from other clients or visitors who annoy him or her.	Avoid deliberate aggravation.
Do not stand in a doorway. Stand off to one side in a relaxed position (feet apart to provide a stable base and arms free).	May perceive this as being cornered.
Avoid placing hands on hips or making a fist.	Hands on hips or fists may be perceived as an attack position.
Place objects between you and client (e.g., bed, chair, table).	Common-sense safety measure.
Avoid being cornered yourself. Stand on the exit side of the room.	
If client has a dangerous article or is moving at you, throw something at his or her face (e.g., sheet, blanket, pillow, garment).	Provides a distraction if escape from area is best choice.
Remove yourself from the situation as quickly as possible or call for help.	Avoid personal danger.

GOAL 3: Will go to room when client thinks that he or she may be losing control.

Intervention	Rationale
When client is calm, teach the client to go to his or her room when losing control.	Most likely to be receptive when calm.
Decide on a cue to assist client in following through, such as, "(client's name), your room."	A technique to assist client to maintain or regain control of self.

COMMUNITY REENTRY GOAL: Client will verbalize needs rather than strike out or fight.

AGGRESSION, VERBAL

GOAL 1: The client will understand that he or she has a choice when dealing with people and situations that provoke verbally aggressive behavior.

Intervention	Rationale
Collect database on verbal aggressiveness. Look for signs of mounting tension in the client.	Nursing process is the basis for intervention.
Intervene and remind client that he or she has a choice in how he or she behaves.	Reminds client that he or she can choose to be in control.

GOAL 2: Will identify four positive, alternative ways to deal with situations that provoke verbal aggressiveness.

Intervention	Rationale
When client is calm, teach the problem-solving approach. Assist in looking at new, alternative behaviors and their consequences. Remind client that the alternatives chosen must fit into his or her life style after discharge.	Most receptive to learning about alternative behaviors when calm. Unusual alternatives are difficult to put into practice and/or maintain.
Decide on a cue to assist client in practicing the new alternatives. For example, "(Client's name), stop!"	Uncomplicated, previously agreed-on cue to support new behavior.

GOAL 3: Will have less than one verbal outburst a day.

Intervention	Rationale
Identify specific reinforcers, depending on the number of outbursts and the time involved.	Specific reinforcers have meaning for client.
When the client has an outburst, ask the following: • "What did you do?" • "Did it help you or someone else?" • "What are you going to do about it?"	Challenge client to think through outcome of behavior and plan next steps.

COMMUNITY REENTRY GOAL: Client will discontinue verbal aggressiveness and deal with feelings in a responsible way, such as:

- Sublimating through physical activity or hobby
- Removing self from situations that provoke verbal aggressiveness
- Talking about feelings and emotional reactions without attacking verbally
- Rethinking the situation and changing the way it is perceived

ANGRY FEELINGS, INAPPROPRIATE EXPRESSION OF

GOAL 1: Will be able to identify his or her anger, such as "I'm angry because my visitors didn't come today."

Intervention	Rationale
Provide observations on nonverbal behavior. Assist client in identifying the source of his or her anger.	Actual examples help identify anger and when it occurred.

Continued

ANGRY FEELINGS, INAPPROPRIATE EXPRESSION OF—cont'd

GOAL 2: Will automatically engage in a favorite sport or activity, such as running, when angry.

Intervention	Rationale
Provide physical outlets for client's angry feelings.	Learn socially appropriate alternative outlets.

GOAL 3: Will show control over angry feelings by eliminating his or her destructive behavior.

Intervention	Rationale
Set limits and give positive reinforcement for appropriate behavior.	Define parameters.

COMMUNITY REENTRY GOAL: Client will deal with angry feelings constructively, through verbalizations and/or physical activity.

BLAMING

GOAL 1: Will identify that he or she is blaming others for problems.

Intervention	Rationale
Develop a sincere, non-punitive relationship with client.	Nonjudgmental attitude.
Encourage client to ventilate feelings about certain things.	
Involve client in assertiveness training.	Learn alternative way of expressing self.

GOAL 2: Will compile a list of personal strengths.

Intervention	Rationale
Assist client in assessing strengths.	Help client get out of victim role.
Encourage client to refer to and add to the list daily.	

GOAL 3: Will use the problem-solving process as a way of taking responsibility for his or her behavior.

Intervention	Rationale
Teach client the problem-solving process.	Practical method of identifying problem and alternative solutions, deciding on alternative, putting it into action, and evaluating result.
Reinforce new behaviors verbally and through special privileges that are important to the client.	Reinforcement supports continuation of desired new behavior.

COMMUNITY REENTRY GOAL: Client will stop blaming others for problems in life by accepting responsibility for his or her own behavior.

DELUSIONS THAT INTERFERE WITH FUNCTIONING

GOAL 1: Will stop talking about his or her delusions.

Intervention	Rationale
Do not agree or disagree with client's delusions.	Agreeing with delusion supports the delusional system.
Calmly and quietly communicate that you do understand what he or she might be experiencing at the time but it is not real.	Empathy for what client is experiencing. Support what is real: an issue of trust.
Divert attention by involving client in simple activity.	Focus client *off* delusions.
Set limits, if necessary, on discussion of delusions. For example, "This topic of discussion does not benefit you" or "If you want to stay out of the hospital, you have to stop talking about these ideas that are not true."	Provides information on what is not socially acceptable.

GOAL 2: Will respond to the following statement (nurse's gentle inquiring tone): "What is it that you wanted and went about getting in a way that others did not approve of that resulted in your hospitalization?"

Intervention	Rationale
Help client identify personal needs and ways to meet them.	Problem solving.
Interrupt anyone making fun of client.	Being made fun of may increase need for delusions.

COMMUNITY REENTRY GOAL: Client will control delusional behavior so that delusions will not interfere with role performance, such as carrying out activities of daily living.

DEMANDING

GOAL 1: Demands on staff will decrease, as reflected in the database, as staff spend more time with client when not demanding.

Intervention	Rationale
Determine what needs client is trying to fulfill through demands.	Data collection becomes basis of intervention.
Spend time with client when not demanding.	Support positive behavior.

GOAL 2: Will increase the tasks that client can do by and for self.

Intervention	Rationale
Help identify one thing client can do by and for self.	Enhance problem-solving skill.

COMMUNITY REENTRY GOAL: Client will make legitimate requests of staff, such as for money to go shopping, rather than unreasonable demands, such as for bringing food from the canteen when client could do it himself or herself.

Continued

DENIAL
GOAL 1: Will actively participate in identifying the problem and exploring alternatives to the situation.

Intervention	Rationale
Establish meaning of situation for client and convey to client that he or she can move through it.	Long-standing denial pattern is difficult to give up.

GOAL 2: Will select and implement an alternative to his or her situation.

Intervention	Rationale
Teach client problem-solving process: • Identify the problem • Explore several alternatives and possible consequences • Choose the best alternative • Evaluate the consequence • If not successful, repeat process	Basis for lifelong solution for problems: that client does have choices. (To do nothing or to deny are also choices.)

GOAL 3: Will evaluate the effectiveness of the alternative that client chooses and pursue the need for further action.

Intervention	Rationale
Evaluate the consequence.	Determine if alternative was achieved.

COMMUNITY REENTRY GOAL: Client will accept the reality of his or her present situation, such as the loss of a loved one, illness, or alcoholism.

DISROBING
GOAL 1: Will keep his or her clothes on while he or she is involved in activities.

Intervention	Rationale
Collect database on disrobing (frequency and precipitating factors).	May be able to establish cause-and-effect relationship.
Dress client in comfortable clothes that fit well and look as nice as possible.	
Fix client's clothes so that he or she cannot remove them easily (choose clothes that open at the back).	Practical, temporary measure.
Make a structured plan to keep the client busy with useful or pleasant work and games.	Structured plan permits all staff to do the same thing with client.
Protect the client from being embarrassed, exposed, or ridiculed. Check client frequently and redress as needed, without comment.	Behavior is to meet a need; nurse should be nonjudgmental and protective as needed toward client.
Attitude is important. Be matter-of-fact. Client must not be punished or shamed.	

COMMUNITY REENTRY GOAL: Client will keep clothes on during the waking hours.

DISTRESSFUL BEHAVIOR THAT INTERFERES WITH FUNCTIONING

GOAL 1: Will practice two ways that have been helpful in the past to reduce distress.

Intervention	Rationale
Encourage client to verbalize feelings.	Verbalization often helps client "see" behavior more clearly.
Explore with client past solutions that have been helpful.	
Support client in practicing old, successful ways of relieving distress that are healthy and appropriate in the setting.	Previous successful methods are often easier to reincorporate into behavior than new ways.

GOAL 2: Will practice one additional new way of dealing with distress.

Intervention	Rationale
Review with client practices regarding the following: • Nutrition • Work habits • Sources of satisfaction • Relaxation • Exercises • Recreation • Rest	Provides baseline for plan to support or modify current health and/or self-care habits.
• Need for information to deal with special stressors, such as finances, interpersonal relationships, assertiveness.	Identify information gaps that have become stressors.
Structure client's day to be involved in appropriate information classes, groups, or one-on-one sessions about topics identified in previous step so that the client learns new ways of dealing with particular distress. Praise client for following plan.	Practical to fill information gaps.

COMMUNITY REENTRY GOAL: Client will use positive ways to relieve distress that can be incorporated into his or her life style. Identify positive ways appropriate for the behavior.

EATING, REFUSAL

GOAL 1: Will eat meals with assistance.

Intervention	Rationale
Talk pleasantly and quietly to client.	Soothing, not challenging or threatening.
Do not criticize client's eating habits or make a fuss about the additional attention needed.	
Remember not to rush client. Seat client next to a client who eats readily. If this does not work, offer a tray on the unit.	Positive modeling by other clients is sometimes effective.
Encourage client to eat.	
Talk about building up physically to get well and go home.	

Continued

EATING, REFUSAL—cont'd

GOAL 1: Will eat meals with assistance.

Intervention	Rationale
Present small portions. Limit choices of food on tray.	Large portions and amounts of food may appear overwhelming.
Help client cut and prepare his food.	
Assist only as needed, using a spoon. Sometimes putting food on the spoon will be enough to encourage client to continue eating. You may need to fill the spoon, put it in his or her hand, and have client continue feeding himself or herself. If necessary, feed the client a few spoonfuls and encourage him or her to continue.	Food preparation, when possible, can stimulate appetite by sight and smell.
Spoon-feed completely only if client is unable to eat with partial assistance.	Give the client an opportunity to assume as much responsibility for self as possible.

GOAL 2: Will eat 50% of meal independently.

Intervention	Rationale
Reinforce desired behavior.	Reinforcement encourages continuation of desired behavior.
Client must not be scolded or punished for not eating.	
Do not threaten the client to force eating.	Threats are counterproductive.
Do not force feed.	Client will not digest food well and may aspirate.
Weigh client daily if part of protocol. Keep doctor informed in case additional measures are necessary.	Objective measure of progress or lack of progress.

COMMUNITY REENTRY GOAL: Client will voluntarily eat his or her meals.

FORGETFULNESS RESULTING FROM A COGNITIVE DISORDER

GOAL 1: Will add information about his or her past to conversation initiated by staff.

Intervention	Rationale
Refrain from asking questions client cannot answer.	Avoid deliberately embarrassing client.
Discuss events from the past that client can share. Use the client's experiences in the past to orient him or her to the present.	Reminiscing often leads to present issues.
If client has forgotten recent events that you know about, help him or her answer questions correctly.	Refresh memory matter-of-factly with clear, short statements.
Do not let other clients tease.	Protect client from embarrassment by others.

FORGETFULNESS RESULTING FROM A COGNITIVE DISORDER—cont'd

GOAL 2: Will recognize own room by a prop such as a framed collage of family pictures secured at eye level to left of doorway.

Intervention	Rationale
Use a collage of meaningful family (or friend) pictures, past and present, to help the client find his or her room. (Some facilities post the client's name in large letters on the door as a prop.)	Pleasant reminder of people meaningful in client's life assists in locating room. Collage can also be used as the following: • A focus for talking about past events • A reminder of recent events such as visits by family members or friends

COMMUNITY REENTRY GOAL: Client will be receptive to methods that will help him or her remember.

GUILTY FEELINGS, INAPPROPRIATE USE OF

GOAL 1: Will be able to verbalize when his or her feeling of guilt started.

Intervention	Rationale
Explore source of guilt verbally and/or nonverbally.	Determine appropriateness of need to feel guilty.
Do not support the client's belief that he or she is guilty.	Avoid reinforcing guilt.

GOAL 2: Will be able to identify that he or she is angry when saying "I'm guilty."

Intervention	Rationale
When client says, "I'm guilty." ask him or her to substitute the words, "I'm angry" or "I resent it," or ask client how long he or she needs to punish himself or herself. Then set a time limit for client to indulge in guilty feelings.	Identify real feeling behind guilt.
Fade out the guilty behavior by gradually decreasing the allotted time for the behavior and increasing the client's involvement outside self, such as assisting with simple chores.	Step-by-step instructions for fading unwanted behavior.

COMMUNITY REENTRY GOAL: Client will identify the constructive alternative that relieves the feeling of guilt.

HALLUCINATIONS THAT INTERFERE WITH FUNCTIONING

GOAL 1: Will admit to the presence of hallucinations.

Intervention	Rationale
Have client name the fact that he or she is anxious or lonely, and connect the hallucinating behavior.	Help provide control over hallucinatory process.

Continued

HALLUCINATIONS THAT INTERFERE WITH FUNCTIONING—cont'd

GOAL 1: Will admit to the presence of hallucinations.

Intervention	Rationale
Develop a one-to-one relationship with client. Discuss real events with client; focus on reality. Refer to voices as "so-called voices." Do not act attentive to discussion regarding hallucinations.	Basis of trusting relationship (relating with group may seem overwhelming). Distract away from hallucinations. Decrease importance of hallucinations.

GOAL 2: Will follow directions for temporary relief of hallucinations.

Intervention	Rationale
Suggest an activity, such as singing, when client hears voices.	Provides temporary relief from the hallucinations.

GOAL 3: Will dismiss voices.

Intervention	Rationale
Teach client to dismiss the hallucinations. For example, instruct client to tell voices to "Go away" or "Leave me alone."	Provide steps to control hallucinatory process.
Reassure client and provide additional attention from staff during this time.	Hallucinations are often frightening and confusing.

COMMUNITY REENTRY GOAL: The client will be able to control hallucinations and respond to the real environment.

HELPLESSNESS

GOAL 1: Will be able to identify use of helplessness and verbalize the reason, such as "I cannot be like you, but I can force you to take care of me" or "If I cannot do it my way, I will not do anything."

Intervention	Rationale
Provide feedback on client's behavior, both verbal and nonverbal.	Help client identify use of helplessness.
Initiate discussion of the underlying feeling experienced before use of helplessness (e.g., anger, jealousy, fear).	Identify underlying feelings that lead to helplessness.
Teach client basics of assertiveness through assertiveness group twice a week.	Alternative behavior pattern provides self-worth and sense of control over self.

GOAL 2: Will show control over helplessness by doing the activity that previously would have been avoided.

Intervention	Rationale
Help identify one daily activity that client can do alone.	Begin with simple steps.
Reinforce independent behavior verbally.	Reinforce achievement.

HELPLESSNESS—cont'd

GOAL 2: Will show control over helplessness by doing the activity that previously would have been avoided.

Intervention	Rationale
Initiate discussion about how client feels when following through with activity.	Get in touch with feeling related to following through.

COMMUNITY REENTRY GOAL: Client will deal with feelings of helplessness constructively by doing things that he or she previously depended on others to do. (Identify specific areas in which client will become independent.)

HOARDING

GOAL 1: Will stop hoarding item because staff will bring item hoarded by client into his or her room daily in specifically increasing numbers.

Intervention	Rationale
Collect database on frequency and amount of hoarding.	Basis for developing and evaluating plan (pinpoint behavior, count behavior).
Move all previously hidden items into client's room (exception is perishable food).	Involve client so he or she knows exactly what is going to happen in behavioral management plan.
Inform client that he or she will receive a specific number of items daily. State exact number.	
Direct client to keep all items in room and not throw or give any away.	Evaluation is ongoing.
Count items daily to be sure they are not being discarded.	

GOAL 2: Will request that the items be removed from his or her room.

Intervention	Rationale
Continue to increase the supply in the predetermined manner until the client requests that all items be removed from his or her room. However, if the hoarded items include food or potentially harmful items such as metal or glass, implement other measures. For example, explain to client that hoarding food is unsanitary because it attracts bugs. Reassure client that he or she will receive plenty of food. Allow the client to keep enough for an evening snack.	Satiation: client receives more than needed without sneaking items. Common-sense restrictions on some items.
Regular cleaning with client is necessary. Be honest with the client when you take the extra food away. The client has the right to know where his or her possessions are, and even though he or she does not like what you are doing, trust will be promoted.	Staff follow steps exactly and matter-of-factly.

COMMUNITY REENTRY GOAL: The client will stop hoarding (specific items).

Continued

IDEAS OF REFERENCE THAT INTERFERE WITH FUNCTIONING

GOAL 1: Will ask for confirmation of what he or she is hearing.

Intervention	Rationale
Reassure client that verbalization or behavior does not apply to him. For example, "No, the police officer is not here to get you. He brought a new client to the unit."	Reduce anxiety.

GOAL 2: Will identify that he or she used to believe that remarks or behaviors applied to self.

Intervention	Rationale
Reassure client that ideas of reference are part of illness. His or her ability to say that he or she "used to believe" shows improvement.	Identifies symptom as part of illness. Suggests sign of improvement.

COMMUNITY REENTRY GOAL: Client will dismiss casual remarks or behaviors as not applying to self.

ILLUSIONS THAT INTERFERE WITH FUNCTIONING

GOAL 1: Will begin to question illusions.

Intervention	Rationale
Be honest with client. Describe carefully what he or she is looking at or listening to, and explain honestly what is real.	Separate what is real from the client's illness symptom.
Do not let others fool or frighten client.	Illusions appear real and can be frightening.
Avoid arguments.	Make matter-of-fact statements of reality. Argument will not change client's perception.
Keep client occupied with work or activities.	
Be calm and reassuring. The client needs to know that this is part of the illness and will subside as he or she continues to improve.	

COMMUNITY REENTRY GOAL: Client will be able to identify correctly what he or she sees and hears.

IMPULSIVENESS

GOAL 1: Will verbalize factors that trigger impulsive behavior.

Intervention	Rationale
Collect data on frequency and precipitating factors of impulsive behavior.	Provides database for planning intervention.
Point out the consequences of impulsive acts.	Cognitive review of whether client or someone else benefits from act.

IMPULSIVENESS—cont'd

GOAL 2: Will request assistance in maintaining control.

Intervention	Rationale
Interrupt any impulsive act and explore alternative behaviors.	Problem-solving process introduced.
Teach client to identify thoughts and feelings before acting on feelings.	Move toward being congruent (thinking, feeling, doing are a match).

COMMUNITY REENTRY GOAL: Client will talk through his or her problems rather than act on his or her feelings.

INABILITY TO FOLLOW DIRECTIONS

GOAL 1: Will follow directions when directions are given before an activity.

Intervention	Rationale
Address client by name. Be sure you have his or her attention. Speak quietly in a low, firm voice. Be unhurried and reassuring. Use statements rather than questions, using "I" instead of "you." For example, "I want you to go for a walk with me." instead of "You should go for a walk."	Even in extreme cases, the last thing a client forgets is his or her name. One's name also separates the person from others.
Be direct. Use short, simple, to-the-point sentences. Give directions before activity.	Simple directions assume nothing: what is said is what is meant.
Ask the client to restate your instructions.	Feedback clarifies possible misunderstanding.
Give client written schedule and/or instructions to support verbal instructions. Observe behavior. If client does not comply, refer to written schedule and review it with him or her.	Written instructions can be referred to as needed.
Prompt client as needed. Make brief, frequent contacts throughout the day. Ask for and answer questions.	Provide opportunity for client to follow through.
Reinforce client verbally when he or she follows directions.	Reinforcers must have meaning for client.

COMMUNITY REENTRY GOAL: Client will follow directions using written directions as a reminder.

INDECISIVENESS

GOAL 1: Will identify each decision-making step he or she gets stuck on.

Intervention	Rationale
Instruct client regarding what to do as a way of teaching new responses.	Indecisiveness may be a way to avoid responsibility and blame for actions. Client may be timid about changing responses.
Using the problem-solving process, explore with client the level at which he or she has difficulty making a decision.	Assists client in identifying difficulty.

Continued

INDECISIVENESS—cont'd

GOAL 2: Will make a decision when offered two choices.

Intervention	Rationale
Reassure the client that it is okay to make a decision and to be wrong.	May resist making decisions because of fear of being wrong.
Offer the client two choices. (Be careful not to choose for client.)	Teach basic steps of problem-solving.
Praise the client for making a choice.	
Insist that the client follow through on the choice he or she has made.	Tendency to not follow through even after choice is made.
Reinforce positively client's success in decision making and follow through.	Reinforcers must be predetermined and of significance to client.

COMMUNITY REENTRY GOAL: Client will make basic decisions, such as what to eat, what to wear, and what activities to engage in.

INSTITUTIONALIZED BEHAVIOR

GOAL 1: Will perform personal care skills with supervision. (This goal should be revised until client performs these tasks without supervision)

Intervention	Rationale
Help identify areas client can control, using a behavior management approach with positive reinforcement.	Long-term institutional living supports having someone do basics for him or her (often by staff who find it easier to "do for" than to encourage or teach the client to "do for self").
Teach client basic skills, such as bathing, care of clothing, table manners.	Changing to a level of independence takes careful planning and follow-through by *all* staff.

GOAL 2: Will approach another client and initiate an activity. (This goal should be revised to move from a one-on-one relationship into a group situation.)

Intervention	Rationale
Through social skills training, teach client to participate actively in personal care.	Client moves from one-on-one with staff to group interaction.

COMMUNITY REENTRY GOAL: Client will live in a less-restrictive setting, such as a community-based residential facility (CBRF).

LONELINESS, FEELINGS OF, THAT INTERFERE WITH FUNCTIONING

GOAL 1: Will develop a relationship with one assigned staff member.

Intervention	Rationale
Develop a relationship with client. Begin with short, frequent visits.	Maintain empathetic, not sympathetic, approach. Sympathetic approach is potentially damaging to both client and nurse.
Always address client respectfully, by name.	
Use touch—shoulders, hand, wrist, or arm—to convey empathy.	
Be alert to your own feelings of loneliness and do not confuse them with client's.	
Discuss with client reason for present loneliness (choice, circumstances, or lack of knowledge of how to make contacts).	Client learns how to seek friendship outside of staff and facility.

GOAL 2: Will attend regularly scheduled activities.

Intervention	Rationale
Explore previous ways client dealt with loneliness successfully.	Previous ways may be worth trying again.
Plan a regular schedule of activities with client that he or she will attend, including occupational therapy and social therapeutic group.	Planned activities provide learning opportunities and interaction with other people.
Initially, attend activities with client and initiate involvement.	Client may initially need one-on-one support.
Ask client to assist with useful activities such as watering flowers, passing trays.	Contrived activities rarely provide the desired outcome.
Encourage client to seek out one other client whom he or she likes and initiate one daily activity with him or her.	Group to one-to-one become next steps.
Listen to client talk about his or her feelings. Reinforce desired behavior.	Opportunity for client to explore feelings and receive reinforcement.
Discuss other possible contacts such as involvement in church, volunteer activities.	Worthwhile activities outside of self provide satisfaction of service to others.

COMMUNITY REENTRY GOAL: Client will deal with feelings of loneliness by continuing group activities and developing a relationship with one other client.

MANIPULATION, DESTRUCTIVE

GOAL 1: Will demonstrate self-control of his or her behavior by not having to be reminded of limits.

Intervention	Rationale
Discuss with client the cause and effect of his or her behavior in relation to his or her environment.	Pattern of behavior usually practiced over a long period of time. May not see harm to others. May question that a direct, honest approach will work.

Continued

MANIPULATION, DESTRUCTIVE—cont'd

GOAL 1: Will demonstrate self-control of his or her behavior by not having to be reminded of limits.

Intervention	Rationale
Be consistent and firm with limits set on client's behavior and with expectations and consequences communicated to client and staff.	
Provide verbal and nonverbal reinforcement when client functions within limits placed on behavior.	Reinforcement needed to support success in modifying behavior.

GOAL 2: Will realistically plan daily activities and adhere to the schedule.

Intervention	Rationale
Teach client to plan daily activities and to concentrate on following the plan.	Client will plan and practice nonmanipulative behavior.

COMMUNITY REENTRY GOAL: Client will eliminate exploitation of others such as "playing one staff member against another."

MASTURBATION IN PUBLIC PLACES

GOAL 1: Will go to his or her room to masturbate with cueing such as "Joe/Jane, go to your room."

Intervention	Rationale
Identify situations in which masturbation occurs.	Determine cause and effect.
Give feedback to client about the uncomfortableness that his or her public masturbation creates in others.	Make client aware of reaction of people who observe his or her behavior.

GOAL 2: Will go to his or her room without cueing.

Intervention	Rationale
Discuss and negotiate ways to provide privacy (e.g., in his or her room with the door closed).	Alternative, private behavior.

COMMUNITY REENTRY GOAL: Client will discontinue masturbating in public.

MISIDENTIFICATION THAT INTERFERES WITH FUNCTIONING

GOAL 1: Will begin to question his or her misidentifications (include specifics).

Intervention	Rationale
Briefly and matter-of-factly tell client correct name of person (or object).	Support reality without emotion.
Avoid arguments with client about misidentification.	Symptoms are real to client; arguing serves to agitate client.

MISIDENTIFICATION THAT INTERFERES WITH FUNCTIONING—cont'd

GOAL 1: Will begin to question his or her misidentifications (include specifics).

Intervention	Rationale
Avoid answering to an incorrect name. Tell client what your real name is and answer to that name.	Maintain honesty and/or reality by all staff.
Be patient and tactful in dealing with client.	Client experiences symptom as part of illness.
Be alert to other clients stimulating client's misidentification. Interrupt if this occurs.	Protect client from those who tease.

COMMUNITY REENTRY GOAL: Client will call people (or objects) by their correct name.

NOCTURNAL WANDERING

GOAL 1: Will decrease wandering pattern by half, as identified in the database.

Intervention	Rationale
Collect database on frequency of wandering.	Count behaviors for database.
Evaluate changes that may indicate a physical problem such as cold, flu, or organic impairment.	Consider physical reasons.
Identify whether client has a problem or need such as the following: • The need to go to the bathroom • Incontinence • Cold • Hunger • Boredom • Anxiety • Disorientation	Identify cause-and-effect relationship if possible.
Deal with the specific problem or need.	Wandering may be unnecessary if need is met.
Use basic nursing techniques to settle the client. For example: • Tighten sheets • Provide extra blanket • Provide small snack or warm milk • Give back rub with warmed lotion • Sit with client • Reassure client • Reorient client, as needed • Provide night light or additional light as needed	

Continued

NOCTURNAL WANDERING—cont'd

If necessary:	If need cannot be met, look for safe alternatives.
• Permit wandering within safe area	
• Involve client in subdued activities	
• Permit client to rest in an easy chair close to unit station	
Continue to use the above-mentioned basic nursing techniques nightly.	Focus on the most successful combination.

COMMUNITY REENTRY GOAL: Client will go back to sleep after awakening at night.

NONASSERTIVENESS

GOAL 1: Will identify the underlying feelings experienced when doing something client does not want to do.

Intervention	Rationale
Interest client in beginning a "Doormat (Poor Me) Journal" and note incidents that happened throughout the day. Suggest four columns called:	Review "victim role" chosen by client.
• What Happened • Outcome (including feelings) • What I Really Wanted to Do • What Stopped Me	
Review the journal once daily with staff.	Follow through on assignment (important if behavior is to change).
Direct client to attend weekly assertiveness group sessions.	Learn alternative response pattern.

GOAL 2: Will succeed in saying "No" to requests that he or she does not want to do and "Yes" to requests he or she wants to do 50% of the time. (This goal should be revised until client is able to say "No" without feeling guilty.)

Intervention	Rationale
Direct client to practice desired responses by writing them down.	Reinforces learning.
Direct client to monitor personal responses throughout the day on the form provided.	
Identify specific reinforcers for 50% success; continue on up to 100% success.	Reinforcers support progress in applying new responses.

COMMUNITY REENTRY GOAL: Client will respond honestly to what he or she does or does not want to do when requests are made.

NONCOMPLIANCE

GOAL 1: Will contribute to a care plan that includes some of his or her choices.

Intervention	Rationale
Attitude of the nurse is important.	Projects that you believe client wants to comply.
Explain in detail the importance of complying with his or her treatment plan, the consequences involved, and the options available.	Fill in information gaps.
Assess client's needs for age, growth, and development level.	Behavior may result from age-related needs.
Assign staff to work with client consistently and develop a relationship.	Develop trusting relationship.

GOAL 2: Will follow a structured daily plan and receive reinforcers for compliance as specified in the plan.

Intervention	Rationale
Encourage client to talk about personal plan. Provide feedback on what is realistic at this time. Develop a structured daily plan and incorporate client's choices as much as possible. Review plan with client. Give client a copy.	Client needs to share responsibility in plan (will not follow through if he or she perceives it as "staff's plan").
Have client attend classes on special needs such as money management, medication, cooking.	Knowledge enhances ability to function effectively.
List specific positive reinforcers for compliance.	Meaningful reinforcers for follow-through.
Contact the follow-up worker for continued support and assistance to client after discharge.	Pattern change needs long-term support.

COMMUNITY REENTRY GOAL: Client will follow through with his or her structured plan of care (include areas of compliance needed).

PHYSICAL SYMPTOMS, INAPPROPRIATE USE OF

GOAL 1: Will express how client feels rather than focus on physical symptoms.

Intervention	Rationale
Collect data on the character, duration, and frequency of symptoms.	Basis for intervention.

GOAL 2: Will use relaxation techniques as a way of handling his or her anxiety.

Intervention	Rationale
Teach client about basic emotional needs and ways they are met.	Learns that needs are universal and that there are healthy ways of meeting these needs.

Continued

PHYSICAL SYMPTOMS, INAPPROPRIATE USE OF—cont'd

GOAL 3: Will assist staff with small tasks such as folding laundry.

Intervention	Rationale
Focus on client when symptom-free and redirect his or her attention outside self.	Reinforce desired behavior.

COMMUNITY REENTRY GOAL: Client will deal with emotional needs constructively in ways such as getting involved in volunteer work.

SECLUSIVENESS THAT INTERFERES WITH FUNCTIONING

GOAL 1: Will accept one-to-one contact with assigned staff.

Intervention	Rationale
Approach client on one-to-one basis for short periods of time.	Less threatening than group approach.
Talk about neutral topics and any topics in which client shows interest. Lengthen contacts as tolerated by client.	
Invite client to play a game or participate in an activity with you.	Support by engaging in activity with client.
Initiate conversation about whom he or she has noticed on the unit and in whom he or she has some interest.	Help client focus outside of self.

GOAL 2: Will join group activities when invited by peers or staff.

Intervention	Rationale
Invite client to watch a group activity. Casually invite him or her to join.	Step-by-step involvement without pressure.
Reassure client if he or she seems tense and encourage him or her to complete the activity.	Careful staff observation permits reassurance, encouragement, or praise as needed.
Praise the client for participation and accomplishment.	

COMMUNITY REENTRY GOAL: Client will join group activities on his or her own.

SEXUAL ACTING OUT

GOAL 1: Will verbalize situations in which his or her sexual acting out behavior occurs.

Intervention	Rationale
Identify situations in which sexual acting out occurs.	Situation will give clues to what triggers behavior.

SEXUAL ACTING OUT—cont'd

GOAL 2: Upon cueing, such as suggesting an activity, client will discontinue inappropriate sexual behavior.

Intervention	Rationale
Openly discuss sexual behavior and clarify any misconceptions about staff/client relationships.	Client may read silence as approval; needs to be dealt with directly and honestly.
Teach client appropriate ways of dealing with sexual impulses.	Client may be unaware of alternative, appropriate ways of dealing with impulses.

COMMUNITY REENTRY GOAL: Client will eliminate inappropriate sexual behavior.

SLEEP, UNSATISFIED

GOAL 1: Will identify usual sleep pattern and needs.

Intervention	Rationale
Monitor and record client's rest and sleep pattern for 2 days.	Baseline on actual observation is important.
Listen to client discuss usual sleep pattern and sleep need.	Input from client regarding perception of sleep.
Provide feedback to client regarding your observation of his or her rest and sleep pattern.	Observation of sleep pattern and client's satisfaction with sleep may be quite different.

GOAL 2: Will identify the kinds of situations that promote or prevent sleep.

Intervention	Rationale
Discuss with client previous pre-bedtime activities.	A previously successful activity may work again.
Discuss with client any changes in pre-bedtime pattern and when the changes began.	Determine cause-and-effect relationship between pre-bedtime activities and stressors taking place.

GOAL 3: Will implement methods to induce sleep.

Intervention	Rationale
Reassure client that it is okay not to sleep.	Trying to sleep increases anxiety. Permission not to sleep reduces anxiety.
Have client refrain from eating shortly before bedtime.	Food shortly before bedtime often disturbs sleep because of digestive process.
Direct client to take a 20-minute warm bath before bedtime.	Relaxation.

Continued

SLEEP, UNSATISFIED—cont'd

GOAL 3: Will implement methods to induce sleep.

Intervention	Rationale
Offer client a back rub after bath.	Further relaxation and feeds need to be touched.
Direct client to follow directions on relaxation tape, being careful to avoid sleeping.	Relaxation is usually the prelude to sleep.
Have client continue this ritual nightly, beginning at the same time each evening.	Repetition reinforces learning.
Instruct client to get up immediately on awakening from sleep rather than staying in bed.	Important to establish routine of time for awakening and going to sleep. Body struggles to reset time clock when pattern is changed.

COMMUNITY REENTRY GOAL: Client will return to previous, satisfying pattern of sleep.

TATTLING

GOAL 1: Will deal directly with the person concerned when accompanied by a staff person.

Intervention	Rationale
Interrupt the behavior.	Begin to change patterning.
Explain to client what you observed happening.	Teach client alternative assertive behavior.
Give client the following information: "I will not deal with the problem you are having with (specific name). However, I will go with you when you talk to him or her about this problem. I will be your silent support."	
If client is unsure how to handle problem, offer the following suggestions:	
• Talk to (specific name) about the feeling you are experiencing in response to what happened.	
• Use "I" centered statements. For example, "I was hurt when you said that I am stupid."	

GOAL 2: Will identify feelings experienced with use of confrontation.

Intervention	Rationale
Encourage venting by having client regard the confrontation in terms of the following:	Encourages dealing directly with fear of rejection and not being liked when confronting someone.
• Risk	
• Feelings	
• Value to client and individual involved	
Praise client for successful follow-through.	

TATTLING—cont'd

COMMUNITY REENTRY GOAL: Client will deal directly with significant people rather than tattling.

TEMPER TANTRUMS

GOAL 1: Will limit temper tantrums to half the number per day identified in the database.

Intervention	Rationale
Collect database on temper tantrums.	Count behaviors (establish baseline). Identify consequences.
Review behavioral guidelines and consequences with client (e.g., a 2-minute time-out or, if client cannot take a time-out, staff will hold him or her). Give client a copy of guidelines.	Involve client in planning.
Make a list of the positive reinforcers client can receive for no time-outs and for certain number of time-outs. Give client a copy.	Reinforcers are meaningful to client.

GOAL 2: Will identify reason for tantrums.

Intervention	Rationale
Develop a trusting relationship with client.	Trust is basis for accepting direction.
Ask client to identify reason for behavior.	Identify behavioral triggers.

GOAL 3: Will go to room and engage in a specific activity, such as playing with drums, instead of having a tantrum.

Intervention	Rationale
Discuss alternative behaviors with client when calm.	Teach problem-solving to client.
Cue client, if necessary, to go to room. Say "(client's name), room."	Work with client to assist in controlling behavior.

COMMUNITY REENTRY GOAL: Client will replace temper tantrums with a constructive way of expressing self.

WORRY, INAPPROPRIATE EXPRESSION OF

GOAL 1: Will determine which worries are past or future and those for which others are responsible.

Intervention	Rationale
Listen to client discuss worries. Have client begin a "worry journal," sorting his or her worries into the following categories: Past, Future, Other's Responsibility, and Legitimately Mine. Review the journal daily with client.	Process assists client to learn which worries he or she can actually do something about.

Continued

WORRY, INAPPROPRIATE EXPRESSION OF—cont'd

GOAL 2: Will discuss feelings experienced when attempting not to worry.

Intervention	Rationale
Listen to client express the feelings experienced. Reassure client that this is to be expected.	Initial attempts may actually increase anxiety.

GOAL 3: Will sign a limited worry contract.

Intervention	Rationale
Discuss the contract with the client as follows: • Determine if the worry belongs to client and if it is in the present. • If the worry does not belong to him or her, have client record it in his or her journal and refuse to worry about it. Tell client to use reminders such as, "That worry does not belong to me!" • If the worry is in the present, have client determine how much time he or she needs for worrying: then tell him or her to limit this amount of time. • Suggest reminders to control returning worry such as "I've already worried long enough about you!" • Gradually decrease the amount of time client uses for worrying about any issue. • Advise client to postpone realistic worry that belongs in the future with reminders such as, "I'll worry about the results of the tests next Friday when I go to see the doctor again." (If necessary, post such dates on a calendar and insist that the client not worry about them until the actual day.) • Review progress with client weekly. Gradually increase the time between reviews.	Steps of contract assist client in learning to own worries directly related to client and dismiss all others.

COMMUNITY REENTRY GOAL: Client will give up constant worrying about situations that cannot be controlled.

SUMMARY

The purpose of this chapter is to provide a resource for behaviors that challenge the nurse. Behaviors that have been developed in a nursing care plan format are aggressive (both physical and verbal), inappropriate expressions of angry feelings, blaming, delusions that interfere with functioning, refusal to eat, forgetfulness resulting from a cognitive disorder, inappropriate use of guilty feelings, hallucinations that interfere with functioning, help-lessness, hoarding, ideas of reference that interfere with functioning, illusions that interfere with functioning, impulsiveness, inability to follow directions, indecisiveness, institutionalized behavior, feelings of loneliness that interfere with functioning, destructive manipulation, masturbation in public places, misidentification that interferes with functioning, nocturnal wandering, nonassertiveness, noncompliance, inappropriate use of physical symptoms, seclusiveness that interferes with functioning, sexual acting out, unsatisfied sleep, tattling, temper tantrums, and inappropriate expression of worry. For each client, the nurse must individualize interventions based on the client's specific behavior.

Critical Thinking Activities

1. Choose one of the behaviors you have experienced and, using the nursing care plan format, develop a goal, interventions with rationale, and plan for evaluation.
2. Choose a behavior that has been challenging to you with a client in the clinical area. Develop a goal, interventions with rationale, and community reentry goal.

Review Questions

Multiple Choice—Choose the best answer to each question.

1. What is a possible intervention with a client who is using denial as a coping mechanism?
   a. Teach the client problem-solving process
   b. Institute limits on discussion of denial
   c. Involve in assertiveness training
   d. Collect database on number of events
2. What is a realistic goal for a client experiencing ideas of reference?
   a. Perform personal skills with supervision
   b. Learn to use quick relaxation techniques
   c. Ask for confirmation of what he or she is hearing
   d. Accept one-to-one contact with assigned staff
3. Which of the following is a possible community reentry goal for the client who is noncompliant?
   a. Eliminate exploitation of others by playing staff against each other
   b. Continue group activities with other clients on a regular basis
   c. Practice constructive activities to relieve feelings of guilt
   d. Follow through with structured plan of care
4. What intervention is needed with a client involved in destructive manipulation?
   a. Be consistent and firm with limits set on behavior
   b. Use touch (shoulders, hand, wrist or arm) to convey empathy
   c. Avoid acting attentive when client initiates conversation
   d. Emphasize that the client must stop the behavior to be liked
5. What intervention may be helpful with a client who is acting out sexually?
   a. Encourage ventilation of feelings of underlying behavior
   b. Teach client to identify thoughts and feelings before acting on feelings
   c. Openly discuss behavior and clarify misconceptions about relationships
   d. Teach client basics of assertiveness through assertiveness group

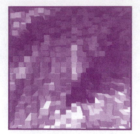

Appendix A
JCAHO Criteria for the Therapeutic Milieu

It is often assumed that staff understand what is meant by "responding to clients' basic physical and physiological needs." To avoid any misunderstanding of how to meet these needs, the Joint Commission on Accreditation of Healthcare Organizations (JCAHO) has mandated the following criteria for the inpatient therapeutic environment. Many of the criteria also apply to outpatient and community treatment settings.

EC.4   The organization establishes an environment of care that enhances the positive self-image of individuals served and preserves their human dignity.

EC.4.1   Waiting or reception areas are comfortable; their design, location, and furnishings accommodate the characteristics of visitors and individuals served, the anticipated waiting time, the need for privacy and/or support from staff, and the organization's goals.

EC.4.2   Restrooms are available for individuals served.

EC.4.3   The design, structure, furnishing, and lighting of the individual environment promote clear visual perceptions of people and functions.

EC.4.3.1   Lighting is controlled by individuals served, when appropriate.

EC.4.3.2   The environment provides views of the outdoors, where possible.

EC.4.3.3   Appropriate mirrors that distort as little as possible are placed at reasonable heights in appropriate places to aid in grooming and to enhance the self-awareness of individuals served.

EC.4.3.4   The environment minimizes distractions that interfere with therapeutic activities.

EC.4.4   The organization promotes awareness of time and season.

EC.4.5   A telephone is available for private conversations.

EC.4.6   Ventilation contributes to the habitability of the environment.

EC.4.6.1   All areas and surfaces are free of undesirable odors.

EC.4.7   Door locks and other structural restraints are used in accordance with the organization's mission and program goals.

EC.4.8   Furnishings and equipment suitable to the population served are available.

EC.4.8.1   Furnishings are clean and in good repair.

EC.4.8.2   Broken furnishings and equipment are repaired promptly.

EC.4.9   Dining areas are comfortable, attractive, and conducive to pleasant living.

EC.4.9.1   Meal and snack times are appropriate

* From JCAHO: Accreditation manual for mental health, chemical dependency, and mental retardation/developmental disabilities services, vol I: Standards. Oakbrook Terrace, IL: Joint Commission on Accreditation of Healthcare Organizations, 1994, pp. 61–63. Reprinted with permission.

to the ages served and facilitate commonly recognized conventions concerning the times when meals and snacks are served.

EC.4.9.2   Depending on the program goals, facilities are available for serving snacks, preparing meals for special occasions, and for recreational activities.

EC.4.9.3   The facilities for serving snacks, preparing meals, and for recreational activities permit participation by the individuals served.

EC.4.10   The dining rooms are adequately supervised.

EC.4.10.1   Staff is provided to assist individuals when needed.

EC.4.10.2   Staff is provided to ensure that each individual served receives an adequate amount and variety of food.

EC.4.11   Sleeping rooms have doors for privacy unless clinically contraindicated.

EC.4.11.1   In rooms containing more than one individual, privacy is provided by partitioning or furniture placement.

EC.4.12   The number of individuals in a room is appropriate to the organization's goals and to the ages, developmental levels, and clinical needs of individuals served.

EC.4.12.1   Except when clinically justified in writing, based on program requirements, no more than eight individuals sleep in a room.

EC.4.12.2   Sleeping areas are assigned based on individual need for group support, privacy, or independence.

EC.4.13   In accordance with the needs of the individuals served, good standards of personal hygiene and grooming are taught and maintained, particularly in regard to bathing, brushing teeth, caring for hair and nails, and using the toilet, with due regard for privacy.

EC.4.13.1   Individuals served have the personal help needed to perform these activities and, when indicated, assume responsibility for self-care.

EC.4.13.2   Incontinent individuals are cleaned and/or bathed immediately after voiding or soiling with due regard for privacy.

EC.4.13.3   The services of a barber and/or beautician are available to individuals served, either in the organization or in the community.

EC.4.13.4   Articles for grooming and personal hygiene that are appropriate to the individual's age, developmental level, and clinical status are readily available in a space reserved near his or her sleeping area.

EC.4.14   Closet and drawer space are provided for storing personal property and property provided for use by individuals served.

EC.4.14.1   If clinically indicated, an individual's personal articles may be kept under lock and key by staff.

EC.4.15   Individuals served are allowed to keep and display appropriate personal belongings and add suitable personal touches to their surroundings.

EC.4.16   Individuals served are encouraged to take responsibility for maintaining their own living quarters and day-to-day housekeeping activities of the program, as appropriate to their clinical status.

EC.4.17   Individuals served wear suitable clothing.

EC.4.18   The organization formulates a policy regarding the availability and care of pets and other animals, consistent with the organization's goals and good health and sanitation requirements.

EC.4.19   Unless contraindicated for therapeutic reasons, the organization accommodates the needs of individuals to be outdoors through the use of nearby parks and playgrounds, adjacent countryside, and organization grounds.

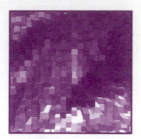

Appendix B
DSM-IV Classification

MULTIAXIAL SYSTEM

Axis I   Clinical disorders
              Other conditions that may be a focus of clinical attention
Axis II   Personality disorders
              Mental retardation
Axis III General medical conditions
Axis IV Psychosocial and environmental problems
Axis V   Global assessment of functioning

              NOS = Not Otherwise Specified.

              An *x* appearing in a diagnostic code indicates that a specific code number is required.

DISORDERS USUALLY FIRST DIAGNOSED IN INFANCY, CHILDHOOD, OR ADOLESCENCE
Mental Retardation

NOTE: *These are coded on Axis II.*

317	Mild mental retardation
318.0	Moderate mental retardation
318.1	Severe mental retardation
318.2	Profound mental retardation
319	Mental retardation, severity unspecified

* From American Psychiatric Association: Diagnostic and Statistical Manual of Mental Disorders, 4th ed. Washington, DC, Copyright © American Psychiatric Association, 1994.

Learning Disorders

315.00	Reading disorder
315.1	Mathematics disorder
315.2	Disorder of written expression
315.9	Learning disorder NOS

Motor Skills Disorder

315.4	Developmental coordination disorder

Communication Disorders

315.31	Expressive language disorder
315.31	Mixed receptive-expressive language disorder
315.39	Phonological disorder
307.0	Stuttering
307.9	Communication disorder NOS

Pervasive Developmental Disorders

299.00	Autistic disorder
299.80	Rett's disorder
299.10	Childhood disintegrative disorder
299.80	Asperger's disorder
299.80	Pervasive developmental disorder NOS

Attention-Deficit and Disruptive Behavior Disorders

314.xx	Attention-deficit/hyperactivity disorder
.01	Combined type
.00	Predominantly inattentive type
.01	Predominantly hyperactive-impulsive type
314.9	Attention-deficit/hyperactivity disorder NOS

312.8 Conduct disorder
313.81 Oppositional defiant disorder
312.9 Disruptive behavior disorder NOS

Feeding and Eating Disorders of Infancy or Early Childhood

307.52 Pica
307.53 Rumination disorder
307.59 Feeding disorder of infancy or early childhood

Tic Disorders

307.23 Tourette's disorder
307.22 Chronic motor or vocal tic disorder
307.21 Transient tic disorder
        Specify if: single episode/recurrent
307.20 Tic disorder NOS

Elimination Disorders

—.—   Encopresis
787.6   With constipation and overflow incontinence
307.7   Without constipation and overflow incontinence
307.6 Enuresis (not due to a general medical condition)

Other Disorders of Infancy, Childhood, or Adolescence

309.21 Separation anxiety disorder
313.23 Selective mutism
313.89 Reactive attachment disorder of infancy or early childhood
307.3 Stereotypic movement disorder
313.9 Disorder of infancy, childhood, or adolescence NOS

DELIRIUM, DEMENTIA, AND AMNESTIC AND OTHER COGNITIVE DISORDERS

Delirium

293.0 Delirium due to . . . *[indicate the general medical condition]*
—.—   Substance intoxication delirium *(refer to Substance-Related Disorders for substance-specific codes)*
—.—   Substance withdrawal delirium *(refer to Substance-Related Disorders for substance-specific codes)*
—.—   Delirium due to multiple etiologies *(code each of the specific etiologies)*
780.09 Delirium NOS
290.xx Dementia of the Alzheimer's type, with early onset *(also code on Axis III)*
  .10   Uncomplicated
  .11   With delirium
  .12   With delusions
  .13   With depressed mood
290.xx Dementia of the Alzheimer's type, with late onset *(also code on Axis III)*
  .0   Uncomplicated
  .3   With delirium
  .20   With delusions
  .21   With depressed mood
290.xx Vascular dementia
  .40   Uncomplicated
  .41   With delirium
  .42   With delusions
  .43   With depressed mood
294.9 Dementia due to HIV disease *(also code HIV affecting central nervous system on Axis III)*
294.1 Dementia due to head trauma *(also code on Axis III)*
294.1 Dementia due to Parkinson's disease *(also code on Axis III)*
294.1 Dementia due to Huntington's disease *(also code on Axis III)*
290.10 Dementia due to Pick's disease *(also code on Axis III)*
290.10 Dementia due to Creutzfeldt-Jakob disease *(also code 046.1 Creutzfeldt-Jakob disease on Axis III)*
294.1 Demeritia due to . . . *[indicate the general medical condition not listed above] (also code the general medical condition on Axis III)*
—.—   Substance-induced persisting dementia
—.—   Dementia due to multiple etiologies
294.8 Dementia NOS

Amnestic Disorders

294.0   Amnestic disorder due to . . . *[indicate the general medical condition]*
         Specify if: transient-chronic
—.—   Substance-induced persisting amnestic disorder
294.8   Amnestic disorder NOS

Other Cognitive Disorders

294.9   Cognitive disorder NOS

MENTAL DISORDERS DUE TO A GENERAL MEDICAL CONDITION NOT ELSEWHERE CLASSIFIED

239.89   Catatonic disorder due to . . . *[indicate the general medication condition]*
310.1   Personality change due to . . . *[indicate the general medical condition]*
293.9   Mental disorder NOS due to . . . *[indicate the general medical condition]*

SUBSTANCE-RELATED DISORDERS

[a]*The following specifiers may be applied to Substance Dependence:*

   With physiological dependence/without physiological dependence
   Early full remission/early partial remission
   Sustained full remission/sustained partial remission
   On agonist therapy/in a controlled environment

The following specifiers apply to Substance-Induced Disorders as noted:
   [1]With onset during intoxication/with onset during withdrawal

Alcohol-Related Disorders
Alcohol Use Disorders

303.90   Alcohol dependence[a]
305.00   Alcohol abuse

Alcohol-Induced Disorders

303.00   Alcohol intoxication
291.8   Alcohol withdrawal
291.0   Alcohol intoxication delirium
291.0   Alcohol withdrawal delirium
291.2   Alcohol-induced persisting dementia
291.1   Alcohol-induced persisting amnestic disorder
291.x   Alcohol-induced psychotic disorder
   .5   With delusions
   .3   With hallucinations
291.8   Alcohol-induced mood disorder
291.8   Alcohol-induced anxiety disorder
291.8   Alcohol-induced sexual dysfunction
291.8   Alcohol-induced sleep disorder
291.9   Alcohol-related disorder NOS

Amphetamine (or Amphetamine-like)—Related Disorders
Amphetamine Use Disorders

304.40   Amphetamine dependence[a]
305.70   Amphetamine abuse

Amphetamine-Induced Disorders

292.89   Amphetamine intoxication
292.0   Amphetamine withdrawal
292.81   Amphetamine intoxication delirium
292.xx   Amphetamine-induced psychotic disorder
   .11   With delusions[1]
   .12   With hallucinations[1]
292.84   Amphetamine-induced mood disorder
292.89   Amphetamine-induced anxiety disorder
292.89   Amphetamine-induced sexual dysfunction
292.89   Amphetamine-induced sleep disorder
292.9   Amphetamine-related disorder NOS

Caffeine-Related Disorders
Caffeine-Induced Disorders

305.90   Caffeine intoxication
292.89   Caffeine-induced anxiety disorder[1]
292.89   Caffeine-induced sleep disorder[1]
292.9   Caffeine-related disorder NOS

Cannabis-Related Disorders
Cannabis Use Disorders

304.30 Cannabis dependence
305.20 Cannabis abuse

Cannabis-Induced Disorders

292.89 Cannabis intoxication
292.81 Cannabis intoxication delirium
292.xx Cannabis-induced psychotic disorder
  .11 With delusions[1]
  .12 With hallucinations[1]
292.89 Cannabis-induced anxiety disorder[1]
292.9 Cannabis-related disorder NOS

Cocaine-Related Disorders
Cocaine Use Disorders

304.20 Cocaine dependence[a]
305.60 Cocaine abuse

Cocaine-Induced Disorders

292.89 Cocaine intoxication
  Specify if: with perceptual disturbances
292.0 Cocaine withdrawal
292.81 Cocaine intoxication delirium
292.xx Cocaine-induced psychotic disorder
  .11 With delusions[1]
  .12 With hallucinations[1]
292.84 Cocaine-induced mood disorder
292.89 Cocaine-induced anxiety disorder
292.89 Cocaine-induced sexual dysfunction[1]
292.89 Cocaine-induced sleep disorder
292.9 Cocaine-related disorder NOS

Hallucinogen-Related Disorders
Hallucinogen Use Disorders

304.50 Hallucinogen dependence[a]
305.30 Hallucinogen abuse

Hallucinogen-Induced Disorders

292.89 Hallucinogen intoxication
292.89 Hallucinogen persisting perception disorder (flashbacks)
292.81 Hallucinogen intoxication delirium
292.xx Hallucinogen-induced psychotic disorder

  .11 With delusions[1]
  .12 With hallucinations[1]
292.84 Hallucinogen-induced mood disorder[1]
292.89 Hallucinogen-induced anxiety disorder[1]
292.9 Hallucinogen-related disorder NOS

Inhalant-Related Disorders
Inhalant Use Disorders

304.60 Inhalant dependence[a]
305.90 Inhalant abuse

Inhalant-Induced Disorders

292.89 Inhalant intoxication
292.81 Inhalant intoxication delirium
292.82 Inhalant-induced persisting dementia
292.xx Inhalant-induced psychotic disorder
  .11 With delusions[1]
  .12 With hallucinations[1]
292.84 Inhalant-induced mood disorder[1]
292.89 Inhalant-induced anxiety disorder[1]
292.9 Inhalant-related disorder NOS

Nicotine-Related Disorders
Nicotine Use Disorder

305.10 Nicotine dependence[a]

Nicotine-Induced Disorder

292.0 Nicotine withdrawal
292.9 Nicotine-related disorder NOS

Opioid-Related Disorders
Opioid Use Disorders

304.00 Opioid dependence[a]
305.50 Opioid abuse

Opioid-Induced Disorders

292.89 Opioid intoxication
292.0 Opioid withdrawal
292.81 Opioid intoxication delirium
292.xx Opioid-induced psychotic disorder
  .11 With delusions[1]
  .12 With hallucinations[1]
292.84 Opioid-induced mood disorder[1]
292.89 Opioid-induced sexual dysfunction[1]
292.89 Opioid-induced sleep disorder
292.9 Opioid-related disorder NOS

Phencyclidine (or Phencyclidine-like)—Related Disorders
Phencyclidine Use Disorders

304.90   Phencyclidine dependence[a]
305.90   Phencyclidine abuse

Phencyclidine-Induced Disorders

292.89   Phencyclidine intoxication
292.81   Phencyclidine intoxication delirium
292.xx   Phencyclidine-induced psychotic disorder
   .11   With delusions[1]
   .12   With hallucinations[1]
292.84   Phencyclidine-induced mood disorder[1]
292.89   Phencyclidine-induced anxiety disorder[1]
292.9   Phencyclidine-related disorder NOS

Sedative-, Hypnotic-, or Anxiolytic-Related Disorders
Sedative, Hypnotic, or Anxiolytic Use Disorders

304.10   Sedative, hypnotic, or anxiolytic dependence[a]
305.40   Sedative, hypnotic, or anxiolytic abuse

Sedative-, Hypnotic-, or Anxiolytic-Induced Disorders

292.89   Sedative, hypnotic, or anxiolytic intoxication
292.0   Sedative, hypnotic, or anxiolytic withdrawal
     Specify if: with perceptual disturbances
292.81   Sedative, hypnotic, or anxiolytic intoxication delirium
292.81   Sedative, hypnotic, or anxiolytic withdrawal delirium
292.82   Sedative-, hypnotic-, or anxiolytic-induced persisting dementia
292.83   Sedative-, hypnotic-, or anxiolytic-induced persisting amnestic disorder
292.xx   Sedative-, hypnotic-, or anxiolytic-induced psychotic disorder
   .11   With delusions
   .12   With hallucinations
292.84   Sedative-, hypnotic-, or anxiolytic-induced mood disorder[1,w]

292.89   Sedative-, hypnotic-, or anxiolytic-induced anxiety disorder[w]
292.89   Sedative-, hypnotic-, or anxiolytic-induced sexual dysfunction[1]
292.89   Sedative-, hypnotic-, or anxiolytic-induced sleep disorder[1,w]
292.9   Sedative-, hypnotic-, or anxiolytic-related disorder NOS

Polysubstance-Related Disorder

304.80   Polysubstance dependence[a]

Other (or Unknown) Substance-Related Disorders
Other (or Unknown) Substance Use Disorders

304.90   Other (or unknown) substance dependence[a]
305.90   Other (or unknown) substance abuse

Other (or Unknown) Substance-Induced Disorders

292.89   Other (or unknown) substance intoxication
292.0   Other (or unknown) substance withdrawal
292.81   Other (or unknown) substance-induced delirium
292.82   Other (or unknown) substance-induced persisting dementia
292.83   Other (or unknown) substance-induced persisting amnestic disorder
292.xx   Other (or unknown) substance-induced psychotic disorder
   .11   With delusions[1,w]
   .12   With hallucinations[1,w]
292.84   Other (or unknown) substance-induced mood disorder[1,w]
292.89   Other (or unknown) substance-induced anxiety disorder[1,w]
292.89   Other (or unknown) substance-induced sexual dysfunction[1]
292.89   Other (or unknown) substance-induced sleep disorder[1,w]
292.9   Other (or unknown) substance-related disorder NOS

SCHIZOPHRENIA AND OTHER PSYCHOTIC DISORDERS

295.xx   Schizophrenia

The following Classification of Longitudinal Course applies to all subtypes of Schizophrenia:
Episodic with interepisode residual symptoms (*specify if:* with prominent negative symptoms)/episodic with no interepisode residual symptoms/continuous (*specify if:* with prominent negative symptoms)

Single episode in partial remission (*specify if:* with prominent negative symptoms)/single episode in full remission
Other or unspecified pattern

.30	Paranoid type
.10	Disorganized type
.20	Catatonic type
.90	Undifferentiated type
.60	Residual type

295.40   Schizophreniform disorder
Specify if: without good prognostic features/with good prognostic features

295.70   Schizoaffective disorder
Specify type: bipolar type/depressive type

297.1   Delusional disorder
Specify type: erotomanic type/grandiose type/jealous type/persecutory type/somatic type/mixed type/unspecified type

298.8   Brief psychotic disorder
Specify if: with marked stressor(s)/without marked stressor(s)/with postpartum onset

297.3   Shared psychotic disorder

293.xx   Psychotic disorder due to . . . *[indicate the general medical condition]*
.81   With delusions
.82   With hallucinations

—.—   Substance-induced psychotic disorder
Specify if: with onset during intoxication/with onset during withdrawal

298.9   Psychotic disorder NOS

MOOD DISORDERS

Code current state of major depressive disorder or bipolar I disorder in fifth digit:
1 = Mild
2 = Moderate
3 = Severe without psychotic features
4 = Severe with psychotic features
   Specify: Mood-congruent psychotic features/mood-incongruent psychotic features
5 = In partial remission
6 = In full remission
0 = Unspecified

The following specifiers apply (for current or most recent episode) to mood disorders as noted:
[a]Severity/psychotic/remission specifiers/[b]chronic/[c]with catatonic features/[d]with melancholic features/[e]with atypical features/[f]with postpartum onset.

The following specifiers apply to mood disorders as noted:
[g]With or without full interepisode recovery/[h]with seasonal pattern/[i]with rapid cycling

Depressive Disorders

296.xx   Major depressive disorder
.2x   Single episode
.3x   Recurrent

300.4   Dysthymic disorder
Specify if: early onset/late onset
Specify: with atypical features

311   Depressive disorder NOS

Bipolar Disorders

296.xx   Bipolar I disorder
.0x   Single manic episode
.40   Most recent episode hypomanic
.4x   Most recent episode manic
.6x   Most recent episode mixed
.5x   Most recent episode depressed
.7   Most recent episode unspecified

296.89   Bipolar II disorder
Specify (current or most recent episode): hypomanic/depressed

301.13 Cyclothymic disorder
296.80 Bipolar disorder NOS
293.83 Mood disorder due to . . . *[indicate the general medical condition]*
Specify type: with depressive features/ with major depressive-like episode/ with manic features/with mixed features
—.— Substance-induced mood disorder
Specify type: with depressive features/ with manic features/with mixed features
Specify if: with onset during intoxication/with onset during withdrawal
296.90 Mood disorder NOS

ANXIETY DISORDERS

300.01 Panic disorder without agoraphobia
300.21 Panic disorder with agoraphobia
300.22 Agoraphobia without history of panic disorder
300.29 Specific phobia
Specify type: animal type/natural environment type/blood-injection-injury type/situational type/other type
300.23 Social phobia
Specify if: generalized
300.3 Obsessive-compulsive disorder
Specify if: with poor insight
309.81 Posttraumatic stress disorder
Specify if: acute/chronic
Specify if: with delayed onset
308.3 Acute stress disorder
300.02 Generalized anxiety disorder
293.89 Anxiety disorder due to . . . *[indicate the general medical condition]*
Specify if: with generalized anxiety/with panic attacks/with obsessive compulsive symptoms
—.— Substance-induced anxiety disorder
Specify if: with generalized anxiety/ with panic attacks/with obsessive

compulsive symptoms/with phobic symptoms
Specify if: with onset during intoxication/with onset during withdrawal
300.00 Anxiety disorder NOS

SOMATOFORM DISORDERS

300.81 Somatization disorder
300.81 Undifferentiated somatoform disorder
300.11 Conversion disorder
Specify type: with motor symptom or deficit/with sensory symptom or deficit/ with seizures or convulsions/with mixed presentation
307.xx Pain disorder
.80 Associated with psychological factors
.89 Associated with both psychological factors and a general medical condition
Specify if: acute/chronic
300.7 Hypochondriasis
Specify if: with poor insight
300.7 Body dysmorphic disorder
300.81 Somatoform disorder NOS

FACTITIOUS DISORDERS

300.xx Factitious disorder
.16 With predominantly psychological signs and symptoms
.19 With predominantly physical signs and symptoms
.19 With combined psychological and physical signs and symptoms
300.19 Factitious disorder NOS

DISSOCIATIVE DISORDERS

300.12 Dissociative amnesia
300.13 Dissociative fugue
300.14 Dissociative identity disorder
300.6 Depersonalization disorder
300.15 Dissociative disorder NOS

SEXUAL AND GENDER IDENTITY DISORDERS
Sexual Dysfunctions

The following specifiers apply to all primary Sexual Dysfunctions:

Lifelong type/acquired type/generalized type/situational type due to psychological factors/due to combined factors

Sexual Desire Disorders

302.71 Hypoactive sexual desire disorder
302.79 Sexual aversion disorder

Sexual Arousal Disorders

302.72 Female sexual arousal disorder
302.72 Male erectile disorder

Orgasmic Disorders

302.73 Female orgasmic disorder
302.74 Male orgasmic disorder
302.75 Premature ejaculation

Sexual Pain Disorders

302.76 Dyspareunia (not due to a general medical condition)
306.51 Vaginismus (not due to a general medical condition)

Sexual Dysfunction Due to a General Medical Condition

625.8 Female hypoactive sexual desire disorder due to . . . *[indicate the general medical condition]*
608.89 Male hypoactive sexual desire disorder due to . . . *[indicate the general medical condition]*
607.84 Male erectile disorder due to . . . *[indicate the general medical condition]*
625.0 Female dyspareunia due to . . . *[indicate the general medical condition]*
608.89 Male dyspareunia due to . . . *[indicate the general medical condition]*

625.8 Other female sexual dysfunction due to . . . *[indicate the general medical condition]*
608.89 Other male sexual dysfunction due . . . *[indicate the general medical condition]*
—.— Substance-induced sexual dysfunction
302.70 Sexual dysfunction NOS

Paraphilias

302.4 Exhibitionism
302.81 Fetishism
302.89 Frotteurism
302.2 Pedophilia
302.83 Sexual masochism
302.84 Sexual sadism
302.3 Transvestic fetishism
302.82 Voyeurism
302.9 Paraphilia NOS

Gender Identity Disorders

302.xx Gender identity disorder
.6   in children
.85   in adolescents or adults
   Specify if: sexually attracted to males/sexually attracted to females/sexually attracted to both/sexually attracted to neither
302.6 Gender identity disorder NOS
302.9 Sexual disorder NOS

EATING DISORDERS

307.1 Anorexia nervosa
   Specify type: restricting type; binge-eating/purging type
307.51 Bulimia nervosa
   Specify type: purging type/nonpurging type
307.50 Eating disorder NOS

SLEEP DISORDERS
Primary Sleep Disorders
Dyssomnias

307.42 Primary insomnia

307.44	Primary hypersomnia
	Specify if: recurrent
347	Narcolepsy
780.59	Breathing-related sleep disorder
307.45	Circadian rhythm sleep disorder
307.47	Dyssomnia NOS

Parasomnias

307.47	Nightmare disorder
307.46	Sleep terror disorder
307.46	Sleepwalking disorder
307.47	Parasomnia NOS

Sleep Disorders Related to Another Mental Disorder

307.42	Insomnia related . . . *[indicate the disorder]*
307.44	Hypersomnia related . . . *[indicate the disorder]*

Other Sleep Disorders

780.xx	Sleep disorders due to . . . *[indicate the general medical condition]*
.52	Insomnia type
.54	Hypersomnia type
.59	Parasomnia type
.59	Mixed type
—.—	Substance-induced sleep disorder
	Specify type: insomnia type/ hypersomnia type/parasomnia type/ mixed type
	Specify if: with onset during intoxication/with onset during withdrawal

IMPULSE-CONTROL DISORDERS NOT ELSEWHERE CLASSIFIED

312.34	Intermittent explosive disorder
312.32	Kleptomania
312.33	Pyromania
312.31	Pathological gambling
312.39	Trichotillomania
312.30	Impulse-control disorder NOS

ADJUSTMENT DISORDERS

309.xx	Adjustment disorder
.0	With depressed mood
.24	With anxiety
.28	With mixed anxiety and depressed mood
.3	With disturbance of conduct
.4	With mixed disturbance of emotions and conduct
.9	Unspecified
	Specify if: acute/chronic

PERSONALITY DISORDERS

NOTE: *These are coded on Axis II.*

301.0	Paranoid personality disorder
301.20	Schizoid personality disorder
301.22	Schizotypal personality disorder
301.7	Antisocial personality disorder
301.83	Borderline personality disorder
301.50	Histrionic personality disorder
301.81	Narcissistic personality disorder
301.82	Avoidant personality disorder
301.6	Dependent personality disorder
301.4	Obsessive-compulsive personality disorder
301.9	Personality disorder NOS

OTHER CONDITIONS THAT MAY BE A FOCUS OF CLINICAL ATTENTION

Psychological Factors Affecting Medical Condition

316	. . . *[Specified psychological factor]* affecting . . . *[indicate the general medical condition]*

Choose name based on nature of factors:

Mental disorder affecting medical condition

Psychological symptoms affecting medical condition

Personality traits or coping style affecting medical condition

Maladaptive health behaviors affecting medical condition

Stress-related physiological response affecting medical condition

Other or unspecified psychological factors affecting medical condition

Medication-Induced Movement Disorders

332.1	Neuroleptic-induced parkinsonism
333.92	Neuroleptic malignant syndrome
333.7	Neuroleptic-induced acute dystonia
333.99	Neuroleptic-induced acute akathisia
333.82	Neuroleptic-induced tardive dyskinesia
333.1	Medication-induced postural tremor
333.90	Medication-induced movement disorder NOS

Other Medication-Induced Disorder

995.2	Adverse effects of medication NOS

Relational Problems

V61.9	Relational problem related to a mental disorder or general medical condition
V61.20	Parent-child relational problem
V61.1	Partner relational problem
V61.8	Sibling relational problem
V62.81	Relational problem NOS

Problems Related to Abuse or Neglect

V61.21	Physical abuse of child
V61.21	Sexual abuse of child
V61.21	Neglect of child
V61.1	Physical abuse of adult
V61.1	Sexual abuse of adult

Additional Conditions That May Be a Focus of Clinical Attention

V15.81	Noncompliance with treatment
V65.2	Malingering
V71.01	Adult antisocial behavior
V71.02	Child or adolescent antisocial behavior
V62.89	Borderline intellectual functioning
	NOTE: *This is coded on Axis II.*
780.9	Age-related cognitive decline
V62.82	Bereavement
V62.3	Academic problem
V62.2	Occupational problem
313.82	Identity problem
V62.89	Religious or spiritual problem
V62.4	Acculturation problem
V62.89	Phase of life problem

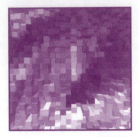

Appendix C
Suggestions for Further Reading

Adams SM, Partee DJ: Hope: the critical factor in recovery. J Psychosocial Nurs 36(4):29–32, 1998.

Alcoholics Anonymous: Twelve Steps and Twelve Traditions. New York, AA Publishing Inc, 1952.

American Nurses Association: Code for Nurses. Washington DC, 1985.

American Nurses Association: Statement on Psychiatric-Mental Health Clinical Nursing Practice. American Nurses Publishing, Washington DC, 1994.

American Psychiatric Assocation: Practice Guidelines for Eating Disorders. Washington, DC, American Psychiatric Association, 1993.

Backlar P: The Family Face of Schizophrenia. New York, GP Putnam's Sons, 1994.

Bereavement: A Magazine of Hope and Healing. Colorado Springs, Colo.

Bonnivier JF: Management of self-destructive behaviors in an open inpatient setting. J Psychosoc Nurs 34(2): 38–42, 1996.

Brookfield SD: Becoming Critical Thinkers. San Francisco, Jossey-Bass Audio Programs, 1987.

Brookfield SD: Developing Critical Thinkers. A workshop led by Stephan Brookfield for health care professionals, educators, and facilitators. University of Wisconsin–Green Bay, April 25, 1995.

Bruch H: The Golden Cage: The Enigma of Anorexia Nervosa. Cambridge, Mass, Harvard University Press, 1978.

Campinha-Bacote J: Transcultural Psychiatric Nursing: Diagnostic and Treatment Issues. J Psychosoc Nurs 32(8):41–46, 1994.

Canfield J, Hansen MV: Chicken Soup for the Soul. Deerfield Beach, Fla, Health Communications, Inc, 1993.

Caraulia A, Steiger L: Nonviolent Crisis Intervention: Learning to Defuse Explosive Behavior. Brookfield, Wis, Crisis Prevention Institute, 1997.

Carlson R: Don't Sweat the Small Stuff . . . And It's All Small Stuff. New York, Hyperion, 1997.

Conversation at the Carter Center: Coping with the Stigma of Mental Illness. Atlanta, Carter Center Mental Health Program, April 1996. (This is a videotape featuring author Kathy Cronkite and actor Rod Steiger sharing their personal experiences of coping with mental illness.)

Cramer C: Emergency! Hypertensive Crisis From Food-Drug Interaction. Am J Nurs 97(5): 32, 1997.

Davis M, Eshelman ER, McKay M: The Relaxation & Stress Reduction Workbook. New York, New Harbinger Publications, Inc, 1995.

Doka KJ (ed): Living With Grief After Sudden Loss—Suicide, Homicide, Accident, Heart Attack, Stroke. Washington, DC, Hospice Foundation of America, 1996.

Donegan KR, Palmer-Erbs VK: Promoting the importance of work for persons with psychiatric disabilities: the role of the psychiatric nurse. J Psychosoc Nurs 36(4):13–23, 1998.

Edelmann RJ: Anxiety Theory, Research, and Intervention in Clinical and Health Psychology. New York, John Wiley & Sons, Inc, 1992.

Edwards J: Guarding against adverse drug events. Am J Nurs, May 97(5):26–30, 1997.

Filley CM: Alzheimer's disease: It's irreversible but not untreatable. Geriatrics 50(7):18–23, 1995.

Fleming MF, Barry KL, Manwell LB, et al: Brief physician advice for problem drinkers. JAMA 277(13): 1039–1045, 1997.

Frank J: Alzheimer's Disease: The Silent Epidemic. Minneapolis, Lerner Publications, Co, 1985.

Gay K: Getting Your Message Across. New York, Macmillan Publishing Co, 1993.

Glasser W: Reality Therapy. New York, Harper & Row Publishers, 1965.

Goldsmith S, Hoeffer B, Rader J: Problematic wandering behavior in the cognitively impaired elderly. J Psychosoc Nurs 33(2):6–12, 1995.

Groetsch M: The Battering Syndrome: Why Men Beat Women and the Professional's Guide to Intervention. Brookfield, Wis, Crisis Prevention Institute, 1997.

Heckheimer EF: Health Promotion of the Elderly in the Community. Philadelphia, WB Saunders Co, 1989.

Hesse-Biber S: Am I THIN Enough Yet? New York, Oxford University Press, 1996.

Hill S, Howlett H: Success in Practical Nursing: Personal and Vocational Issues, 3rd ed. Philadelphia, WB Saunders Co, 1997.

Hirschmann JR, Munter CH: When Women Stop Hating Their Bodies. New York, Fawcett Columbine, 1995.

Johnson B: So, Stick a Geranium in Your Hat and Be Happy. Dallas, Word Publishing, 1990.

Kirkpatrick H, Landeen J, Byrne C, et al: Hope and schizophrenia: clinicians identify hope-instilling strategies. J Psychosoc Nurs 33(6):15–19, 1995.

Kosten TR: Generic and polydrug use disorders. In: Tasman A, Kay J, Lieberman J: Psychiatry, vol I. Philadelphia, WB Saunders Co, 1997.

Kovach C, Henschel H: Planning activities for patients with dementia. J Gerontological Nurs 22(9):33–38, 1996.

Kubler-Ross E: On Death and Dying. New York. Macmillan Publishing Co, 1969.

Lang NM, Kraegel JM, Rantz MJ, et al: Quality of Health Care for Older People in America. Washington, DC, American Nurses Association, 1990.

Larson L: Practical application of newer antipsychotic agents, J Care Management, Mason Medical Communications, Sept 1997, pp 36–39.

Lerner HG: The Dance of Anger: A Woman's Guide to Changing the Patterns of Intimate Relationships. New York, Harper & Row Publishers, 1985.

Mace N, Rabins P: The 36-Hour Day. Baltimore, The Johns Hopkins University Press, 1991.

Madow L: Anger: How to Recognize and Cope With It. New York, Charles Scribner's Sons, 1972.

Malone J: Milieu and Part Time Nurses: A Contradiction? An Editorial. J Psychosoc Nurs and Mental Health Serv 32(7), 1994.

Managing Managed Care for Publicly Financed Mental Health Services. Washington, DC, Brazelon Center for Mental Health, 1995.

McGivney SA, McGivney JH: Eternally Young: A Guide to Aging Well. New York, Ageless Publishing, 1989.

McKay GD, Dinkmeyer D: How You Feel Is Up To You. San Luis Obispo, Calif, Impact Publishers, 1994.

Meltsner S: Body & Soul: A Guide to Lasting Recovery From Compulsive Eating and Bulimia. Center City, Minn, Hazeldon Educational Materials, 1993.

National Advisory Mental Health Council: Parity in Coverage of Mental Health Services in an Era of Managed Care. Department of Health and Human Services, National Institutes of Health, National Institute of Mental Health, April 1997.

Nihart MA: Understanding psychosis and the role of newer antipsychotics. J Care Management. Mason Medical Communications Sept 1997, 29–34.

Oldham JM (ed): Personality Disorders: New Perspectives on Diagnostic Validity. Washington, DC, American Psychiatric Press, Inc, 1991.

Pardue SF: Decision-making skills and critical thinking ability among associate degree, diploma, baccalaureate and master's prepared nurses. J Nurse Educ 26(9):354–361, 1987.

Paris J (ed): Borderline Personality Disorder: Etiology and Treatment. Washington, DC, American Psychiatric Press, Inc, 1993.

Plante TG: Getting physical: does exercise help in the treatment of psychiatric disorders? J Psychosoc Nurs 34(3):38–43, 1996.

Rapoport JL: The Boy Who Couldn't Stop Washing: The Experience and Treatment of Obsessive-Compulsive Disorder. New York, New American Library, 1989.

Report of the Federal Force on Homelessness and Severe Mental Illness: Outcasts on Main Street. Washington, DC, Interagency Council on the Homeless, 1992.

Rogers S: To work or not to work: that is not the question. J Psychosoc Nurs 36(4):42–46, 1998.

Rubin TI: The Angry Book. New York, Collier Books, 1969.

Sheehan S: Is There No Place on Earth for Me? New York, Vintage Books, 1982.

Skinner BF: Science in Human Behavior. New York, Macmillan Publishing Co, 1953.

Slavinsky A: Psychiatric nursing in the year 2000: from a nonsystem of care to a caring system. J Nurs Scholarship Winter 17–20, 1984.

Stein MB: Social Phobia: Clinical and Research Perspectives. Washington, DC, American Psychiatric Press, Inc, 1995.

Substance Abuse and Mental Health Services Administration (SAMHSA): Before You Label People, Look at Their Contents. DHHS Publication No. 96–3118, Washington, DC,

The National Resource Center on Homelessness and Mental Illness: ACCESS 8(1):1–8, 1996.

The President's Commission on Mental Health Report. Washington, DC, US Government Printing Office, 1978.

Torrey EF: Nowhere to Go: The Tragic Odyssey of the Homeless Mentally Ill. New York, Harper and Row Publishers, 1988.

Torrey EF: Surviving Schizophrenia: A Family Manual. New York, Harper & Row Publishers, Inc, 1988.

Ungvarski P: Update on HIV infection. Am J Nurs 97(1):44–51, 1997.

Ward-Collins D: "Non-compliant": Isn't there a better way to say it? Am J Nurs 98(5):27–31, 1998.

Watkins J: Hearing Voices. The Richmond Fellowship of Victoria, PO Box 30, Brunswick West, 3055 Victoria, Australia, 1993.

Weil A: Spontaneous Healing. New York, Ballantine Books, 1995.

Weiner-Davis M: Change Your Life and Everyone in It. New York, Fireside, 1996.

Yager J, Gwirtsman HE, Edelstein CK: Special Problems in Managing Eating Disorders. Washington, DC, American Psychiatric Press, Inc, 1992.

Yi ES, Abraham IL, Holroyd S: Alzheimer's disease and nursing: new scientific and clinical insights. Nurs Clin North Am, 29(1):85–99, 1995.

Zimmerman PG: Emergency! Tricyclic antidepressant overdose. Am J Nurs, 97(10):39, 1997.

Zola S: Memory: A Seminar For Health Professionals by Mind Matters Seminars. Green Bay, Wis, 1997.

Zuckerman D, Debenham K, Moore K: The ADA and People with Mental Illness: A Resource Manual for Employers. Washington, DC, American Bar Association, and Alexandria, Vir, National Mental Health Association, 1993.

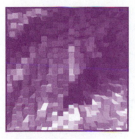

Appendix D
Evaluation Exercises

This appendix is intended to help the student apply the material presented in the textbook. Two types of exercises are offered to meet the student's learning style. In the first exercise, the student is asked to respond to illustrations of behaviors found in people who have psychiatric disorders described in the book. This exercise can be used as a pre-evaluation and/or post-evaluation tool. The second exercise is a crossword puzzle that covers certain aspects of the material presented in the textbook.

EXERCISE 1
INTERACTIONS WITH CLIENTS

The following situations illustrate behaviors found in people who have psychiatric disorders. Study the scenario and illustration for each situation. Then state your immediate feeling response to the situation and appropriate verbal and nonverbal responses to the client.

Responses will be evaluated based on understanding of behavior:

- The responses should indicate the use of positive approaches suggested in the book.
- The responses should not support the client's pathological behavior.

Guidelines with some possible answers to the illustrated behaviors are listed at the end of the exercise.

Situation A

Miss Eldridge is a 30-year-old woman with many physical complaints. All of her laboratory tests have been negative. She continuously paces back and forth. As she meets you in the hallway, she relates the following:

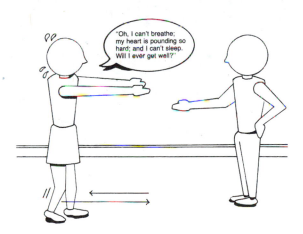

1. Give your immediate feeling response to the above situation.
2. Give appropriate verbal and nonverbal responses to the above situation.

Situation B

Mrs. Cannon is a 28-year-old woman who sits on the floor in the corner of the room and seldom speaks to anyone. Periodically, she turns her head as if listening to someone and then speaks, al-

353

though no one is present. You are approaching her to take care of her needs.

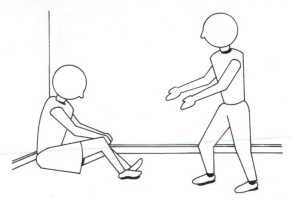

1. Give your immediate feeling response to the above situation.
2. Give appropriate verbal and nonverbal responses to the above situation.

Situation C

Mr. Hensen is a 19-year-old man who is very argumentative. He does not accept the fact that he is in the hospital. As you approach him, he makes the following comment:

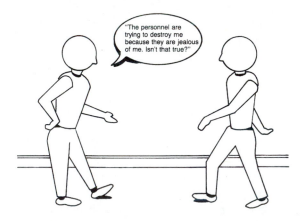

"The personnel are trying to destroy me because they are jealous of me. Isn't that true?"

1. Give your immediate feeling response to the above situation.
2. Give appropriate verbal and nonverbal responses to the above situation.

Situation D

Mrs. Jordan is a 42-year-old woman who sits in a chair all day and repeats over and over again how

unworthy she is. You decide to sit with her. As you approach her, she makes the following comment:

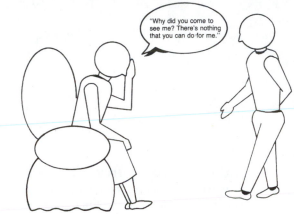

"Why did you come to see me? There's nothing that you can do for me."

1. Give your immediate feeling response to the above situation.
2. Give appropriate verbal and nonverbal responses to the above situation.

Situation E

Mr. Barton is a 36-year-old salesman. He is always on the go, talking loudly and critically about what is going on. As you enter his room, Mr. Barton makes the following comment:

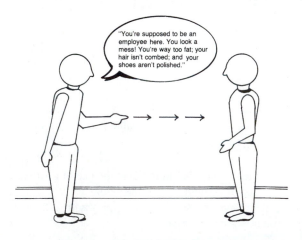

"You're supposed to be an employee here. You look a mess! You're way too fat; your hair isn't combed; and your shoes aren't polished."

1. Give your immediate feeling response to the above situation.
2. Give appropriate verbal and nonverbal responses to the above situation.

Situation F

Mr. Tuttle is an 80-year-old man who is disoriented as to time and place. He has trouble finding his room and the bathroom. He still thinks that he is back on the farm. As you approach him, he makes the following request:

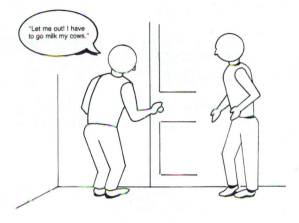

1. Give your immediate feeling response to the above situation.
2. Give appropriate verbal and nonverbal responses to the above situation.

Situation G

Mr. Felton is a 35-year-old man who has just been admitted for the twelfth time for alcoholism. While you are admitting him, he relates the following:

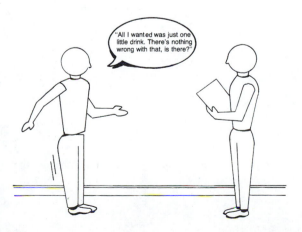

1. Give your immediate feeling response to the above situation.
2. Give appropriate verbal and nonverbal responses to the above situation.

Situation H

Molly McGee is a 38-year-old woman who is mentally retarded and emotionally disturbed. She sits in her rocking chair all day, cuddling her doll. As you approach her, you notice a large puddle under her chair.

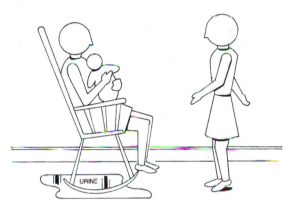

1. Give your immediate feeling response to the above situation.
2. Give appropriate verbal and nonverbal responses to the above situation.

SUGGESTED RESPONSES FOR EXERCISE 1

Situation A

Responses should support reality and not focus on the client's complaints. For example: "I know at this time you probably feel you'll never get well. However, the symptoms are part of your illness. As you continue to work on your problem, your symptoms will gradually disappear."

Situation B

Responses should keep the client in contact with reality and offer direction, as necessary, to meeting activities of daily living. For example: "Mrs.

Cannon, I'm Mrs. Troxel. It is time for dinner. I will walk with you to the dining room."

Situation C

Responses should neither agree nor disagree with the client's ideas but should present reality in a matter-of-fact way. For example: "I can understand why you have this idea at this time, but this is not what is really going on."

Situation D

Responses should not support the client's negative view of self but should attempt to help the client function and focus outside of self. For example: "Perhaps there is nothing that I can do for you right now, but I would appreciate it if you could help me fold the laundry." (If the client follows through with this task, be sure to express your gratitude.)

Situation E

Responses should not be defensive, challenging, or retaliating but should indicate an attempt to channel the client's overactivity constructively. For example: "You might have a point there. It's a nice day. How about the two of us going for a walk?"

Situation F

Responses should reflect orientation to time, place, and person, and should utilize the client's past to orient him to the future. For example: "Mr. Tuttle, you are in the hospital now and not on the farm. But tell me about when you were a farmer and did your own milking. How early did you have to get up to start the milking?"

Situation G

Responses should be nonjudgmental. For example: "Obviously, Mr. Felton, you did not have just one drink for you to be admitted to the Mental Health Center."

Situation H

Responses should not reprimand the client but should include alternatives. For example: "Molly, you are wet. Let's go to your room and change your clothes." (Start Molly on a regular bathroom schedule. Take her to the bathroom every 2 hours.)

EXERCISE 2
UNDERSTANDING MENTAL HEALTH CROSSWORD PUZZLE

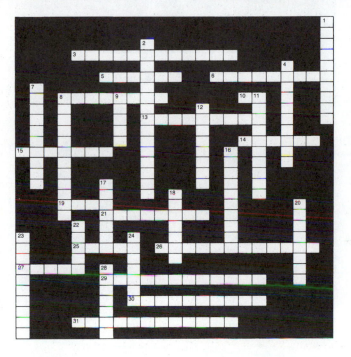

Across

3. Transfer of feelings to a less threatening object
5. Original support group
6. Plusses in a person's life
8. Opposite of listening
10. Abbreviation for delayed intellectual development
13. Undivided attention in conversation
14. Rejection of things as they actually are
15. Imaginary achievement
19. A biological, social, or psychological hole in a person's life
21. Prevention from reaching a goal
25. An antagonistic feeling
26. Exaggerating a desirable trait
27. An aspect of caring
29. Attitude or behavior when secure with oneself
30. Channeling anxiety into physical symptoms
31. Incorporation of another's standards so that they are not external threats

Down

1. Unconscious forcing of unpleasant experiences into the unconscious
2. Giving a logical-sounding excuse that conceals the real reason
4. Attacking behavior in response to frustration and hostile feelings
7. Moving away from reality
8. Inpatient facilities for care
9. A way of taking care of oneself
11. Retreating to earlier patterns of behavior
12. Activity to fulfill a need
16. Inner perceptions perceived as having origins outside of self
17. Negative actions canceled out by other actions
18. Chemical coping
20. Specific plan of action
22. Measurable and attainable achievements
23. Morbid sadness
24. Physical impairment of the brain
28. Vague, uncomfortable feeling
Answers to Crossword Puzzle on next page

ANSWERS TO CROSSWORD PUZZLE

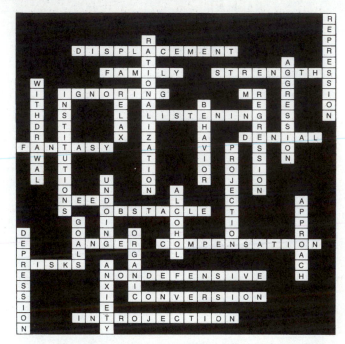

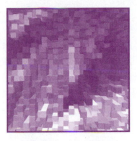

Glossary

Abnormal Involuntary Movement Scale (AIMS) Includes an examination procedure and a way to document findings of possible tardive dyskinesia.

Action for Mental Health 1961 report by Joint Commission on Mental Illness and Health. Placed strong emphasis on community-based services; called for reduction in size of large state hospitals and development of mental health services in local communities.

active listening Nurse tries to understand what client is feeling or what verbal or nonverbal message means. Nurse rephrases client's words and reflects them back for clarification. Client and nurse determine whether return message or feedback was clear.

ADA Americans with Disabilities Act, signed into law by President George Bush on July 26, 1990.

adult family home A residence in which care and maintenance above the level of room and board, but not including nursing care, are provided to one or two residents by a person whose primary domicile (home) is that residence (some states certify three or four residents).

advocacy Representing the needs of a certain group by supporting their cause through being active on committees, boards, etc.

aggression An action, verbal or physical, for dealing with frustration and anxiety caused by not achieving a desired goal.

agitation State of being disturbed, upset, excited; apparent in face or movement of involved person.

agnosia Failure to recognize or identify objects despite intact sensory function.

Alcoholics Anonymous (AA) model A method of sobriety that includes a 12-step program and complete abstinence from alcohol.

all-or-none thinking Additional data will not be considered because the person has already made up his or her mind.

alogia Restriction in fluency and productivity of thought and speech.

alternate personality Subpersonality that recurrently takes control of behavior in dissociative identity disorder.

alternative living settings Settings that provide an opportunity for clients to achieve independence while providing support and training.

antisocial personality disorder Previously known as *psychopathic, sociopathic,* or *dysocial personality disorder.* Pervasive pattern of disregard for and violation of rights of others; begins in early childhood or early adolescence and continues into adulthood.

apraxia Impaired ability to carry out motor activities despite intact motor function.

assertiveness Expressing feelings, needs, and ideas without violating rights of others.

associative looseness Words and thoughts do not hang together.

attention-deficit disorder Developmentally inappropriate degrees of inattention, impulsiveness, and hyperactivity.

autism Preoccupation with self.

avolition Restriction in the initiation of goal-directed behavior.

359

behavior management The application of behavior principles to modify behavior.

behavior principle A rule describing the relationship between what a person does and a specific condition.

behavior procedure The application of behavior principles to bring about behavior change.

bereavement Emotional and behavioral state of thoughts, feelings, and activities that follow a loss.

binge eating Episodic, uncontrolled, rapid ingestion of large quantities of food over a short period.

biological model Includes genetic, inherited potential, and nutritional factors, as well as infections and biochemical changes.

bipolar disorder Formerly known as *manic-depressive disorder.* Person has experienced a manic, depressive, or mixed episode.

body dysmorphic disorder Preoccupation with an imagined defect in appearance where there are no obvious abnormalities. Usually focuses on a facial defect; interferes with functioning.

body language Nonverbal communication; includes facial expressions, eye contact, posture, gestures, touch, personal space, and appearance.

burnout A process marked by physical, emotional, and behavioral symptoms.

CAGE questionnaire Assessment tool for substance use. Composed of four questions related to acronym. Two or more positive answers suggest diagnosis of substance use disorder; three or more confirm it.

coached memories False memories that result from statements and questions made by the therapist to the client.

Coalition on Mental Health and Aging An organization formed in 1991 to address the mental health service needs of older people.

cognitive behavioral therapy A combination of cognitive therapy and behavioral therapy. Teaches client new problem-solving skills and new behavioral skills for dealing with the client's environment.

cognitive dysfunctions Include disturbance of both higher and lower functions. Higher cognitive dysfunctions may include reduced interest in activities or subjective feelings of low self-worth, poor health, helplessness, and hopelessness. Lower cognitive dysfunctions may include poor concentration and attention and dementia-like symptoms.

cognitive therapy (CT) Attempts to change a client's automatic negative thoughts that cause or perpetuate depression through use of homework assignments and exercises that help identify, test, and challenge these maladaptive assumptions.

community reentry goal A post-hospitalization goal for continuity of treatment in a community setting.

community support program (CSP) Community care and treatment of people with severe mental illness.

compulsion An undesired, repetitive behavior symbolic of unresolved problems. Used to lower feelings of overwhelming anxiety.

continuum Imaginary line between mental health and mental illness. People move within the continuum throughout a day and a lifetime, depending on personal needs. Movement along the continuum may be sharply distinct or a subtle evolution of reactions to stress.

conversion disorder Separating anxiety-producing problems from awareness by developing motor or sensory symptoms that symbolize the unresolved problems.

coping The way a person handles a threatening or challenging situation.

crisis facility A safe environment for people as an alternative to inpatient care.

deinstitutionalization (1960s) Large numbers of mental patients began to be moved out of state hospitals and into the community. Many chronically ill patients became homeless, or if they needed rehospitalization, would go to nursing homes.

delusion of grandeur Unrealistic belief or idea of one's own importance or identity.

dementia Loss of intellectual abilities, memory impairment, and other brain dysfunctions because of organic causes; impairs daily functioning.

denial A coping mechanism whereby the individual refuses to recognize the existence of a personal problem; a major coping mechanism of alcoholism.

depersonalization Person experiences a sense of unreality; may feel that he or she is seeing self from distance or as if in a dream.

destructive manipulation Feelings and needs of others disregarded as manipulative client treats other people as objects to fulfill needs.

dissociation Coping mechanism. Painful ideas, situations, or feelings are separated from awareness.

distorted thinking Negative, incorrect thinking that shapes the client's view of the world. This includes seeing everything as black or white or good or bad, jumping to conclusions, etc.

distractibility Short attention span; easy to change topic or behavior through suggestion.

diversional activities Used to entertain or divert client's thoughts from stresses of life or to fill time.

drug holiday Planned days off from taking long-term medications. Increased compliance and reduced side effects.

dysthymia Chronically depressed mood, sometimes expressed as irritability.

echolalia Repetition by a person of words spoken to him or her.

echopraxia Spasmodic and involuntary imitation of the movements of another.

ego Conscious part of personality. Operates on reality principle; mediates between id and superego.

egocentrism Me, myself, and I: The person's entire focus centers around himself or herself.

elation Emotional excitement marked by acceleration in mental and bodily activity.

electroconvulsive therapy (ECT) Electrical stimulation used to induce convulsions and to treat severe depression, mania, and acute schizophrenia.

emotional dysfunctions May include the classic depressed affect plus anxiety or irritability. Client may appear apathetic.

empowerment Mental health consumers become active and have a political, social, and cultural voice in matters that concern their cause.

environmental deprivation Lack of social and intellectual stimulation during early developmental years that results in mental retardation.

escape The withdrawal from undesirable behavior in an attempt to end the behavior.

extinction The discontinuation or withdrawal of positive reinforcement for a specific behavior.

extrapyramidal side effects (EPS) All involve muscle control. Most common include dystonia, parkinsonism, and akathisia.

family therapy Family is viewed as a system with subsystems, boundaries, rules, alignments, and power. Therapeutic changes within the family system affect the environment and behavior of others within the family.

fugue Altered state of consciousness. Involves both memory loss and traveling away from one's home or work. Client assumes new identity and has no memory of past.

generalized anxiety disorder Excessive worry that something terrible is going to happen (natural disaster, illness, harm to self or loved one). Client is aware of extreme worry and tries to conceal it.

generic approach Based on certain recognized patterns of behavior that are present in most crises, such as bereavement, disaster, or chronic illness.

gentle self defense Specific defensive techniques to protect oneself and/or others against injury from a client who is acting out physically and poses a danger to self or others.

grief process Learning to cope with a specific loss. Mourning and bereavement are a part of the process.

group homes Homes for people who need supervision, care, and service in addition to board and room.

group therapy Form of psychotherapy that uses peer as well as professional relationships in a

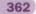

collaborative, structured, time-limited format. Can result in symptom relief and resolution of interpersonal problems.

hallucination A false sensory perception that is real to the person and cannot be changed by logic. Hearing and seeing are most common hallucinations. Can also involve touch, taste, or smell.

humanistic theory A belief that how a person moves through the life cycle depends on how he or she deals with the specific needs of the cycle.

hypochondriasis Person preoccupied with fears of having a serious illness; no physical basis.

id Unconscious part of personality includes the primitive urges and instincts such as sexual desires and aggression. Considered to have an observable effect on the person's thinking, feeling, and actions.

ideas of reference Identifying behavior of others as referring to self.

imagery A useful tool for relaxation by visualizing positive images.

individual approach Focus on the unique needs of the person and the events that caused the crisis.

interpersonal psychotherapy (IPT) Problem-focused therapy on one of four interpersonal areas: grief, role dispute, role transition, or interpersonal deficit.

intra-aggression Anger turned inward so that it no longer poses an external threat to the individual.

involuntary commitment (civil commitment) Admission to psychiatric hospital initiated by police, family, or someone other than person needing help.

JCAHO Joint Commission on Accreditation of Healthcare Organizations. In 1994, published guidelines for criteria for therapeutic milieu for mental health, chemical dependency, and mental retardation/developmental disabilities services.

KISS Acronym for "Keep It Short and Simple."

La Belle indifference Lack of concern about physical symptom when symptom is used to lower anxiety.

learning disabilities If brain function results in cognitive difficulties, it is called a *learning disorder* according to DSM-IV. The public school system refers collectively to learning disorders, motor difficulties, and language disorders as *learning disabilities*.

leisure counseling Classes on the effective use of leisure time, focusing on recreational activities that can be performed throughout the life span.

lethality As used in this text, refers to the seriousness of a suicide threat and the degree it is likely to result in death.

life skills training Educational classes that help mental health consumers continue to live in the community.

light therapy Full-spectrum light and bright white light used to treat seasonal affective disorder (SAD).

love and belongingness Stage 3 of Maslow's Hierarchy of Needs. Person feels a need to belong to a group, to have companionship, and to give and receive love.

major depressive disorder A serious disorder of mood characterized by sleep disturbance, change in appetite, weight gain or loss, loss of energy, fatigue, feelings of worthlessness, slowed thinking, and suicidal ideation.

mania Person experiences feelings of excitement, elation, or extreme irritability.

maturational crisis Includes the many issues that arise in progressing from one stage of development to the next.

mental health consumers A term used to describe former psychiatric patients/clients, psychiatric survivors, or ex-patients.

Mental Health Parity Act of 1996 Attempted to provide equality in annual and lifetime limits by insurance companies for mental health services and general medical illnesses.

Mental Health Systems Act (1980) Encouraged each state to review and revise its laws to ensure that mental health patients receive the protection and services they require.

milieu Total environment.

milieu therapy Using the total environment as a therapeutic mechanism.

MINDS Minneapolis detoxification scale developed at the Minneapolis Veterans Affairs Center by M. Willenbring and N. Dillon. Protocol is currently in the process of being validated.

moderation management A "reducing harm" focus for alcohol abusers. Limits number of drinks per day, number per week, and never permits drinking while driving.

music therapy The functional application of music toward the attainment of specific therapeutic goals.

National Mental Health Act (1946) Provided federal aid for research, training, and community service.

negative reinforcement A combination of escape behavior and avoidance. The behavior of "giving in" has been strengthened because it turned off something aversive.

neurosis A minor mental illness in which the client is in touch with reality. Currently called *anxiety disorder.*

nonassertive behavior Person does not express own feelings and needs when rights are infringed on deliberately or accidentally; ends up feeling hurt, misunderstood, and often angry.

normalization Making available conditions of everyday life that resemble, as closely as possible, the usual patterns of living for the general population.

object constancy Capacity to hold constant and real a person or object of importance when that object is not present. Begins developing at toddler age and is completed at school age.

OBRA (1987) Omnibus Budget Reform Act. Prevented inappropriate placement of people with mental illness in nursing homes. Each state received a designated amount of money to cover alcohol, drug abuse, and mental health services. How and where money was spent was determined by states.

obsession Recurrent, persistent thoughts, impulses, or images experienced as intrusive and that cause marked anxiety.

obsessive-compulsive disorder Persistent feelings and thoughts that result in repetitive acts to relieve anxiety.

pain disorder Pain continues after extensive evaluation determines there are no physical findings to account for pain and its intensity. Pain causes significant difficulty in important areas of functioning.

panic disorder Overwhelming anxiety that results in the person's inability to function in an appropriate way. Client has unexpected, recurrent panic attacks.

paraphilias Socially destructive sexual behaviors. Some are sexual crimes; some are not.

parkinsonism Characterized by tremors, rigidity, masked facies, "pill-rolling" motion of fingers, shuffling gait.

personality disorder Behavior and inner experience of a person are markedly different from the expectations of his or her culture.

pleasure principle Desire for immediate gratification.

positive symptoms Outward, serious symptoms. Most likely to improve with antipsychotic medication.

possession In dissociative trance disorder, client believes he or she has been taken over by a spirit or other person.

progressive relaxation The tensing and relaxing of muscle groups from head to toe or toe to head, resulting in deep relaxation.

projection A coping mechanism whereby an individual attributes his or her own weaknesses to others.

psychiatric treatment team Mental health and other professionals within the psychiatric hospital and community who are involved in client care.

psychogenic Psychological.

psychoanalytic therapy Intensive exploration of the inner self, including repressed emotions.

psychological autopsy After a client's suicide, members of the psychiatric treatment team share feelings and insights. They look at what could have been done differently, any signals that were missed, and what was done correctly.

psychosocial theory   Theorists, including Erickson, Sullivan, and others, believed that social experience with significant people helps mold identity.

psychosurgery   Surgery on the brain that has an effect on the client's psyche.

psychotherapy   Commonly referred to as *talk therapy.* Involves individual, group, and family therapies.

psychotic   Out of touch with reality; experiencing a major mental illness.

random thinking   Incomplete thoughts come and go with no particular purpose.

reaction formation   A coping mechanism during which a person disguises from the self an unacceptable desire or drive by developing its exact opposite to an exaggerated degree.

reality orientation   A way of orienting clients who are disoriented to time, place, things, and person; involves staff on a 24-hour basis.

regression   A coping mechanism during which the individual reverts to behavior characteristic of a less stressful time in life.

response cost   An aversive technique for reducing undesirable behavior by withdrawing specific positive reinforcers.

rumination   A way of going through same thoughts again and again without determining a course of positive action to solve the problem.

rummaging   Searching for something familiar for security. Client is confused about environment.

scapegoat   The identified "sick one" who acts out the family dysfunction and brings the family into therapy.

schizophrenia   A group of psychotic disorders characterized by severe interference in thinking, feeling, and doing.

seclusion   The involuntary confinement of a person alone in a room where the person is physically prevented from leaving.

selective serotonin reuptake inhibitors (SSRIs)   A category of antidepressants that affect the neurotransmitter serotonin.

self-help group   A group of people who meet to work on one specific problem area that they all have in common.

sensory stimulation group   Purpose is to stimulate senses of clients who lack usual sensory stimulation because of illness or age.

separation anxiety disorder   Excessive anxiety when separated from home or from people to whom child is attached (usually a parent).

serotonin   Neurotransmitter that appears to be primarily involved in anxiety, schizoaffective disorders, mood disorders, and violence.

serotonin syndrome   A potentially serious side effect related to combining SSRI with other serotonin antagonists or taking SSRI too soon after another drug has been discontinued.

shaping   The procedure used to teach a complex behavior using small steps.

situational crisis   Develops from an external event such as an accident, loss of job, death, illness, retirement, or financial troubles.

social phobia   Persistent fear of social or performance situations.

somatization   Client expresses psychological stress on an unconscious level through physical symptoms; symptoms relieve anxiety.

somatoform disorder   Physical symptoms without a known organic cause. Symptoms are not intentional; results in distress or impairment of functioning.

specific phobia   Excessive fear that is more than for normal age.

splitting   Primitive defense. Person sees self and others as all good or all bad; fails to integrate positive and negative qualities of self and others into cohesive whole.

stigma   Characteristics that mark a person as different from others.

stigmatization   Stigma selected by a social group to imply that a person is flawed.

stress   Body's reaction to demands made on the person. Stress is not an event, but the perception of an event.

substance abuse   Maladaptive use of alcohol and/or other drugs.

substance dependence   Client needs more of

substance to get desired effect. Use of alcohol and/or other drugs continues even with awareness of related physical or psychological problems.

substance intoxication Reversible maladaptive behaviors or psychological changes that develop during or shortly after substance abuse.

sundowning Cannot see well in dim light and becomes confused. Confusion and restlessness occur because brain can no longer sort out cues in environment.

superego According to Freud, who described three parts of personality, the superego is primarily unconscious, incorporates the values of human society, and acts as sensor for the id. Sometimes referred to as *conscience*.

support group A group of people who meet to talk about how to cope with a specific problem or illness. The group is often facilitated by a professional.

supportive apartment living Individual apartments or cooperative apartments that are contracted or owned by a private or public mental health agency. Mental health consumers maintain independence by paying rent and performing housekeeping chores.

talk down The managing of verbal threats by redirecting the person toward a calmer state-of-being.

talk up A way of handling manipulative behavior by sharing the person's behavior with staff and informing them of what the person is trying to do.

therapeutic activities Activities used to attain a specific care plan goal or objective.

time-out Refers to time-out from positive reinforcement.

trance Altered state of consciousness in which client has a selective or limited response to environmental stimuli.

transference The client responds to the therapist as though experiencing the early event.

transitional objects People or articles (toys, blanket) that provide support to a person during changes that he or she goes through.

transorbital lobotomy A form of psychosurgery, no longer used, that involved introduction of a sharp object into the brain to sever an intended connection.

unilateral treatment Placement of electrodes during ECT on nondominant side only.

verbal de-escalation Another term used to describe talking down.

voluntary admission Initiated by a person seeking help for his or her problems.

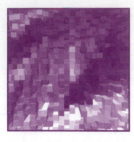

Index

Page numbers in italics indicate illustrations; t indicates tables.